OCCUPATIONAL THERAPY
in Rehabilitation

Occupational Therapy

in Rehabilitation

A Handbook for Occupational Therapists,
Students and others interested in
this aspect of reablement

FOURTH EDITION

Edited by

E. M. MACDONALD, M.B.E., B.Litt., T.Dip.

Honorary Fellow of the British Association of Occupational Therapists and of the World
Federation of Occupational Therapists

with the help of

G. MacCAUL, M.B.E., Dip. Bedford P.T. College, T.Dip., F.B.A.O.T.

L. MIRREY, M.B.A.O.T.

E. M. MORRISON, M.B.A.O.T.

and others

Foreword by

The Right Hon. Lord Amulree, M.A., M.D., F.R.C.P.

Physician, University College Hospital, London, 1949-1966. President, Geriatric Society
Past President, Association of Occupational Therapists

LONDON
BAILLIÈRE TINDALL

A BAILLIÈRE TINDALL book
Published by Cassell Ltd

35 Red Lion Square, London WC1R 4SG
Sydney, Auckland, Toronto, Johannesburg

The Macmillan Publishing Company Inc.
New York

First published 1960
Third edition 1970
Fourth edition 1976
Reprinted 1978

ISBN 0 7020 0577 0

Spanish edition (Salvat Editores, Barcelona) 1972
Japanese edition (Ishiyaku Publishers, Tokyo) 1972

© 1976 Baillière Tindall

PRINTED IN GREAT BRITAIN AT
THE UNIVERSITY PRESS
ABERDEEN

Contributors

Miss R. H. ANDERSON, S.R.O.T., M.B.A.O.T.
Ex Head Occ. Therapist and Tutor in Play Therapy, Institute of Family Psychiatry, Ipswich, 1959–69. Occ. Therapist, Child and Family Guidance Service, Bath. Postgraduate Course in Play Therapy. Speaker at W.F.O.T.* Congresses 1962, 1966.

Miss N. BERRINGTON JONES, M.B.A.O.T.
Head Occ. Therapist, Liverpool Health Department.

Miss S. M. BLENCOWE, S.R.O.T., M.B.A.O.T.
Superintendent, Centre for Spastic Children, Cheyne Walk, London, 1966–73. Formerly Senior Occ. Therapist, Centre for Spastic Children, Cheyne Walk, London, 1961–63, and King George VI Children's Rehabilitation Centre, Bulawayo, Rhodesia, 1963–65.

Miss E. B. L. BUSHELL, R.N.M.S., S.R.O.T., M.B.A.O.T., T.DIP.
Formerly Principal, School of Occ. Therapy, and Chief Supervisor of Training, Botley's Park Hospital, Chertsey, Surrey.

Mrs P. CHAPLIN, M.B.A.O.T.
Head Occ. Therapist, Smith Hospital for Autistic, Psychotic and Emotionally Disturbed Children, Henley on Thames. Course in Pre-school Play Groups and Nursery Schools.

Miss E. D. COOK, S.R.O.T., M.B.A.O.T.
Occ. Therapist, Child Guidance Clinic, Cheltenham. Formerly Head Occ. Therapist, Park Hospital for Children, Oxford, and Coney Hill Hospital, Gloucester.

Miss J. E. FORD, S.R.O.T., M.B.A.O.T.
Head Occ. Therapist, Cowley Road Hospital, Oxford, since 1958. King Edward VII Hospital Fund for London, Essay Prize Winner. Memorial Fund Scholarship to write a book on Occupational Therapy for Geriatric Patients.

Mrs E. M. GROVE, S.R.O.T., M.B.A.O.T.
Group Occ. Therapist, St George's Hospitals, Hyde Park Corner, and Tooting, also of the Atkinson Morley Hospital and Wolfson Medical Rehabilitation Centre, London.

Miss R. HALLIDAY, DIP.O.T.(N.S.W.) AUSTRALIA
Staff Therapist, N.S.W. College of Occ. Therapy, Australia. Formerly Assistant Head Occ. Therapist, Royal Alexandria Hospital for Children, N.S.W., Australia. Visiting Staff at Atkinson Morley Hospital, Wimbledon, and at the Workmen's Compensation Board Rehabilitation Centre, Canada.

Miss E. M. HOLLINGS, S.R.O.T., HON. FELLOW B.A.O.T.
Research Therapist, Oxford Rehabilitation Research Unit, Nuffield Orthopaedic Centre, Oxford. Formerly Head Occ. Therapist, Nuffield Orthopaedic Centre and the Mary Marlborough Lodge, Oxford.

Miss P. E. JAY, S.R.O.T., M.B.A.O.T.
Formerly Head Occ. Therapist, Farnham Park Rehabilitation Centre, Slough, Bucks. Co-author of *Help Yourselves*, a Handbook for Hemiplegics, London, 1966. Author of *Coping with Disablement*, Consumer's Association, 1974.

Miss B. Johnson, s.r.o.t., m.b.a.o.t.
Head Occ. Therapist, Lewisham Hospital, London.

Miss G. MacCaul, m.b.e., hon. fellow b.a.o.t., t.dip., dip. bedford physical training college
Formerly Head Occ. Therapist, King's College Hospital Group, London.

Miss E. M. Macdonald, m.b.e., b.litt. (oxon), s.r.o.t., t.dip., hon. fellow b.a.o.t., hon. fellow w.f.o.t.*
Formerly Principal, Dorset House School of Occ. Therapy (Bristol, Bromsgrove and Oxford). Pilgrim Trust Grant to study Occupational Therapy in the United States (1938). Organiser, Ministry of Health Emergency Medical Service Occupational Therapy Courses, World War II. Research under aegis of University of Oxford into Development of Occupational Therapy and Allied Services, with relation to future expansion. First Chairman, Occupational Therapists' State Registration Board. First Occupational Therapy Representative, Council for Professions Supplementary to Medicine.

Miss M. S. Malthouse, s.r.o.t., m.b.a.o.t.
Head Occ. Therapist, Mount Vernon Hospital, Middlesex.

Miss M. A. Mendez, o.b.e., s.r.o.t., hon. fellow b.a.o.t.
Head Occ. Therapist, Queen Mary's Hospital, Roehampton. Present Chairman, Occupational Therapists' State Registration Board. Occupational Therapy Representative, Council for Professions Supplementary to Medicine. President, World Federation of Occupational Therapists, 1972–76.

Mrs L. M. Mirrey, s.r.o.t., m.b.a.o.t.
Head Occ. Therapist, Cane Hill Hospital, Coulsdon, Surrey. Formerly Head Occ. Therapist, Claybury Hospital. Public Relations Officer to the Association of Occupational Therapists, 1963–65. One year extramural course in Psychology, Cambridge University. University Extension Diploma in History of Art.

Miss J. Northcote Green, s.r.o.t., m.b.a.o.t.
Formerly Tutor-Librarian, Dorset House School of Occupational Therapy, Oxford. Formerly Head Occ. Therapist, St Bartholomew's Hospital, London, and Headington Hill Hall Rehabilitation Unit, Oxford.

Miss J. H. Pitts, s.r.o.t., m.b.a.o.t.
Day Care Manager, Social Services Department, London Borough of Brent. Formerly Senior Occ. Therapist, Sherrard's Industrial Rehabilitation Unit, Welwyn, Herts. Research Assistant, Industrial Engineering Department, Hatfield Polytechnic.

Miss B. Watson, s.r.o.t., m.b.a.o.t.
Head Occ. Therapist, Claybury Hospital, Essex. Formerly Head Occ. Therapist, Cane Hill Hospital, Coulsdon, Surrey. Formerly Occ. Therapist, Queen Elizabeth's Training College for the Disabled, Leatherhead. Attended Administration and Management Courses. W.F.O.T. Delegate to N.A.M.H. World Congress.

Miss J. Whitlock, s.r.o.t., m.b.a.o.t.
Head Occ. Therapist, Park Hospital for Children, Headington, Oxford.

Miss E. S. Wilson, m.b.a.o.t.
Occ. Therapist, Schieffelin Leprosy Research Sanatorium, S. India (since 1964).

Foreword

When Miss Macdonald asked me, in 1960, to write a foreword to the first edition of her book, *Occupational Therapy in Rehabilitation*, I was delighted to do so: I had known Miss Macdonald for a long time, and of her work for even longer. I had always admired the training given at Dorset House, the oldest training school for occupational therapists in the country, whose work is known throughout the world. Now, I am very pleased to bless the launching into the world of the fourth edition of this book.

The field and scope of occupational therapy is expanding every year, and its influence is nowhere more important than in the field of medicine with which I have been associated, that of geriatrics. Here, the occupational therapist no longer keeps strictly to the ward or to her own department. Much exploring needs to be carried out in a patient's home to find out what modifications are necessary before the patient can return there, and who is better able to carry out this exploration than the intelligent and skilled occupational therapist? In the treatment of elderly patients it is often difficult—even if desirable—to decide who plays the most vital and important role: all we know is that without the work of the occupational therapist many old people would not now be leading the useful, normal and independent lives that they are. The same applies to the young, as any one who has watched the progress made by those children who are known as the Thalidomide babies, knows.

When I wrote a foreword to the first edition of Miss Macdonald's book I mentioned that Sir Ludwig Guttman, the director of the Spinal Injuries Centre at Stoke Mandeville, maintained that he did not regard his treatment of a patient completed until he was once again paying his Income Tax. This is far too great an ideal to be lost sight of, so I unashamedly bring it forward again. It is from the work of students and practitioners who have read this book, and learned from it, that this ideal has become realisable and it is good to know that much of Miss Macdonald's teaching has influenced the development of work in many foreign countries—I have particularly in mind South America, where advance has been encouraged and helped by the I.L.O.*

I wish Miss Macdonald all success with her new edition.

AMULREE
London, 1975

Preface

The first edition of this book was published in 1960, and the second, in 1964. The third edition, coming out in 1970, was very radically revised in the light of the recent and rapid developments in all treatment services. In this latest revision, reference will be found to the new structure of the Health and Social Services, to the many useful investigations and reports made on the Remedial Professions and, in relation particularly to occupational therapy, to the extension of the use of psychological testing and other valuable tests for fulfilling the responsibility of adequate assessment of the patients for treatment and resettlement.

The book is still designed, as were its forerunners, to give an outline of occupational therapy in rehabilitation as currently practised. It is introduced by an account of the development of this particular form of treatment throughout the centuries, culminating in the State recognition of the profession in this country.

The Professions Supplementary to Medicine Act was passed in October 1960 and was followed in 1961 by the setting up of the Council for the Professions Supplementary to Medicine, with representatives from the Privy Council, the Health Ministers, the Secretary of State for Scotland, the Minister of Health and Local Government of Northern Ireland, the English Colleges, the Scottish Corporations, the General Medical Council, and the professions to be registered. The Registration Board for Occupational Therapists started work in February 1962. Applications for the first registration were invited for September 1963. The years between 1960 and 1975 have seen the integration of the profession and the forging of closer links between it and allied treatment services. There are now 4,035 State Registered Occupational Therapists in Great Britain, and a further number working overseas. The professional association is lively and forward-looking, with a membership of about 5,000, and provision has been made for extension of the work by advanced study and research.

In the preparation of this book it has been assumed that readers have some knowledge of the basic subjects required for the direction and application of the treatment and that present or intending occupational therapists will have a knowledge of certain activities and techniques, and of methods of analysing and guiding their use appropriately. No attempt has been made to indicate precise activities for precise disabilities, although, undoubtedly, certain activities have greater treatment value and versatility than others.

While contributions to the text have come from experts in all fields, it is intended that the book be viewed as a whole, and read consecutively. Information given in one chapter has relevance to another. The whole book has been put together to fill an urgent need. It is an attempt to indicate clear aims, and to prevent diffusion of thought in what is, inevitably, a diffuse subject. Although it covers a vast number of treatment aspects and methods, it is intended only as an introduction to the wide variety of fields in which the occupational therapist works. It has always been the hope of the editors and contributors that the specialised sections of the work will become the subjects of more specialised and separate books.

Although the many reports on, and recent developments in, the Health and Social Services, and their organisation, is having considerable influence on the structure and practice of the profession, it is interesting to note that, even as the techniques and aspects change, and as the profession extends its spheres the basic philosophy and principles of the treatment remain very much the same as they have been throughout history. The primary needs of man are still for acceptance, recognition, and security, in home and job, but modern man must be given treatment in a modern way. There is, then, a call for the use of progressive, specialised, and rationalised techniques, in keeping with the thought and living of this fast-moving age. The challenge to the occupational therapist is to be observant, ingenious, and up-to-date in outlook and practice; to be well informed, adaptable and versatile; to create and foster the appropriate therapeutic relationships, and to communicate and co-operate increasingly with other members of the rehabilitation teams, and with government and voluntary agencies.

E. M. MACDONALD, *September, 1975*

Acknowledgements

I would like to begin my list of acknowledgements with a particular note of thanks to Lord Amulree, one time President of our Association and now a Vice President and a good friend, who gives the profession unfailing help and encouragement.

Dr J. Sommerville, F.R.C.P. is another helpful supporter of our work. He was a member of the Occupational Therapists' Registration Board, and Medical Director of the Camden Road and Consultant to Wolfson Rehabilitation Centres, in London (N.W. and S.W. respectively). He has contributed the most explicit and succinct opening paragraphs in Chapter I.

I would also like to thank my collaborators and sub-editors, Miss G. MacCaul and Mrs L. M. Mirrey, who, in addition to their editing functions, have contributed major sections (other than those of which special mention is made below), to the *physical* and *psychiatric* chapters of the book, and Mrs B. Morrison, also a sub-editor, for extensive help in collation and preparation of all contributions and supporting data. Thanks are also due to their respective helpers, Miss P. Jay and Miss B. Watson; to Mrs A. Hughes and Mrs E. Newlands for typing—and retyping—with care and patience; to Miss O. Chubb and Mrs M. Sage for help with the diagrams; and to Dr and Mrs Mirrey, the photographic department of King's College Hospital, Miss B. Johnson, of Lewisham Hospital, Miss E. Rogers and the Medical Photography Department, Nuffield Orthopaedic Centre, Oxford, and Miss M. Cooper of the Bristol Royal Infirmary for the preparation of a new set of photographs.

We are grateful, too, to the following for their special contributions to and/or advice on particular sections, indicated below in chapter order.

Miss J. Northcote Green, Help, Benefits and Resettlement (chapter 4).
Miss E. M. Hollings, Assessment and Reporting (chapter 6).
Miss P. E. Jay and Miss L. Cheshire, Splints (chapter 8).
Mrs E. M. G. Grove, Head Injuries and Parkinsonism (chapter 10).
Miss B. Johnson and Miss S. Lawton, Rheumatoid Disease, Osteo-arthrosis and Ankylosing Spondylitis (chapter 11).
Miss J. E. Edwards, Pulmonary Tuberculosis (chapter 11).
Miss M. A. Mendez, Amputees (chapter 11).
Miss S. M. Malthouse, Burns (chapter 11).
Miss E. S. Wilson, Leprosy (chapter 11).
Miss E. B. L. Bushell, Mental Subnormality (chapter 16).
Miss R. Anderson, Mrs P. Chaplin, Miss E. D. Cook and Miss J. L. Whitlock, Children and Adolescents with Psychological Disorders (chapter 17).
Miss R. Halliday, Children with Physical Disorders (chapter 18).
Miss S. Blencowe and Miss J. Pitts, The Cerebral Palsied (chapter 19).
Miss J. E. Ford, Geriatric Patients (chapter 20).
Miss N. Berrington Jones, Miss B. Anstice and Mr J. Chick, Occupational Therapy in the Community (chapter 21).
Miss B. Watson, Industrial Work in Rehabilitation (chapter 22), and, with Mrs M. Davies, Communication and Management relating to an Occupational Therapy Department (chapter 23).

Our debt to the following for their advice and help must also be acknowledged.

Dr P. J. R. Nichols, Director of Physical Medicine, Nuffield Orthopaedic Centre, Oxford, and Butterworth and Co. Ltd for permission to reproduce check lists 1 and 2 (chapter 6) from *Rehabilitation of the Severely Disabled*.
Dr J. Burrows, Director of Physical Medicine, Mundesley Hospital, Norfolk, for help on the chapter on the Upper Limb (chapter 6).
Dr B. E. W. Mace, Lewisham Hospital, for help with the section on Rheumatoid Disease, Osteo-arthrosis and Ankylosing Spondylitis (chapter 11).
Miss E. S. Robertson, Queen Mary's Hospital, Roehampton, for advice re Amputees (chapter 11).
Dr S. G. Browne, O.B.E., Director, The Leprosy Study Centre, London. Consultant Advisor in Leprosy to the Department of Health, for advising on the Leprosy Section (chapter 11).
Dr J. G. Howells, Institute of Family Psychiatry, Ipswich, and Dr C. Ounsted, The Park Hospital for Children, Oxford, for comments and help on the section on children with Psychological Disorders (chapter 17).
Dr E. F. Mason, M.B.E., Director of Physical Medicine, United Oxford Hospitals, and Miss E. Dallas, Formerly Director, St Andrews School of Occupational Therapy, Northampton (former contributor), for advice and contributions to chapter on Children with Physical Disorders (chapter 18).
Miss M. Mort, a former contributor to the section on Geriatric Patients (chapter 20).
Mr J. J. Lowe and Mr D. W. Sutton, of the United Oxford Hospitals, and Mr H. L. Dennison, Bursar, The Dorset House School of Occupational Therapy for advice on finance and other aspects in the organisation of an occupational therapy department (chapter 23).

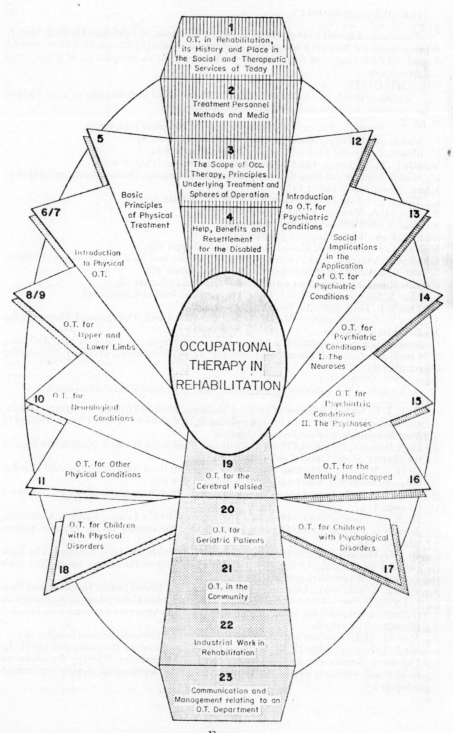

1
O.T. in Rehabilitation, its History and Place in the Social and Therapeutic Services of Today

2
Treatment Personnel Methods and Media

3
The Scope of Occ. Therapy, Principles Underlying Treatment and Spheres of Operation

4
Help, Benefits and Resettlement for the Disabled

5
Basic Principles of Physical Treatment

6/7
Introduction to Physical O.T.

8/9
O.T. for Upper and Lower Limbs

10
O.T. for Neurological Conditions

11
O.T. for Other Physical Conditions

12
Introduction to O.T. for Psychiatric Conditions

13
Social Implications in the Application of O.T. for Psychiatric Conditions

14
O.T. for Psychiatric Conditions I. The Neuroses

15
O.T. for Psychiatric Conditions II. The Psychoses

16
O.T. for the Mentally Handicapped

OCCUPATIONAL THERAPY IN REHABILITATION

19
O.T. for the Cerebral Palsied

20
O.T. for Geriatric Patients

21
O.T. in the Community

22
Industrial Work in Rehabilitation

23
Communication and Management relating to an O.T. Department

18
O.T. for Children with Physical Disorders

17
O.T. for Children with Psychological Disorders

FIG. 1.

Bold figures indicate chapter numbers.

Contents

Chap.   PART FIVE   *Page*

PART SIX

Part One

CHAPTER 1

Occupational Therapy in Rehabilitation, Its History and Place in the Health and Social Services of Today

The planning which lies at the heart of successful rehabilitation must be directed towards a well-defined end. The level of optimum function to which a patient may aspire is a highly individual matter, being determined by all the circumstances of the individual case and not merely by the physical or psychological limitations which confront both the patient and the therapist responsible for treatment. This optimum function will be represented by a point on a scale between normality and complete dependence.

This book deals with the principles of treatment, and it will be apparent that the essence of medical rehabilitation is activity and that the patient must do the work under the supervision of the therapist.

The planning of a programme for the individual patient requires considerable knowledge, skill, and the ability to keep this programme under constant review. The object should be, at any one time, to produce a situation which represents a challenge to the patient—a challenge which can be accepted and achieved. To set too high a target produces frustration and even despair. To set too low a target produces boredom and apathy, and prolongs the rehabilitation process unnecessarily. Programme planning must result in a series of activities in logical sequence which are designed to produce the best possible total situation rather than merely influence—say—the range of movement in one particular joint, or a particular psychiatric symptom.

For physical conditions the specific effects of exercise consist of improvement in muscle power, range of joint movement, coordination, endurance and speed. For psychiatric conditions an activity may be used specifically to improve working capacity and normal personal and social habits. Also, the relationship established between patient and therapist through the activity may be used to help the patient understand and resolve specific psychiatric problems. At the same time properly prescribed and controlled activity provides valuable information concerning the functional capabilities of the individual patient, and so contributes to the planning of the patient's future management and resettlement. There are significant and valuable side-effects to specific exercise. Cardiac and respiratory reserve and general physical fitness are improved by such treatment. Furthermore, the effect of such improvement is reflected in the patient's mental state and results in better motivation, and so helps to speed up the rate of progress. Likewise, stimulation of the mind through purposeful activity can improve psychological performance.

One of the services which contributes to the rehabilitation of the patient is occupational therapy, which has been described as 'an active method of treatment with a profound psychological justification'. [1] This may appear a generalisation. It is nevertheless true, applied as it is to a treatment service which has so many facets and so few boundaries.

The responsibility and aim of the occupational therapist is, through careful assessment of the patient's problem, and the use of appropriate situations and activities, to help the patient to recover or to develop competence [2] in the physical, psychological, social and economic aspects of his life—competence to communicate, to make personal adaptations and relationships, to become adequate or proficient in work and recreation, competence to take his appropriate place in life in an appropriate way.

The term occupational therapy is often, and quite wrongly, applied to any occupation in which the disabled person may be engaged. It is not denied that this occupation may have a therapeutic effect, but it may have the opposite. It is only true therapy if it is medically prescribed and expertly applied for the definite purpose of dealing with the specific socio-medical problem of the individual. Hence the need for the therapist to have a knowledge of disease and disability, of social problems as they affect the person receiving treatment, of occupational and vocational opportunities and of the physical and psychological demands and effects of these [3].

The occupational therapist of early history was the 'doctor' himself. Later, with increasing claims on his time, and as the advantages of the treatment became more apparent, causing it to be more widely used, he had to call in the help of other experts, and the occupational therapist of today gradually came into being as a medical worker. This occupational therapist is now a trained specialist who, through a study of particular aspects of certain sciences, and of practical methods of ability assessment, together with an analysis of the elements of a number of activities and of their value in rehabilitation, guides, under the prescription of the doctor, the occupational treatment of the patients referred to her. She may, in fact, be termed an Occupational Therapy Consultant, in that her emphasis is on the therapeutic uses of the occupation so as to bridge the gap between disability and ability. Because of the diversity of activities which may be needed, and because of the persistent shortage of those with her therapeutic expertise, it may be necessary for her to become even more of a consultant and to direct or advise, and forge closer links with experts in activity techniques.

The early history of occupational therapy is closely related to that of physiotherapy and remedial gymnastics, and, less closely, but also quite distinctly, with the work of the orthoptist, speech therapist and social worker. From a study of their combined development one point of particular interest emerges. Almost all early forms of exercise, medically prescribed, had a social implication and a mental *and* occupational interest. Exercise was seldom used without the 'diverting' element. Stress on the importance of body and mind persisted throughout the ages [4], and this consideration of mental, physical and social interdependence has remained one of the fundamental rules in applying occupational therapy.

It is necessary to recognise that the development of rehabilitation by occupation could only follow the progress of the sciences which contribute to all forms of medical treatment. Those particularly relevant to occupational therapy are anatomy, physiology, psychology and pathology; mathematics and mechanics. As these came to follow an accepted scientific pattern, occupational therapy, like other treatment services, also developed. Meanwhile its 'occupational' aspects were evolved from the arts, crafts and trades of the different centuries, and the story of their use as treatment makes fascinating and enlightening reading, sobering only in the fact that it has taken a very long time to put to good use the wisdom and recommendations of the rehabilitation experts of earlier years.

Although treatment by occupation may have a history dating back earlier than written records, some of the first references to its use appear in the period of magic (before 600 B.C.). Aesculapius is said to have quieted delirium 'with songs, farces and music' [5] and Homer tells of the 'noble craftsman god', Hephaistos, who, lame and disowned by his mother, was rescued by Thetis and Euronyme and given the equipment for forging 'much cunning handiwork' [6], becoming, thereby, established in a 'gainful' occupation.

Following the period of mythology and magic came that of scientific experiment (600 B.C. to A.D. 200). Pythagoras and Thales, like Aesculapius and Orpheus, used music as a remedy, and Hippocrates, emphasising the body-mind link in all treatment, recommended wrestling, riding, and 'labour', meaning, so we are told, 'strong Exercise, or Exercise turned into a business' [7], except for acute conditions.

It was during this time that marked strides were made in the scientific study of the correlated subjects. Dissection, although sporadic, became a basis for the understanding of anatomy, and the *causes* of disease were sought. The subjects of mathematics, and of leverage and movement were also pursued and for these such names as Eudoxus, Euclid and Archimedes are remembered.

Cornelius Celsus, besides contributing to the study of anatomy and medicine, recommended what may perhaps be termed 'occupational exercise' for maintaining health, i.e. sailing, hunting, handling of arms, ball games, running and walking. He prescribed 'clara lectio', or reading aloud, for a weak stomach,[8] and wrote 'of several kinds of madness and their cures', recommending the use of occupation 'suitable to the temper of each'. He suggested that this be applied, for some conditions, indirectly, a method which in modern treatment terms might be called 'behaviour and environmental engineering' or 'behaviour therapy'. He also urged the *combined* use of treatment techniques.

Another outstanding name of this period is that of Galen, who promoted treatment by occupation, suggesting such activities as digging, ploughing, fishing; house, ship or plough building; in fact, anything by which a skilled or unskilled worker earned his livelihood. This stresses, even at that early date (A.D. 130–200), a vital element which has to be, but is not sufficiently, remembered in applying occupational therapy today, i.e. the importance of directing the treatment on realistic vocational and resettlement lines.

In the ensuing period, that of the Dark Ages (A.D. 200–1250), progress almost ceased, but at intervals, and particularly at the end of the period, certain events, important to this history, and indeed to the history of other, allied professions, occurred. Some of the most striking were the experiments of Caelius Aurelianus, a fifth-century neurologist, who wrote of passive and active treatment of all kinds for all types of paralyses. He included massage, poulticing, baths (wax and others), graded exercises and speech therapy. Exercises against resistance and with the aid of slings and pulleys [9] are fully described and read like an account of modern combined treatment [10], the patient being exhorted to share in the effort of rehabilitating himself.

From A.D. 1100, and with the founding of many of the universities of Europe, came a revival in scientific study. One of the most significant factors of this time was the institution of medical examinations, and of state control and licensing of medical practice [11], a pattern which has been followed, if only recently, for this and a number of allied professions.

Between A.D. 1250 and 1700 there followed considerable progress. Medical studies were more profound, and greater attention was given to detail. Attention was redirected, too, to anatomical and physiological study and that of philosophy and psychology. Hospitals were set up, although treatment, particularly of the mentally ill, still left much to be desired.

During this period attention was directed to analysis of movement, and Leonardo da Vinci, Descartes and Francis Bacon (Lord Verulam) became interested in industrial physiology, taking especial note, as did Ramazzini later, of rhythm, posture and expenditure of energy, while Sanctorius Sanctorius, influenced by Descartes, Harvey and Galileo, developed his theories on metabolism.

Occupational exercises and recreations, for 'toughening up', and for enjoyment, were recommended by physicians and educationalists of the day. The prescriptions of Thomas Sydenham included riding—(for gout, colic, diarrhoea, constipation and asthma)—and to those who had no horses, he lent his own. Riding and hunting for children of the upper classes, and rural work, such as ploughing, digging and carrying loads, for those less well-to-do, were prescribed by Nicolas Andry, famous orthopaedic surgeon and Professor of Medicine in Paris.

Ramazzini, 'Professor of Practical Medicine' at Padua, stressed the importance of prevention rather than treatment, and of observing the patient-worker in his workshop. He noted particularly the value of weaving (a trade of the times) as exercise, and refers to cobbling, tailoring and pottery. In spite of the apparent appreciation of the value of treatment by occupation during this period, however, there is little evidence of consistency in experiment or of systematised assessment, analysis and 'prescription'.

From 1700 to the present day the development of the profession falls into two fairly distinct periods. Between 1700 and 1850 there were further advances in psychology, anatomy and physiology, including the mechanics of respiration. Discoveries relating to the action of the nervous system, and to the differentiation between reflex and volitional action, were made. All this tended to cause treatment to become more complex and specialised. Closer links were developed between European countries, more medical books were published, and the Industrial Revolution gave wider publicity to health and social problems. More hospitals were established, and the beginnings of improved treatment, particularly in the mental field, became apparent.

Electricity came, during this period, to be more closely linked with medical practice, and it is important and interesting to note that this was one of the factors which influenced the gradual separation of the exercise treatment group, consisting, as it did, of the overlapping techniques of occupational and physiotherapy, and remedial gymnastics. Electricity brought a change to the emphasis of physiotherapy itself, and the significant feature of this was that much of the exercise given as treatment gradually lost its occupational or mental interest. The body continued to receive treatment but the mind interest of the exercise was not wholly maintained. All the attributes, which had been merged in the rather general form of occupational and exercise therapy, were still needed, but became separated. This brought specialisation to each group, and the different treatment entities began to emerge as separate professions, with less in common between their methods and techniques.

Before the separation, which was gradual, there were, however, a number of instances of the use of the combined forms of treatment during this period. Francis Fuller, in his *Medicina Gymnastica* [12], gave great support to the use of exercise and made more definite recommendations for the treatment of specific diseases by these various methods than had been given hitherto. He pleads for 'Exercise . . . to be taken as a common Aid to Physic' for 'Exercise . . . is to Physic as a Bandage is to Surgery, an assistance or Medium', and discusses riding, wrestling, exercises with a hanging ball, and other activities and their medical application.

In 1780 C. J. Tissot classified occupational exercise as *active*, *passive*, and *mixed*, and among the activities he recommended were sewing, playing the violin, sweeping, sawing, bell-ringing, hammering, chopping wood, riding and swimming. Sir John Sinclair (1806), in several publications [13], also recommended exercise through work, and prescribed, for an advancing society in which fewer of its members would need to do manual work,

> 'that species of voluntary labour which is generally accompanied with some degree of pleasure as well as toil, which goes by the name of EXERCISE'.

Dr Buchan, in his *Domestic Medicine* (1774), stressed the advisability of men learning some mechanical employment, and of making 'masterly specimens of their own workmanship, for the maintenance of health', while John Shaw (1792–1827), head of a medical school in London, recommended *graded exercises*, particularly for scoliosis.

The recognition of the value and need for occupation for the maintenance of health was also subscribed to in the psychological field. Philippe Pinel, and after him William Tuke and Vizencio Chiarugi, had their patients freed from chains, and provided occupations for them. In a *Description of the Retreat. The Modes of Treatment and a Statement of Cases* published in 1813, and dedicated to William Tuke, by his grandson, Samuel Tuke, there is, in speaking of mania, reference to the 'beneficial effects of exercise and variety of objects' and the 'advantage of regular labour in some cases'. 'The different kinds of amusing employments adapted to different classes of Patients' are also referred to, as is the introduction of books, the importance of arresting attention, and the difficulty of devising suitable employment. Reading, writing, drawing, and playing at ball, chess, and draughts are all mentioned, and reference is made to a patient who applied himself to mathematics 'with which he had been well acquainted in his youth'. In a later *Manual of Psychological Medicine* published in 1879, and written by John Charles Bucknill and Daniel Hack Tuke, the following occupations are also listed: balls, visits to theatres, and theatrical entertainments. They say:

> 'Work, no doubt, has also a moral influence, and in that regard we may call it Occupation, and consider it together with Recreation',

and continue:

> 'It appears to us that women in our public asylums ought to share with men the advantage of outdoor work. . . . Some of them are kept too stringently to the monotonous and not very wholesome labour, that of the wash-tub, for example',

adding:

'It certainly ought to be laid down, as a rule, that no lunatic patient should be permitted to engage in work except under medical sanction.'

These are all points still relevant to the application of occupational therapy today.

Henri Monnier, describing A. Grohmann's *Work Institute for the Nervously Ill* in Zurich [14] refers to the debilitating effects of inactivity, and to the importance of interesting the patients in an occupation which might, later, help them to earn a livelihood. He lists gardening and woodwork, stressing the strengthening quality of these; and typography, modelling, and art, as therapeutic, and possibly vocational, activities.

The history of occupational therapy from this time on, and relating particularly to its development in Europe and later in America is well and fully told by Dr S. Licht, in his *Occupational Therapy Source Book* [15]. The succeeding account here is limited, therefore, to the factors which particularly influenced its development in this country.

From 1850 onwards there was the gradual emergence of the various supplementary treatment services as professions and between then and now came the formation of associations, the institution of training courses, and of recognised examinations and qualifications. In the latter part of the nineteenth century women were taking up careers and, at the turn of the century, were being accepted into the professions. The Crimean War hastened the establishment of nursing, the First World War of physiotherapy (although some occupational therapy was also carried on), but it was in the Second World War that occupational therapy in this country really came into its own.

The main trend of expansion in the early part of the period had been in the psychological field, and by the end of the nineteenth century occupational therapy was practised, although in rather different forms, in this country, in Ireland, the United States, France, Germany, Switzerland, Austria, Norway and Portugal, and in Belgium at Gheel. In Great Britain the best-known centres were at The Retreat, York, and at Hanwell Asylum, now St Bernard's Hospital, Southall.

There was, at this stage, and particularly in the United States, considerable speculation as to what the best name for the service should be, and who would be the best person to administer it. The treatment suffered from fluctuating popularity and acceptance, partly because of its apparent simplicity, and partly because it depended, as it still does, too much on the enthusiasm of particular doctors. In 1914, Eva Charlotte Reid suggested calling it 'Ergo therapy', [16] and 'moral [17] treatment', 'manual work', and 'invalid occupations', were other proposals, none truly descriptive of its therapeutic aims. Finally George Barton, of Clifton Springs, originated the term 'Occupational Therapy', and taken in its fullest and widest sense (which is not always done) it is difficult to find a better.

The problem of the worker remained. Nurses were primarily interested in nursing, particularly of the acutely ill. In any case the nursing approach is not really applicable in this work. It is eminently important in giving the patient specialist care and a 'home base' in the hospital setting, and even for providing, as is done in a home, occupational and social interests and this *is* the function of the nursing profession. For the application of true occupational therapy, however, the visiting or visited occupational therapist is the person to direct the treatment for those who need it—and this is not necessarily every patient—approaching the patient, as she does, from a totally different and specialised angle.

On the other hand, vocational instructors were seldom 'treatment minded', although there is no doubt that their technical expertise can contribute usefully to the occupation of patients, and to 'therapy', if working in appropriate collaboration with the 'consultant' therapist. Doctors themselves were too busy, and, without a greater knowledge of a wide range of activities and of the physical and psychological implications of these, could often do no more than recommend 'occupation' in very general terms. Who, then, was to carry out these rather wide and unprecise prescriptions with sufficient medical and technical skill, and with due care and understanding? By a process of evolution and experiment it became apparent that the person should combine some of the qualities of both nurse and instructor, should have a vital interest in people, organising ability, and a knowledge of mental and physical illness, and of activities and their therapeutic possibilities. After selection and training on these lines the *Occupational Therapist* of today emerged.

Although the main impetus came to occupational therapy during the Second World War, the treatment was also used during the First. In this Canada took the lead, closely followed by the United States. In Great Britain the eminent surgeon, Sir Robert Jones, showed his appreciation of occupational therapy, and prevailed upon the War Office to set up 'Orthopaedic Centres'. At one he established the first curative workshop of its kind. He wrote:

'Our first experiment in devising work having a direct curative bearing upon the recovery from injuries was started . . . at Shepherd's Bush Military Orthopaedic Hospital [18]. The Plan was rapidly extended to other centres. It has proved a very valuable adjunct. . . . Theoretically we have the power to compel men to adopt this curative agent. In practice the power is never needed. We depend largely upon the psychological element to help in the recovery. . . . Those of us who have any imagination cannot fail to realize the difference in atmosphere and morale in hospitals where patients have nothing to do . . . from that found where, for part of the day, they have regular, useful and productive work. If a patient's former trade or employment is a suitable one he is put to use tools he understands. Otherwise some occupation *suitable for his disability and curative in character* is found for him.' [19]

This is an admirable description of the meaning of occupational therapy. It is distressing, however, that in the last war, although the use of the treatment was far more widespread in the Emergency Medical and other Service Hospitals, it was often not possible to use the more realistic occupations because of trade prejudice. Treatment activities were limited, therefore, to the field of crafts. This was frustrating to those who had to carry out the prescriptions, and gave quite a wrong emphasis to the occupational aspect of the treatment. It seriously affected the doctors' appreciation of its possibilities and had a narrowing effect on training, in that students could not be taught what they were not able to practise. This state of affairs has however vastly improved in the last decade.

It is notable that the spurt of interest shown in the 1914–18 war was not maintained. Until the late 1920s occupational therapy continued to be used mainly in mental hospitals, although the system of application of the treatment, as such, had not been very clearly defined. Some of the first demonstrations were given by Dr D. K. Henderson, in Edinburgh, and by Dr J. Iveson Russell, at the North Riding Hospital, Yorkshire, the latter publishing the first English book on *The Occupational Treatment of Mental Illness* [20].

The first school of occupational therapy in Great Britain was started at Bristol in 1930, [21] at a treatment centre for neurotic and early psychotic patients. A curative workshop for out-patients requiring physical treatment was also opened there in 1938, to demonstrate the value of occupational therapy for physical disabilities. It was in great part this demonstration, coupled with that of the Shepherd's Bush experiment that encouraged the Ministry of Health to establish the rehabilitation workshops in their Emergency Medical Service [22] hospitals, referred to above, during the Second World War.

1930 to 1940 was a decade of progress and integration which merged into the expansion of the following years. In 1934 the first English conference of occupational therapy was held, and in 1936 the Association of Occupational Therapists in England was formed (the Scottish one, having been started in 1932, was re-formed in 1946). In 1938 the first public examinations of the English Association were held, and with the war came a hurried and somewhat hectic expansion in the physical field. War-time courses were organised for those with allied qualifications, such as nurses, physiotherapists, and experts in certain occupational techniques. These were 'grafted on' to the full-time courses.

In 1943 the Association in England (which also covered Wales and Northern Ireland) became incorporated, and in 1974 it and the Scottish Association joined to become the *British Association of Occupational Therapists*. In 1951 the *World Federation of Occupational Therapists** was formed, and has held International Congresses in Edinburgh (1954), Copenhagen (1958), Philadelphia (1962), London (1966), Zurich (1970) and Vancouver

(1974). This World Federation has forged links for the profession with the World Health Organisation.

This account will not be complete without some reference to the effect of the National Health Service on the profession, and to the place of occupational therapy in the socio-medical framework of today. With the implementation of the National Health Service Act in 1948, came a greater awareness of the components of that service, among them occupational therapy and its allied professions. In 1949 the Minister of Health and Secretary of State for Scotland set up eight committees under the chairmanship of Mr (later Sir) Zachary Cope, one of which was:

'to consider the supply and demand, training and qualification of Occupational Therapists in the National Health Service, and to make recommendations.' [23]

The findings, published in 1951, were not satisfactory, the members of the profession itself dissenting from others on the committee and being forced to issue a minority report. Because of lack of unanimity on the whole report, it was dropped.

In 1954 the Ministers set up a combined Working Party in an attempt to resolve the deadlock. This move had been preceded by the passing of 'The National Health Services (Medical Auxiliaries) Regulations' in January of the same year, defining 'the qualifications required for employment as medical auxiliaries in the National Health Service'. The Ministers gave the assurance that these regulations would 'in no way prejudice the possible introduction of statutory registration', declaring them to be a temporary measure, pending further negotiations. The Ministers have, undoubtedly, a responsibility for making proper provision for the functioning of the National Health Service* and for distinguishing, for this purpose, the qualified from the unqualified. The members of the profession also have a responsibility. This is first to their clients, the patients, whether their contact with them is through the National Health Service or in some other field [24]. They have also a responsibility to the organisations in, or through which, they work. As members of a treatment team, and in company with others in the team, occupational therapists had already developed standards of ethics, training and qualification as a guarantee of a high level of service. The introduction of State Registration under the Professions Supplementary to Medicine Act of 1960 has given official recognition to this and allied professions, and has, through each Professional Board, linked state and professional interest and responsibilities for 'promoting high standards of professional education and professional conduct' [25] in the Health and Social Services. It is recognised that the exercise of the profession of Occupational Therapy calls for certain special qualities of character and temperament and makes persistent demands upon the physical and mental resources of the practitioner.

How, then, does occupational therapy stand in the medico-social treatment framework today? Like others, it is now a distinct profession, with its professional association, interested not only in the ethics and qualification referred to above, but in further study and development. Although, as with other treatment services, its application was, at first, empirical, there is an increasing awareness of the necessity for the testing of hypotheses and the formulation of theory. Only by doing so can the profession extend its usefulness beyond the limits of the repetitive and somewhat non-progressive application which was apparent in its early history.

In addition to achieving state registration, the Cope Committees and the subsequent Working Party have brought the different professions into clearer focus, and helped to create greater understanding between them. This has undoubtedly led to closer cooperation, if only indirectly, and this, in its turn, has contributed to improved treatment. The medical profession, too, understands more of the purpose of occupational therapy and is better able to prescribe and use it.

The late 1960s and the early 1970s have brought a spate of government and other reports, all of which have had varying degrees of influence on the systems and work of the profession [26]. The most important of these, in relation to occupational therapy, and to its links with allied workers, were the following:

(1) 1966 *The Salmon Report*, on senior nursing staff structure.

(2) 1968 *The Seebohm Report*, many recommendations of which are implemented through the *Local Authority Social Service Bill, 1970*.

(3) 1970 *The Oddie Report and Recommendations of the Remedial Professions' Committee of the Council for the Professions Supplementary to Medicine*.

(4) 1972 *Rehabilitation*, the Report of the Subcommittee of the Standing Medical Advisory Committee of the Central Health Services Council, Chaired by Sir Ronald Tunbridge, O.B.E.

(5) 1972 *Statement by the Committee on the Remedial Professions*, set up by the Department of Health and Social Security in 1969, also chaired by Sir Ronald Tunbridge, O.B.E.

Although the remedial professions had been discussed fairly fully in the last three of the reports listed above, there was concern that there were not enough constructive proposals to encourage further collaboration and development, so two more committees were set up to produce the following reports:

(6) 1973 *Report of the Remedial Professions Committee* (a successor to that chaired by Dr Oddie, see (3) above), now chaired by Dr Burt and also produced by the Council for Professions Supplementary to Medicine.

(7) 1973 *The Remedial Professions*, a Report by a Working Party set up in March 1973 by the Secretary of State for the Social Services, under the

chairmanship of E. L. McMillan, Esq., of the Department of Health and Social Security.

The profession was represented in all but (1) and (2) above, and valuable recommendations were made, especially in (7), in connection with the following:

Inter-professional relationships   Career structure
Relationship with the medical profession   Training
Relationship with the nursing profession   Research
Relationship with social workers
Relationship with other staff concerned with
remedial therapy

The latest influence on the functioning of the profession has been the *Reorganisation of the National Health and Social Services* on 1 April 1974. An outline of the new structures is given below.

Under the *National Health Service Act of 1946* it became the duty of the Minister of Health [27] 'to promote the establishment in England and Wales of a comprehensive Health Service designed to secure improvement in the physical and mental health of the people in England and Wales and in the prevention, diagnosis and treatment of illness' [28].

This act, together with the *National Health Service Act (Scotland) of 1947* (with similar provisions for Scotland), came into effect in 1948. These Acts, and the *National Assistance Act of 1948* [29] also gave increased powers and responsibilities to local authorities to provide for the care of the sick and disabled people living at home, either directly, or through voluntary agencies [30]. *The Disabled Persons Employment Acts 1944 and 1958* and the *Mental Health Act 1959* were other forms of legislation which contributed to the reorganisation and development of schemes for the treatment and rehabilitation of the disabled.

The provisions of the National Health Service Act and of the National Assistance Act are now implemented, in different ways, through the *National Health Service Reorganisation Act (1973)* and the *Social Services Act (1970)*, supported by the Disabled Persons Employment Acts and the Mental Health Act, referred to above, and *The Chronically Sick and Disabled Persons Act (1970)* and the *Employment and Training Act (1973)*.

The 'Ministry of Labour', which became the 'Department of Employment and Productivity' is now called the *'Department of Employment'* only, in the terms of the Employment and Training Act.

The structure of the new Health Services [31] (England and Wales) now comprises:

(1) *The Department of Health and Social Security**, which covers the former Ministries of Health, Pensions, National Insurance and the National

Assistance Board. The Department is run by a Secretary of State, and two Ministers of State, one responsible to the Secretary for Health and the other for Social Security.

(2) Fourteen *Regional Health Authorities**, members of which are appointed by the Secretary of State, and are answerable to him/her.

(3) *Area Health Authorities**, conforming to the new local authority metropolitan and county divisions. Teaching Hospitals come under these. The Chairmen are appointed by the Secretary of State, and the members by the Regional Health Authorities, local authorities and universities with which they are connected. They are responsible to the Regional Health Authorities. The *Family Practitioner Committees** of the Area Health Authorities will administer the *Family Practitioner Services**. Area and Regional Authorities will also set up *Professional Advisory Committees**.

(4) *Districts**. A District is defined as 'a population served by the community health services supported by the specialist services of a district general hospital'. Local operational schemes will be planned and coordinated by a *District Management Team*. Each District will have a *District Medical Committee**, a *Health Care Planning Team** and a *Community Health Council**, through which the community will be able to express feelings about the services, to the Area Health Authorities or others.

Community Medicine will come under the District Management Team, with a *District Community Physician**, whose duties will involve him in Preventive Medicine, Health Education and in creating a liaison with the social services of the local government and helping them to deal with their health problems.

In Scotland the organisation differs somewhat. The Department of Health and Social Security is parallelled by the *Scottish Home and Health Department**. There are no Regional Health Authorities. The next in line are 15 *Area Health Boards**, with boundaries conforming to those of local authorities. The next level is the *District**, and, under the Area Health Boards there are 5 *Teaching Districts*. Each District has a *District Executive Group** and the parallels of the Health Care Planning Teams* and the Community Health Councils* have yet to be established. *Community Physicians* are appointed in Districts; they liaise with local government authorities but are not in local government employment.

The function of the occupational therapist has become more clearly defined. Occupational therapists work in an ever-increasing variety of spheres. These are indicated by the contents list of, and the recommendations in, this book. Although it is proper for occupational therapy students to have a basic training course—(and it is encouraging to hear of experiments for sharing this with students of other professions)—there is need, too, for specialisation and research, after qualification, within the profession. Schemes have been devised for advanced work and it is important that therapists should be prepared to detach themselves sufficiently from their immediate claims to make use of these proposals and facilities, in the interests of improved treatment and extension of the service.

In closing this chapter on the development of the profession and its links with members of other professions it is not, perhaps, out of place to mention other groups which claim to apply different forms of occupational 'therapy'—'work or industrial therapists', 'music or drama therapists', 'art therapists' and the like. If trained in an occupation and in *therapy*—with emphasis on the therapy—they are, in fact, occupational therapists. If not trained in therapy, however, they can only, surely, claim to be specialist teachers or instructors in their particular subjects, and as such should clearly cooperate fully in all treatment considerations with trained therapists. It should be more widely appreciated, however, that a particular occupation is not, in itself, therapeutic. It is its careful selection and appropriate and specialist application which is the key to the therapy. Occupational therapists use music, art and industrial work of all kinds in their treatment, and many are highly proficient in these and other specialist techniques.

The relation of the occupational therapist to the nurse, especially in mental hospitals, must be that of the closest cooperation, and from experience it has been found that, given good leadership from the doctors, there can be excellent teamwork. The recommendations of the Salmon Report are likely to influence future planning, but in any re-orientation it is vital that the patient should not become the subject of contention rather than attention, or a pawn in a game in which enthusiasm for experiment, for expansion of spheres or for status, are the most important elements.

In all the considerations of the health and social services of today occupational therapy is recognised as an integral part of them and has an increasingly important contribution to make to them, in collaboration with other health and social service experts. 'Health' and 'Service' are as important today as they were to the early pioneers in what has now become the distinct profession of Occupational Therapy [32].

REFERENCES

1. Clark, D. Stafford, *Psychiatry Today*, p. 169. London, 1952 (Now available as a Pelican Book).
2. See Fiske, D. W. & Maddi, S. R. *Functions of Varied Experience*. Illinois, 1961 (chapter 5, p. 106).
3. In co-operation with social workers.
4. See Reeves, J. W., *Body and Mind in Western Thought*. London, 1958.
5. Le Clerc, D., *History of Physick*, trans. Drake and Baden. London, 1699.
6. Homer, *The Iliad*, Book XVIII.
7. Strother, E., *An Essay on Sickness and Health*. London, 1725.

8. Celsus, C., *Of Medicine*, trans. Grieve, revised Futvoye. London, 1837.
9. See Drabkin's (I. E.), translation of *Caelius Aurelianus on Acute Diseases*. Baltimore, 1951.
10. See Hollis & Roper, *Suspension Therapy in Rehabilitation*, 2nd ed. London, 1965.
11. This precedent has since been followed for dentistry and nursing and is now established for occupational therapy and other allied professions.
12. Or, *Every Man his own Physician*. London, 1740.
13. Sinclair, J., *A Collection of Papers on the Subject of Athletic Exercise*, and *The Code of Health and Longevity*. London, 1806.
14. Leipzig, 1898.
15. Baltimore, 1948.
16. '*Work Therapy*', Greek '*Ergon*' = work or effort.
17. See this chapter, p. 6, quotation 2.
18. In March 1916.
19. Watson, E., *The Life of Sir Robert Jones*. London, 1934. (Italics ours.)
20. London, 1938.
21. By Dr Casson, Elizabeth, *The Dorset House School of Occupational Therapy*. (This moved to the midlands during the war, and then to Oxford, where it now is.)
22. This Service was an experimental forerunner of the present National Health Service.
23. See *Reports of the Committees on Medical Auxiliaries*, pp. 1–71. H.M.S.O.*, 1951. The other Committees dealt with Almoners, Chiropodists, Dietitians, Laboratory Technicians, Physiotherapists and Remedial Gymnasts, Radiographers, and Speech Therapists.
24. Independent hospitals, local authority health or educational services, or in private practice, etc.
25. *Professions Supplementary to Medicine Act*, 1960.
26. In addition to the Reports listed in this chapter there have been the following reports:
1968 The Zuckerman Report, for and about hospital scientific and technical services and staffs.
1972 The Briggs Report, on the role and education of nurses in the hospital and community.
27. And the Secretary of State in Scotland, and the Minister of Health and Local Government in Northern Ireland.
28. *National Health Service Act 1946*, Part I (1).
29. *National Assistance Act 1948*, Part III (29).
30. *National Assistance Act 1948*, Part III (30).
31. See *Reorganisation of the Health Service 1974*. N.E. Met. R.H.B., Oaklea, 47 Whitehall Lane, Buckhurst Hill, Essex. How the Health Service will be reorganised in 1974. *Occ. Ther.* 35, no. 9, 1972. Progress of N.H.S. reorganisation. *Occ. Ther.*, 36, no. 5, 1973. Interpretational relationships in the Health Service. *Occ. Ther.*, 36, no. 7, 1973.
32. Occupational therapists are advised to read Nokes, P., *The Professional Task in Welfare Practice*, London, 1967, and Rehabilitation in the Re-organised National Health Service. *Occ. Ther.*, 37, no. 7, 1974.

* See *Glossary*, pp. 454–5.

CHAPTER 2

Treatment Personnel, Methods and Media

Occupational therapy, although registered as a Profession Supplementary to Medicine, is one of the special disciplines which have, in the medical team headed by the doctor, an important contribution to make in the treatment of the patient. It has more than a supportive function. It has a dynamism of its own in the contribution it makes to re-education for living—for living with, or through, a disability—and to prevention.

Because occupational therapy depends so much on the involvement of both therapist and patient, and because the techniques, which are subordinate to the therapy, are only a part of the philosophy [1] of treatment, it would seem best to discuss, first, the agent applying the treatment, the Occupational Therapist. The aims, methods and location of treatment will be considered next, and some reference will be made to occupations and techniques which may be used therapeutically. Almost any activity can be used. What matters is the *aim* of its use, and whether it achieves, or is suitable to achieve, the purpose for which it is employed.

The Occupational Therapist

Occupational therapists could never function adequately without the combination of knowledge of psychological and medical subjects, of methods of assessment, of social interaction and conditioning, and of various occupations and skills. They must have the capacity to use certain facets of their own personalities in the treatment situation, to evaluate the use of a variety of other media and to develop their work on increasingly scientific lines. At the same time they must not exclude the intuitive approach, which should in turn, be analysed, criticised and evaluated.

Much of the success of this treatment devolves on the occupational therapist herself, on her professional manner and objectiveness and on the 'rapport' she makes with the patient. The therapeutic relationship is all important, and sometimes a patient may have to be transferred from one occupational therapist to another if this relationship cannot be established.

Empathy [2], better than sympathy, is perhaps the key. For this work a well-integrated personality is needed, as is careful training, through example, precept and practice. Although some of the necessary qualities may be innate, others will have to be acquired, and training and practice are no less important for the occupational therapy student than they are for the doctor, nurse, or person who is proficient in some other skilled profession.

An occupational therapist should be perceptive, and will learn, in the course of training and practice, and in working with the doctors and others in the rehabilitation team, what importance to attach to the results of this perception and observation. She should in no way over-impose her will or intention. Some firmness may be necessary and some persuasion called for, but these should be tempered with good judgment, a genuine interest in people and in life in general, a happy disposition, and a sense of humour, all kept in good perspective. The need for an occupational therapist to be an organiser, administrator and teacher, as well as a therapist, is also important, and it will be clear from the succeeding chapters that these qualities are essential for achieving satisfactory results. Training in imparting information [3] clearly and systematically, and with full consideration for the personal, physical and psychological implications of the situation, is a vital part of a student's course and constructive critical help in this is needed from the occupational therapists who take students for clinical practice.

Adaptability is an essential quality for an occupational therapist, because, as the field is so wide, the adequacy of the work has to be clearly demonstrated. By virtue of her training in interpersonal relationships she may be able to find workable solutions, particularly if new and perhaps unorthodox ideas have to be tried out. There will always be the necessary limitations of organisation and finance to be met, and the occupational therapist may, at times, have to accept these. The emphasis should, however, be on 'necessary' only; the occupational therapist should never use these limitations as an excuse for accepting, too easily, poor facilities and conditions. If she is consulted, as she should be, on the form her work should take in a particular situation, and if she is ready to cooperate with the problems of that situation, better treatment for the patient should result. So often, in applying for a post, an Occupational Therapist fails to familiarise herself with the circumstances and problems of the 'set-up' and is then disappointed with conditions or limitations undiscovered before she accepted the post. At the same time, idealistic concepts should give way to realistic ones, and even difficult situations should be seen as a challenge.

The Aims, Methods and Location of Treatment

The question arises as to whether occupational therapy can be described as a science or developed as one. The answer to the first is—hardly yet, and to the second—yes, we believe so. It is, clearly, important for doctors, psychologists, therapists and others to explore further the possibilities of this treatment. Hypotheses should be formed, controls devised where possible, and findings tested and recorded [4]. Only in this way can the more scientific application of the treatment be developed. In any case, what is expected from the treatment must be stated and the choice of method geared to this.

The following objects, clearly related to the concept of competence already advanced [5], are some of the immediate aims of occupational therapy, and form the framework for more specific direction of treatment:

(1) The 'reablement' [6] of the patient for restoration to former life and work.

(2) Where this is not possible, the maintenance of existing function and the use of this in re-establishment of the patient in former work or in a new occupation.

These aims apply both physically and psychologically. That the patient can remain, or become, independent and can earn a living, is of paramount importance. In the event of this being impossible, the aim should be:

(3) The use of activities to help in a happier adjustment to limitations, personal and in the home, with, perhaps, the possibility of occasional earnings.

Referral of Patients

The first necessity for successful treatment is the referral from the doctor in charge of the case. An occupational therapist may be put into touch with patients through others, such as social workers, health visitors, etc., but it is a part of her ethical code to treat only on medical 'prescription'. This cannot, in itself, be detailed or precise in its reference to a particular occupation or to a certain technique of an activity, but must indicate the medical and social needs of the patient.

The essential features of referral are:

(1) Provisional diagnosis [7].
(2) Important medical information, relative to treatment.
(3) Treatment aims. (This is the core of a good prescription.)
(4) Contra-indications or precautions, if other than those normally associated with the diagnosis.

To these should be added essential social information about the patient and other items of importance for particular types of disability. If forms are used some indication should be given on these of the scope of treatment activities available. (See following form for referral of patient for physical treatment.)

REHABILITATION CENTRE
Occupational Therapy

NAME	AGE
DIAGNOSIS	OCCUPATION

AIMS OF TREATMENT	WORKING POSITION

AIMS OF TREATMENT

1. Assessment: ADL { a. Personal / b. Domestic
2. To build up muscle power in specific area
3. To improve range of movement in specific joint
4. To improve balance and coordination
5. Assessment: Resettlement and Work Capacity
6. General toughening

SPECIAL INSTRUCTIONS

Doctor's signature..............

WORKING POSITION

1. Standing
2. Sitting
3. Limb in elevation

DEGREE OF WORK

1. Heavy
2. Medium
3. Light

Date..............

The following is a sample of a useful form of referral for psychiatric treatment.

OCCUPATIONAL THERAPY

DATE OF ADMISSION	MARITAL STATE	AGE	WARD	NAME: Mr Mrs Miss

Previous
occupation and work record

Diagnosis and presenting symptoms

Emotional stability

Aim of treatment: (Doctor prescribes in consultation with team.)

1. Return to previous environment and work.

2. Prevocational guidance

3. Work in hospital utilities

4. Any other aim

Specifically in:*

1. O.T. Depts.—Admission
   —20-30 group
   —middle age group
   —psycho-geriatric group
2. Ward class
3. Typing pool
4. Cookery and housewifery
5. Dressmaking
6. Art class
7. P.T. class
8. Industrial unit

Other treatments received:

Precautions and/or special instructions:
Reports required every day/week/month
O.T. Dept.
Hospital

Doctor's signature
Date

* This can be adjusted to suit local requirements.

Methods of referral will vary from hospital to hospital or centre to centre, but it is essential for the occupational therapist to have the medical referral in some form, and to recognise that unless she has this she is effecting a breach of etiquette and responsibility. If serious results occur only she could be held responsible, with resulting serious professional, and possibly financial consequences [8].

There are several ways of implementing the advice and instructions given. The occupational therapist must first assess the needs of the patient. Then, with the aims of treatment in mind, help the patient to select the form of activity which will be most valuable as treatment. She may need to offer suitable incentives to gain the cooperation of the patient, and must see that interest, effort and satisfaction are maintained during treatment, so that he finds, not only satisfaction in attaining the goal, but has justifiable opportunity for zest and pleasure in the process.

In a psychiatric therapeutic community the selection of the activity may be the subject of discussion by all staff and patients, this discussion and the reasons for the choice being instruments of treatment in themselves.

It must be remembered, however, that even if occupational therapy has, as is rightly claimed, 'a profound psychological justification', the activities used should not necessarily always coincide with the choice and interests of the patients. Indeed, if limited thus, the occupation might in some instances be the opposite of therapeutic.

Reading Case Histories and Taking Notes

Personal and medical information included in the prescription or referral form may be brief. The occupational therapist should augment this by discussion with the medical officer and other members of the treatment team, and by reading case histories and reports. Certain case histories are available to her; others, sometimes in mental hospitals, may be seen by the doctor only. It is important that the patient can feel that personal information he discusses with his doctor can be regarded as confidential, nor are all details relevant to the treatment provided by the occupational therapist, or members of allied medical services.

If case histories are not available a summary of the essential information must be sought verbally or in writing, and the occupational therapist herself must indicate what is, in fact, necessary. In some instances, the head or senior occupational therapist only may have access to the case histories, and she will extract details required by the other members of her department. No occupational, or any other trained therapist, can work without information concerning her patients, but information, whether obtained from a case history or from discussion in clinics or ward rounds, is completely confidential. No patient should ever be discussed by name with any persons except those directly responsible for his treatment.

Reporting on Treatment [9]

The value of occupational therapy does not end with the successful involvement of the patient in a therapeutic activity. A further important function of the occupational therapist is to keep in close touch with the doctor and other members of the rehabilitation team and to draw up appropriate reports for them. These need not be extensive, unless this is especially requested, but should be trenchant and couched in professional terms and should give a realistic picture of the patient's competence, in the fullest sense in which this term is being used [10]. Forms which may offer useful suggestions are shown in the section on Assessment and Reporting (chapters 6, 7 and 19) but the occupational therapist is advised to discuss with the doctor and other treatment colleagues in her particular centre, the angle and aim of her work and of theirs, before deciding upon the points to emphasise in reporting. It is possible that she may not, at first, get sufficient help in this because of lack of understanding of the possibilities of occupational therapy and of its use in collaboration with other treatments. The first task of the occupational therapist may, therefore, be one of interpretation and she may have to devise her first forms herself [11]. She should emphasise, however, that these are only experimental and, as soon as possible, forms should be planned by the whole team.

Location of Treatment

The organisation of occupational therapy in ward or workshop, the type of equipment necessary, and other administrative considerations are discussed in chapter 23. The differences in organisation for physical, psychiatric, and other centres will also emerge from other chapters. For the purpose of considering the planning of treatment in correct perspective it is necessary, however, to make brief reference here to the differences in location of the treatment.

Treatment in the ward. Because short-term patients do not require occupational therapy in the acute stages, and, with advances in medicine are able to return home more quickly, occupational therapy for ward patients has lessened considerably. Once prescriptive considerations permit or require it, however, it should be started in its simplest form, if only conversational. Ward work calls for considerable preparation and, although time consuming, is important for specific cases, such as some psychiatric, neurological and child patients. Even if the treatment given is in the form of diversion or indirect treatment, the foundation of the necessary personal relationship and 'pattern' for later more specific treatment may be laid at this stage. This is true for all types of hospitals.

The Occupational Therapy Department or treatment room. Many hospitals have some occupational therapy centre attached to the ward (as in psychiatric hospitals), or in physical hospitals, in a separate unit, adjacent to other treatment units and, where possible, with access to space for outdoor activities. Out-patients as well as in-patients may attend these units. In the workshop there is greater opportunity for participation in group work, or for work more akin to the patients' own jobs. The best use needs to be made of the working atmosphere and of the opportunity for variation and progression in treatment.

From the hospital treatment department many patients may be able to return to their own work or to undertake a new job. An industrial workshop attached to the hospital may offer a transition or an alternative for those who have to remain in medical care. Where work in the open community is impossible, it may be necessary to arrange it under sheltered conditions or in the home.

Discussion of methods of retraining and resettlement will be found in chapters 4, 7 and 22. It is sufficient therefore to refer only briefly here to the sheltered workshop and to treatment in the home [12].

The sheltered workshop. The different types of sheltered work conditions, ranging from Remploy* factories to day centres, are discussed in chapters 4, 21 and 22. In the sheltered workshop conditions of work are geared to the needs and problems of the workers, and the transition from hospital to a day centre or sheltered workshop is preferable to relegation to being what is termed 'homebound'. A workshop has the advantage of offering wider social contacts and the fact of going out to work has a normalising effect. As in the hospital industrial unit, it also offers the possibility for each person to work at a section or unit of production, within his capabilities, instead of having to complete the whole of an article with varying degrees of difficulty in the techniques needed. It is true of course that production can be 'broken down' for various homebound workers so that each does a section, but the incentives of working with others, and of seeing the various stages being done, and the finishing of the object, are lacking.

A report on the considerations of workshops in hospitals, by the *Standing Mental Health Advisory Committee* [13], stated:

> 'The Committee recommended that industrial schemes in hospital should be contained within separate units in which the regime should approximate to that of outside industry. Patients should have "a modest financial incentive to engage in work designed to re-establish social capacity". The Committee also considered that industrial work in a unit which conforms to the less exacting hospital pattern might be done by patients, especially the subnormal, who are likely to remain in hospital for the rest of their lives.'

The place of the occupational therapist in such schemes may vary. In the hospital she may, in fact, be the supervisor, or she may, in cooperation with the doctor, be the assessor and consultant. Any occupational therapist contemplating working in collaboration with a sheltered work scheme would be advised to visit some of the experimental centres [14]. She should also undertake a course of work study.

Work for patients in their homes is provided by community occupational therapists of the health or social services departments of the county local authorities. It is difficult to organise and is time consuming, but, after initial problems have been overcome, is most rewarding and increasingly important in the concept of community care. It requires a great deal of ingenuity, imagination, experience, energy and integrity. It should not be viewed by patient or therapist as a permanency. Many patients who have been given treatment in their homes, with, perhaps, little hope of progression, have been able, later, to go to work in sheltered conditions, with the social assets that accompany this.

In the future the occupational therapist may have a particularly valuable supportive role to play in both hospital and community situations, helping parents, particularly mothers, through the period of shock, acceptance and initial care of physically and mentally subnormal children. A knowledge of child development from an early age, experience with infants, young and older children, and the ability to transmit sympathy and confidence are essentials for this much needed work.

The above discussion on location of treatment has brought to the fore the consideration of individual and group work. Each has its place in the application of occupational therapy.

Individual and Group Treatment

The mobility of the patient, and the particular physical and/or psychological aims of the treatment may dictate whether it should be given individually or in a group. The group offers the security of 'belonging', of incentives for self-testing, self-expression, communication and achievement, and in all occupational therapy, with the emphasis always laid on reintegration and resocialisation of the patient the group situation can itself be considered a therapeutic medium.

At times, however, there is a strong case for careful individual treatment for certain people, and much specific physical treatment has to be given individually, although often in a group setting. The balance of individual and group work receives special reference in chapters 5 to 11 for physical cases and in chapters 12 to 16 for those who are mentally ill, and is also discussed in subsequent chapters.

Patients' Reactions to Occupational Therapy

A patient's reaction to treatment is important and can indicate something of his attitude to life and work. Before being able to give treatment successfully the therapist must seek an explanation of these attitudes. The patient needs, too, to be encouraged to share in the planning and implementation of his treatment. Because of the variety of media which can be used, and because it is often applied through 'everyday activities', rather than through new and unknown rituals and techniques, there is perhaps a greater variety of reaction than to many therapeutic methods. Bearing all these points in mind various factors have to be taken into consideration.

Work for men or women, the adult or the child. Prescriptive requirements sometimes call for light work for men, or heavy work for women, or for what may be looked upon as a childish activity. The occupational therapist should see that self-esteem is not damaged by ill-considered planning or lack of imagination in proposing or presenting an activity to a patient. Too much care or apology can, of course, have the reverse of the desired effect.

Practical versus intellectual interests. Too often an occupational therapist fails to offer sufficient choice of activity to her patients, when the prescriptions would allow for a choice, particularly for the patient with more cultural interests. This is often due to pressure of work but is seriously detrimental to the value of the treatment. Time should be found to open up new lines of interest and possibilities, and reference books and information on these should be made available.

Other attitudes which the occupational therapist has to recognise and deal with are those of the meticulous person, the 'slap-dash', the patient or impatient, the persistent or the one who is easily discouraged. Whatever the disability to be treated, these and all other personal attitudes should be taken into account. They may at times have to be accepted, and treatment planned in accordance with them, or they may be qualities which in themselves call for treatment. The adage, that 'it is as important to know what patient the illness has got, as what illness the patient has got' is abundantly true for the occupational therapist. Even in the treatment of physical disability the psychological 'overlay' may first need therapeutic attention. Similarly, in considering treatment for the psychiatric patient, assessment of the physical condition of the patient is of real consequence.

Other points of importance in planning treatment are:

Warmth, comfort, good light and good posture for the patient.
Efficiency in preparation of work and apparatus.
Length of working time and rest periods.
Compatibility of companions.
A good choice and supply of materials, books, etc.
Sufficient help, instruction and encouragement.
Regular attendance of patient, and of staff to patient.
Assurance through attention to requests and needs.
Consideration of general independence of the patient.

Activities which may be Used as Treatment Media

Having stated the importance of the interpersonal relationship between occupational therapist and patient, and of the location, method and circumstances of treatment, it is now possible to indicate various groups of activities which may be used therapeutically, remembering always that these do not in themselves represent treatment. The range is far wider than can be discussed here, or than any one occupational therapist can offer; the variety is unlimited. A considerable amount of necessary and satisfactory treatment may be given through non-productive activities in contrast to those in which articles are made for pleasure or sale, i.e. in retraining for competence in activities of daily living. In the productive occupations the emphasis should not be wholly on the product but on the effect of the production on the patient. Emphasis *should* be on as high a standard as possible except for patients for whom this is clearly contra-indicated, and if earnings are to depend on the article produced (as against a possible return to former employment after treatment) the occupational therapist may, at some stage, call upon a technical specialist to help the patient to achieve a marketable standard of work. This is as it should be. The occupational therapist may not have the time or expertise to complete the technical teaching, nor in many cases need she do this, although in others she may be the only person capable and trained to do so.

Activities, then, are the treatment media of the occupational therapist, but the aim of treatment can never be stated in terms of what is made, what is played, what is done or what is sold. This is not to suggest that the finished product, or the degree of efficiency achieved, are not important, especially if the aim of treatment includes emphasis on these aspects. The value lies in the use the patient has been able to make of the activity and the degree to which this has furthered the progression of his rehabilitation.

The activities which may be used therapeutically may be listed under the following headings:

(1) Personal Activities of Daily Living.
(2) Expressive and Creative Activities.
(3) Intellectual and Educational Activities.
(4) Industrial and Vocational Activities.
(5) Recreational Activities.

Personal Activities of Daily Living* [15]

The first urgent personal need of the patient is to dress and undress, to deal with his toilet, to be able to feed himself, and to be able to move around his home if possible. Added to these basic activities are those of 'everyday doings' in some form, reading, writing, doing household chores or going out for recreation or to earn a living. The first aim of occupational therapy should be directed to maintaining or establishing this independence.

To help to achieve success in these activities various aids have been developed. An important rule, however, is that if a person can achieve a movement with reasonable ease, or by learning a new method, a gadget is not needed. On the other hand, to allow or encourage exhausting effort, when the help of an aid could preserve energy for something more important, is poor economy. In certain cases, however, i.e. for the arthritic, some effort is almost certainly necessary to maintain function.

Expressive and Creative Activities

There has been a tendency, in the last few years, to swing away from the use of these activities for treatment. This has, in part, been brought about by the mistaken interpretation of occupational therapy as 'giving the patients something to do', resulting in a series of unattractive rugs, unoriginal and badly-made felt toys, or baskets or embroidery of poor design or in poor-quality materials. The swing has gone over almost too far to production, and 'industrial work' or 'out work' on contract is considered a more up-to-date form of treatment. It cannot be claimed that one or other activity is more therapeutic and/or economic. Problems and abuses arise in the use of either and both have their place in the application of treatment. In both cases care must be taken that the patients are not exploited; in the former, in making things for staff or hospital sales; in the latter, in providing cheap labour for concerns outside the hospital.

It is important to consider for a moment why art and craft-work, used properly came to fill such a valuable role in occupational therapy. One fact is that it offers an outlet for emotional and creative qualities in a way that no single industrial process can. Again, there is usually an unhurried approach to work of this nature which is seldom the case in a more formalised industrial or group activity. There are times when this more leisurely aspect has value in treatment. Dr M. E. M. Herford, writing in the *Lancet*, says:

'In rehabilitation much has been said about the importance of returning the individual to "a work environment". .... It is in this direction that it seems a creative social function of rehabilitation may be lost.' [16]

He goes on to plead the case for 'the joy of creation' which, through the introduction to a new craft or interest, may at the same time bring improvement in function beyond that which might have been achieved by too early a return to the workshop atmosphere. He adds:

'It seems that there is a thread in a pattern which might be, for industrial workers, compensation for dull routine and monotonous mass-production work.'

It is quite clear to the occupational therapist that in certain cases art and craft-work can be as useful, or more so, than any other activity. Training in craft-work, too, forms the basis of the skill, dexterity, ingenuity and precision that are so essential for many jobs, and, in fact, for an occupational therapist herself.

Something should be said here, too, about standard and design, both particularly relevant to this group of activities. Emphasis should be on the simplicity of technique and design, which may help in the production of an acceptable article by a worker who has no great ability. It must be remembered, however, that at times it is almost impossible to achieve what could be termed 'a good standard' in the eyes of a buying public, but this does not necessarily indicate a poor result in treatment. Again, what a patient and his relations consider 'acceptable' may be the very opposite of what is, in terms of the highly trained expert, good design. The occupational therapist can do much to control the situation by showing attractive samples and patterns, and by controlling the supply of materials, colours, and designs available. 'But', one is asked, 'should she, in fact, control it?' This is a part of what she herself has to judge from the therapeutic angle, and the basis for the decision must be the possible effect on the patient, and his need, if need there is, to produce a marketable article. There is a tendency, however, to use the therapeutic emphasis as an excuse for accepting a low standard of work which *could* be better. This is a poor compliment to, and poor business for, a patient who genuinely needs to earn, and who needs the stimulation of finding that his goods are in demand. When possible, it is best to encourage patients to practise before attempting to make saleable goods, but even the practice work should be attractively presented and progression should be planned carefully.

Intellectual and Educational Activities

These, and vocational activities, may be geared to the ultimate establishment or re-establishment of the patient in some earning capacity, or they may be used to develop or continue some interest unrelated to a job. 'Intellectual activities' are hard to define, but are here taken to mean those which cannot be called productive, in the terms of making an article, but productive of interest and zest. Those which fall into this category are in the nature of 'hobby studies' and might include such subjects as the history of art or architecture, some form of historical, geographical, mathematical, scientific, or similar study, or research, the learning of a language or of sketching or painting for interest rather than for vocational use, the study of music, musical form, the history of music, etc.

The occupational therapist should recognise that not everyone wants to do practical or productive work. Some may welcome the opportunity to engage in an intellectual pursuit which has been crowded out of a busy life. Too often the type of patient who would enjoy this form of occupation is exhorted to make something which, unless necessary for treatment, is unacceptable or uninteresting, and may detract seriously from the value of occupational therapy in the eyes of doctor or patient. A knowledge of the library facilities available is necessary, as is a readiness to seek the help of other experts or enthusiasts in subjects outside the range of those of the occupational therapist herself or her staff.

Children and young people who have to be hospitalised for long periods, and for whom study is *not* contra-indicated, should be interested, as far as treatment aims allow, in educational activities. These can be introduced indirectly, through games, competitions, etc., or approached quite directly as a desirable and useful way of utilising the period of hospitalisation. In hospitals where young children are treated as long-term cases there is usually a hospital school, and the occupational therapist would confine her activities to specific treatment. It has been thought that the latter would not then be necessary. This is not the case. The school teacher and the occupational therapist have totally different functions and one is needed as much as the other.

There are some hospitals which cater for children but do not have large enough numbers to warrant the employment of a teacher. Here it may be on the fringe of the occupational therapist's function to help to employ and educate the child, in collaboration with nurses and voluntary workers or parents, and to supply the necessary books, materials, etc. The need for this should not be ignored.

For older patients courses can sometimes be arranged with local teachers who may be willing voluntarily to help an individual, or through classes organised with the Local Education Authority for which, if the group is large enough, instructors can be provided. Correspondence courses can also be arranged through the Preparatory Training Bureau* of the British Council for Rehabilitation* [17]. It is important to realise that those applying for these must be carefully assessed for ability and 'stick-ability'. To benefit from what is, of necessity, a difficult course, in that work on one's own requires great application and interest, both qualities are necessary. It is sometimes possible to increase the value of such a course by the use of a voluntary teacher, as suggested above.

Industrial [18] and Vocational Activities

This fourth group of activities covers an almost limitless range. No occupational therapist can be proficient in all, but she must be capable of assessing their value to and with the patient and must prepare herself to undertake advisory or supervisory responsibilities in relation to them. It is important too, that she should be able to work well with the other experts whom she may have to advise or supervise.

If the occupational therapist is to act in either capacity she must know even more than she does at present of the needs of her patients in terms of health, intelligence, interests, aptitudes, attitudes and values. She must recognise the importance of individual and group incentives, of competition, goal attainment, and of reward, in short, of the value of the group situation as a rehabilitative factor. She needs more appropriate and specialised knowledge in the industrial field. She needs to develop better methods of assessment; she needs to know more of the problems of the worker at first hand, of individual and group pressures, and of method and motion study. If she is to undertake actual supervisory responsibility in an industrial workshop she will need to add to this a knowledge of contract work, costing, layout, bookkeeping, packaging, despatching, etc.

The 'lead out' to more competitive industrial or vocational work in the occupational therapy department itself may be achieved through the use of such activities as household tasks; outdoor activities such as gardening, bricklaying, etc.; industrial activities, such as work on a lathe or press; office tasks, such as typing and audiotyping or computer operating, and draughtsmanship; activities requiring dexterity, such as switchboard work, packaging, or assembling large or small items; and certain forms of craftsmanship, such as sewing, weaving, wood and metal work, basketry, pottery, etc. Handprinting, photography, shoe-repairing, watch and clock repairing, hand bookbinding, commercial art, illustration and lettering are further activities with a vocational bias which can be used as treatment.

The therapist, through a knowledge of these, or the capacity to recognise what is involved in their execution, should be able to treat her patient with some activity akin to the work to which he is to return, or to use this knowledge to assess him for some alternative job. Regional variants should also be taken into consideration. There are great differences between rural and urban work activities, and considerable imagination and ingenuity may be needed in devising appropriate treatment, particularly for the former. The therapist may, at some stage, pass the patient on to technical experts for specialist instruction and retraining. This shared responsibility is entirely in keeping with her function and theirs.

Study courses in many of the subjects listed here, as in the foregoing section, can be arranged through the Preparatory Training Bureau* of the British Council of Rehabilitation*. In some cases the social worker may collaborate and undertake the necessary negotiations. In others the occupational therapist has to do so. She should, in any case, share in the planning of the occupation with and for the patient and do any assessment necessary prior to training.

In a psychiatric hospital an introduction to vocational work can be given through allocation of patients to hospital industries or administrative departments, such as the sewing rooms, laundries, kitchens, paint and repair shops, stores, accounts or clerical departments, farms and gardens. In hospitals where there are 'industrial' sheltered workshops the occupational therapist should have the closest consultative liaison with the supervisors if she is not responsible for them. All industrial and vocational allocation of patients should be arranged on a planned basis and always for the benefit of the patient through consultation between psychologists, doctors, nurses, occupational therapists and departmental supervisors, and where possible with the patients themselves. A serious weakness of many present schemes is the lack of cooperation and cohesion, resulting in interdepartmental competition instead of cooperation. Here again much depends on the medical leadership of the team.

Recreational Activities

If a patient can, even to a limited extent, manage his daily or work activities another urgent need is for recreation. The method has to be tempered to the need. Occupational therapists are trained to help patients to organise physical and/or general recreations of all kinds and to give instruction in a number of activities which can be developed as hobbies. Here the help of voluntary workers or the Friends of the hospital can often be enlisted, as can experts in various games, sports, music or drama, etc.

In studying any of the skills used in treatment the student is expected to develop:
(1) An appreciation of the importance of the establishment or re-establishment of the patient to the fullest degree possible in personal independence, in the home, in a job and/or with some hobby or interest.
(2) An appreciation of good design, a knowledge of handling, shaping and controlling materials, a knowledge of handling tools, caring for them and working with them on materials.
(3) An appreciation of the value of intellectual and cultural pursuits, and of study and training courses for the disabled, and of how to link patients with, or organise, these.
(4) A knowledge of the elements of work study and of industrial conditions.

The occupational therapy student also studies the subjects of *Anatomy and Physiology, Psychology, Medical and Surgical Conditions treated by Occupational Therapy; Psychiatry; Occupational Therapy and Resettlement for Medical, Surgical and Psychiatric Patients; Communication and Management* [19]. After obtaining her basic qualification she is expected, through post-graduate work, to continue to extend her knowledge and experience in some specialised field or fields. There is still much to be done in experiment and research to enable occupational therapy to render its full contribution to the re-establishment of patients.

REFERENCES

1. ... 'That which deals with the ultimate reality or with the more general causes and principles of things', *Concise Oxford Dictionary*.
2. 'Empathy is akin to sympathy, but whereas sympathy says "I feel as you do", empathy says "I know how you feel". .... Empathy allows us to appreciate another person's feelings, without becoming emotionally involved with him.' Armstrong, R. W., 'Empathy', *Nursing Times*, 12.10.56, p. 1006.
   And see: The nature of involvement. *Occ. Ther.*, 35, no. 1, 1971.
3. The word 'teaching' can be used provided it is not taken by the students to imply *school* teaching, which has the danger, for the inexperienced, of suggesting too much 'managing'. This is out of place in occupational therapy.
4. A possible order of investigation might be: *Observation; Hypothesis; Experiment; Evaluation of Hypothesis; Re-check of findings.* And see *General Notes on the Preparation of Scientific Papers*, The Royal Society. London, 1957.
5. See chapter 1, p. 2 and ref. 2.
6. *Reablement* is taken, in this book, to mean the 'making of the patient able', physically and mentally, i.e. the development of actual function to the fullest possible degree. *Reconditioning* is another term for the same process.
   Rehabilitation includes both of the above, but is used in the wider sense, signifying 'the whole of the process of restoring a disabled person to a condition in which he is able ... to resume a normal life'. (*Report of the Committee of Inquiry on the Rehabilitation of Disabled Persons*, H.M.S.O.*, 1956, 5.)
   Resettlement is taken to mean the training and/or placing of a patient in employment. This is a part of rehabilitation.
7. Often the occupational therapist is required to contribute to a diagnosis through her observations and reports. Reference to the chapters on treatment will indicate how the diagnosis is, in itself, an indication of the treatment required.
8. As in other professional associations, Members of the British Association of Occupational Therapists can insure against claims, but this, although a wise precaution, cannot mitigate the results of non-professional behaviour.
9. See chapter 6.
10. See ref. 5 above.
11. The occupational therapist should study those of well-developed departments, although modification for her particular needs will almost certainly be necessary.
12. See chapter 21.
13. *Hospital and Social Services Journal*, 13.6.58, p. 620.
14. See chapters 4, 21, 22.
15. See chapter 7.
16. Herford, M. E., *The Lancet*, 13 December 1950.
17. See chapter 4.
18. See chapter 22.
19. See *Manual for the Diploma Course and Examination of the British Association of Occupational Therapists*.
* See *Glossary*, pp. 454-5.

The Scope of Occupational Therapy, the Principles underlying Treatment and the Spheres of Operation

The Scope and the Patient

The scope of occupational therapy is indicated by its four aims. It contributes to the physical, psychological, social and economic rehabilitation of the patient. These apply in all cases of treatment, but vary in relation to the needs of a particular patient, and the disability from which he is suffering.

Before considering the general physical and psychological principles involved, it is advisable, briefly, to consider the situation in which patients may find themselves. Few have any knowledge of anatomy or physiology, fewer have more than a rudimentary idea of the illnesses from which they are suffering or of the operations which they have to undergo. They may have little insight into the treatment they are receiving and are often unable to interpret the technical language which they hear. In addition to feeling ill and having to adjust to separation from family, friends and habitual surroundings and routine, they have also to adjust to strangers, to a totally new and unaccustomed environment and to a routine which is mainly centred on physical needs. Meanwhile, they are to some extent deprived of the satisfaction of their normal psychological ones. For some, a return to their previous way of life will be impossible, and long cherished ambitions and hopes may have to be modified or completely foregone. For others the period in hospital is short and relatively undisturbing.

Emotional involvements may include some or all of the following:

Apprehension: pending investigation and diagnosis.

Relief: at being able to admit illness, and have this confirmed, after perhaps resisting it.

Fear: of the unknown and unexplained, or perhaps of the return of pain, as in heart cases.

Anxiety: for the welfare of the family, for job, etc.

Despair: expecting the worst—(few do this).

Self-consciousness: over disability and, perhaps, over lack of privacy in hospital.

Lack of adjustment: to hospital, to treatment and/or to disability, and to results of interruption in the normal living routine of sleep, meals, etc.

Some patients (i.e. the hemiplegic or accident case) may be severely shocked and their reaction to hospital and treatment may be seriously complicated by this. The majority can, however, overcome these difficulties, provided they are given time and a reasonable amount of explanation of what they must expect, even if it is to be unpleasant. They need also to be helped to have peace of mind about their families [1], and to understand that treatment will continue until no more is needed. They must also be helped to understand that the occupational therapist is one of a team of treatment workers, and that occupational therapy is a supportive complement to other treatments, e.g. chemotherapy. Patients must be encouraged to cooperate and to share responsibility for the treatment, where it is necessary and possible. On the whole patients are cooperative and philosophical.

Among the different types of patients there may be some, however, who may blame their environment for their misfortune and appear hostile towards staff and other patients [2], or who blame themselves and appear depressed and overanxious, attemping to assuage their guilt feelings by an almost compulsive helpfulness, being continually worried lest they are being a nuisance to the staff [3]. Others minimise the situation, appear to luxuriate in dependence, gradually becoming apathetic and unwilling to face the future when they will have once more to meet the realities of normal daily living [4]. Not only must the occupational therapist give appropriate treatment: she must take into consideration all these personal factors remembering, as has been said before, that there may be a psychological overlay even in physical illness or injury.

Unless contra-indicated, occupational therapists should expect a high standard of effort and work from their patients. They should give reasons for what is being done and should avoid wrapping up the treatment so that the patients do not recognise it as such. Patients *want* treatment and are usually prepared to accept it. In this way the occupational therapist can contribute to the security and stability of the patient and to the dispelling of emotional stress.

General Principles of Treatment

Occupational therapy may be used in a number of different ways:

1. As a Means of Assessment [5]

If a patient is unable to return to his previous work, occupational therapy may be used to help to assess his mental and physical competence for resettlement in some other type of work. The assessment of the patient's residual capacities may be as important as the assessment of deficit. The occupational therapist cannot, however, do this full assessment alone: it should be the result of observation, tests and factual knowledge on the part of the 'reablement' team, but the part she has to play is important.

Assessment of the patient is not an end in itself and careful consideration must be given to the reasons for doing it. Can a patient return to his particular job? Is he likely to benefit from a course of training in a particular skill? Reports on his ability to mix with others, to tolerate frustration, or to adjust to authority may be needed, or advice may have to be given on the choice of the hospital industry or sheltered work which will suit him best. It may be necessary, if he is likely to be homebound, to assess the patient's capacity for working alone, and his ingenuity or patience in extricating himself from difficulties or his inability to do so.

2. As a Means of Restoring General Health and Function

After long illnesses return to work is a slow and difficult process. A planned course of occupational therapy can build up the patient's general health and function, and resistance to fatigue, by accustoming him, gradually, to regular and increasing hours of work under conditions as similar as possible to those to which he will return. The occupational therapy department should, therefore, be a place in which the patient can reorientate himself by maintaining habits of punctuality, orderliness and care of equipment, and by working towards the standard of physical strength, and psychological adjustment and confidence, necessary for successful and unstrained performance. Where possible the therapeutic occupation should approximate to the patient's normal work, involving the use of muscles needed for his habitual employment, and/or the mental concentration and precision akin to that of his former job. Convalescence will thus be shortened, and successful return to work facilitated.

3. As a Means of Restoring Local Function (in a Physical Sense)

Occupational therapy contributes to the recovery of local function in a physical sense, by means of specific treatment. This should be planned to increase joint mobility, and to improve muscle strength, coordination and endurance in such a way that the patient learns to make the best use of the gradual improvement in anatomical function in his usual everyday activities. The demands of the patient's life and work should be kept continually in view so as to refit him to return to it as fully and quickly as possible.

4. As a Means of Helping the Permanently Disabled to Become Independent

Through occupational therapy the patient who is left with a residual disability is able to learn how best to manipulate his environment to suit his handicap, and to what degree he can adapt himself to conditions in the social and economic settings to which he will be discharged. Permanently disabled people who are living below their full capacities can be helped towards personal independence in the activities of daily living, and in social adjustment to their disabilities. This is discussed further in later chapters, but it is important to stress here the value of occupational therapy in this field, for old as well as young people.

5. As a Prophylactic Measure

In considering the value of occupational therapy in prevention of disease, emphasis is placed (*a*) on the value of exercise for maintaining general physical health, and (*b*) on psychological considerations in alleviation of over-introspection, boredom and anxiety.

In addition to preserving a healthy mental outlook during illness, much can be done to conserve joint action and muscle strength after injury, and to preserve function.

Patients, particularly long-term ones, have always to make their own adjustments to the situations in which they find themselves. They must be helped to understand something of their problems and the way to modify or resolve them, and to assess their abilities so as to decide how, in the circumstances, these may be developed best. The occupational therapist, with others in the medical team, should give patients the sense of security in which these problems can be worked out in an objective way, undistracted by anxiety, morbid preoccupations and unimpaired by apathy. Situations must be provided for them to test their abilities themselves and to relate their progress to future goals. This use of introspection can have positive results. Introspection which leads to reinforcement of psychopathological tendencies may, however, retard a patient's recovery. For such cases occupational therapy is used, not only prophylactically, but also therapeutically.

In acute illness energy will be absorbed in the struggle for survival, or a period for recovery from post-operational shock may be required. Eventually most patients reach a state in which they are able to turn their attention to the external environment and it is at this stage that occupational therapy may be prescribed. Once the routine in hospital, and in treatment is familiar, patients may find it boring. Boredom is a condition which simulates fatigue. If the patient has found his occupational therapy monotonous and uninteresting, although the period of work may have been relatively short, his attention will wander, his efficiency become impaired, and he may complain of tiredness or headache. Unless he can be diverted to something which gives him new experience, his energy may be misdirected and his progress delayed.

A patient absorbed in an occupation is less likely to attend to his symptoms. Nevertheless, attention may shift rapidly from one focus to another.

It is not enough, therefore, merely to occupy the patient, if he is to be distracted from preoccupation with self or anxiety about the future. Before the occupation can become therapeutic the patient must be helped to feel that it has some intrinsic interest, value and particular personal relevance. He must also understand its therapeutic aim. The occupation should appeal to his immediate needs or be of use to him in the future. The most satisfactory occupation is one which covers these points. The patient will then be motivated to perform it for one or several of the above reasons.

Work should never become habitual unless this in itself is an aim of the treatment, as in the habit training of the deteriorating patient. As the patient progresses, his physical and psychological abilities must be increasingly exercised. Without constant observation of the patient's state and a *pari passu* grading of his occupation, no progress can be made or demonstrated to him. The latter is of importance in that people are unwilling to work in a situation where there is no means of knowing whether or not they are improving. This is particularly true in cases of obvious physical impairment.

In dealing with physically ill patients, it must be remembered that, while most are well adjusted, a few may be neurotic before they come to the hospital. Some physical illness may, in fact, precipitate psychological disturbance. A normal anxiety is, however, often reasonably easily relieved and the patient looks forward actively to discharge. It is vitally important that this attitude be maintained.

The Importance of a Comprehensive Treatment Plan

Any occupational treatment plan must relate to the physical and psychological state of the patient, the hospital routine and the other treatments being given. The patient's past experience, condition, and behaviour, and possibilities for his future must also be considered. A smooth progression of work and interest must be arranged to fit him for a return to his job or to prepare him for a new one. A typist with a fractured humerus will return comparatively easily to sedentary work, but a house-painter with the same injury will lose his job if his whole arm and physique are not strong enough for him to do ladder work safely and continuously. He will need additional exercise, through *general* work as well as local treatment, to ensure his full return to normal endurance and mobility.

Each patient's plan must be arranged to gain the maximum benefit from each treatment. Physiotherapy may well be followed by occupational therapy, while free and active movements are at their optimum, but when physiotherapy is strenuous and active, occupational therapy may be more beneficial if given during another part of the day.

Treatment intended to alleviate psychological disturbance must also relate to the patient's physical state and to other treatments which are being given. The plan for occupational therapy will involve consideration of the patient's entire day, his meal times and those of exercise, work, relaxation and rest. This will require cooperation between medical, nursing, occupational therapy, technical, administrative and other staffs because, without it, periods may be wasted which might have been used to the patient's advantage.

Occupational Therapy for Patients with Special Needs

Ward-patients

The occupations used in treating patients will vary according to the environment and the disability at each stage of treatment. The occupational therapist working in a ward is a visitor in someone else's department and should seek the help and cooperation of the sister-in-charge. Care should also be taken to fit visits in with the normal routine of the ward. Bed-patients in both physical and psychiatric hospitals are few. In the former only long-term cases are bed-fast, in the latter, only extreme senile and organic cases, or those recovering from neurosurgery are kept in bed. If treatment is given in these conditions comparatively light activities should be used free from heavy or noisy equipment, and care must be taken to avoid untidiness, by providing containers in which to keep materials and tools, and adequate protection for clean beds. Light crafts are suitable, and games and puzzles and educational courses are invaluable.

Posture, comfort and a good light are all important. When occupations are needed for a patient whose position is restricted, variety can be introduced with some ingenuity and extra equipment. Frames are obtainable, or can be made, to hold working boards on to the back of the bed, or to fix other equipment at a suitable level and angle. Patients lying in the prone position or on one side usually have a better view of anything that they wish to do; but their exact positions and degree of mobility vary so much that each one must be considered and planned for separately. Awkward positions are always tiring, so that the activity chosen must be one that can be handled easily, and is not too large. The same points are important for patients who are immobilised, e.g. nothing must lean against or interfere with traction cords and weights. Work for the one-handed patient must be well supported and fixed, and for this magnets and a magnetic board may be used.

In a psychiatric hospital ward, patients may be confused and restless and only simple occupations should be planned. The time should be used in trying to form some relationship with them, or in allaying restlessness through simple repetitive tasks.

In treating neurosurgical cases the occupational therapist will be guided by the surgeon and psychiatrist in charge of the patient. Emphasis will be on the social aspect of the visit, the care of personal appearance and the fresh start that the patient is about to make.

Ambulant Patients

Ambulant patients on treatment should come to an occupational therapy department whenever possible, so that the range of their activities may be more extensive than in the wards. These may include games, such as table tennis and skittles; occupations needing special equipment, e.g. cookery, pottery, clerical techniques and photography; and heavier occupations such as wood or metal work. It may even be possible to assign them to a sheltered workshop to do some form of productive work, or gardening.

Patients who are mobile only with the aid of sticks, crutches and chairs, are limited in their choice of activity but a patient in a wheel-chair can play skittles and table tennis and do woodwork, while the patient with a leg in plaster can do wood-turning on a treadle lathe if he has a suitable seat, and support for the injured leg.

In some psychiatric hospitals, or in psychiatric units in general hospitals, the occupational therapy departments are often on, or adjacent to the wards. When patients are too ill or disabled to attend a more distant unit, classes can be held here.

Patients in Differing Groups

Patients in varying groups, i.e. age groups, social groups, intellectual groups, urban groups and rural groups, have different needs, interests, and diffi-culties. As the methods and problems of giving occupational therapy to patients of varying age groups are considered in detail in later chapters, reference to them here is limited to a reminder that they need special con-sideration. Treatment for groups with social and intellectual differences have certain elements in common. Recognition of divergences is necessary, as is a capacity to 'weld' the differing personalities. Awareness of the varying competencies and claims of each is essential in planning treatments, and this also applies to thought for the urban and rural patients. Imagination, ingenuity and a wide knowledge of social and industrial factors is called for.

The Long-term Disabled

The problem of the long-term disabled lies to a great extent in their own and their families' attitude towards their disabilities. The occupational therapist can do much to help them, if their treatment is first used as a means of making an accurate assessment of their capabilities so that false hopes are never raised. They can then be encouraged and helped to become as inde-pendent as possible in the activities of daily living, and finally, when feasible and necessary, led on towards training and work. As always, the occupational therapist must take into account the other treatments which her patient is having and she must know what precautions may be necessary.

The Spheres of Operation

The spheres of operation of the occupational therapist are indicated in the foregoing and following chapters. They include the hospital settings, in hospitals of all kinds, i.e. physical (general and specialised), psychiatric, for acute and long-term cases and for the mentally handicapped, hospitals for children and for geriatrics. They also include the community setting, in special centres and the patients' homes. This latter is increasing substantially and is becoming an important extension of the scope of occupational therapy [6].

The discussion in these first three chapters has been introductory, aimed at 'setting the stage' for the more detailed and specific descriptions and instructions in the succeeding chapters. It will be noted that all aspects of treatment are complementary and interrelated, as well as being specific and specialised. The occupational therapist will, after the basic training, extend her knowledge and experience in a field of her choice.

REFERENCES

1. This comes mainly into the province of the medical or psychiatric social worker but the occupational therapist can be a valuable ally.
2. Rosenzweig's 'Extrapunitive' reactions.
3. Rosenzweig's 'Intropunitive' reactions.
4. Rosenzweig's 'Impunitive' reactions.
5. See Chapters 6 and 7. And see Davies, B. M., Organisation of occupational therapy in the new Health and Social Services. *Occ. Ther.*, 37, no. 4, 1974.
6. See opening paragraph of this chapter and chapter 21.
   And see:
   Patient, Doctor and Society, Nuffield Provincial Hospitals Trust, London 1972.
   Hedley, P., *Overcoming Handicap*, London, 1972, concerning teaching home economics and needlework to the handicapped.

CHAPTER 4

Help, Benefits and Resettlement for the Disabled

Medical rehabilitation leading to resettlement in some form is the aim of all occupational therapy. This, clearly, cannot be done by the occupational therapist alone. Throughout this book emphasis has been laid on team work, and the combined efforts of the team should culminate in the satisfactory reestablishment of the patient. It is important that the occupational therapist dealing with rehabilitation and resettlement should make a careful study of the provisions of all relevant legislation and should study memoranda and pamphlets issued by government departments [1] and other agencies.

Statutory Services

The Department of Health and Social Security: The Health and Social Services

In all areas the Health Services [2] cover:

(1) Hospital and specialist services for all types of illness.
(2) General practitioner services; dental, ophthalmic and pharma-ceutical services.
(3) Environmental health services, preventive medicine, maternity, child and old people's welfare, care and after-care, home nursing, health visiting and ambulance services.
(4) The supply of nursing equipment for the home, surgical appliances, wheel-chairs and invalid cars.

The Social Services [3] cover, for the disabled:

(1) Home helps, social worker visits, provision of meals-on-wheels, home aids and adaptations, telephones, television, radio, visiting library and recreational services.
(2) The keeping of registers of 'substantially and permanently handi-capped persons' [4].

(3) The provision of Day Centres, hostels and homes for handicapped workers and residential accommodation for those needing care and attention [5], but not hospital treatment.

Occupational therapists are involved in many aspects of both Health and Social Services*.

The Department of Health and Social Security, National Insurance, Pensions and Benefits

Up-to-date information on all kinds of pensions and benefits is given in leaflets obtainable from post offices or the local offices of the Department of Health and Social Security [6]. Benefits are based on *compulsory insurance contributions* paid by employer and employee for men of 15 to 65 and for women of 15 to 60 in three main classes:

(1) Employed persons.
(2) Self-employed persons.
(3) Non-employed persons.
(There are special provisions for married women and widows.)

Exemption from payment is made under certain conditions, e.g. during a period of unemployment, incapacity, full-time education and apprenticeship, or if below a certain income level.

Pensions may be provided from different sources:

(1) National Insurance retirement pensions.
(2) Pensions available through employers' superannuation schemes.
(3) Private insurance pension schemes.
(4) Supplementary pensions or payments through government or charity grants.

The following benefits and allowances may be of particular relevance in dealing with the rehabilitation and resettlement of the disabled:

(1) *Sickness Benefit* [7] is paid if a patient cannot work because of illness or disablement, provided he has worked and paid National Insurance contributions. After 28 weeks of illness this may be changed to invalidity benefit. After the first 8 weeks in hospital National Insurance benefits are reduced, and after one year (52 weeks) the patient is paid on a 'pocket money' rate. If there are family commitments these are dealt with individually. The earnings rule forbids those receiving sickness benefit from working and earning more than the hours or sum per week, laid down, without forfeiting part or all of their benefit.

(2) *The Industrial Injuries Scheme* [8] provides benefits and allowances for those who are incapacitated or disabled because of an industrial accident or prescribed industrial disease. Injury benefit covers a maximum of 26

weeks and when this ends, if disablement persists, disablement benefit is available, 'depending on the degree of disablement resulting from the accident or disease'. The earnings rule does not apply to disablement beneficiaries, and those with severe residual disability may apply for further financial help.

(3) *Supplementary Benefits* [9] provide extra financial help to those whose incomes fall below a fixed ceiling, assessed according to individual need. For those under pensionable age they are known as Supplementary Pensions. Those who are disabled or self-employed may also be entitled to supplementary benefits, and there are extra allowances available under certain conditions for heating, rent and rates rebate, free prescriptions, dental treatment and glasses, free welfare milk, etc. An earnings rule is in force for those receiving supplementary help. On admission to hospital, supplementary benefits may cease. If, however, the patient has dependents, adjustments are made regarding benefits affecting them.

(4) *A Family Income Supplement* [10] may be payable where the total family income amounts to less than a fixed ceiling and there are dependent children.

(5) *The Constant Attendance Allowance* [11] is a tax-free benefit for people living at home and needing constant attention, and for supervision to avoid substantial danger to themselves or others.

There are further allowances available for Industrial Injury [12] and for War Pensioners.

The Department of Employment

Since the Employment and Training Act 1973 the Department of Employment [13] has set up a Manpower Services Commission [14] to deal with employment needs of all kinds. It has two executive branches, the Employment Service Agency and the Training Service Agency. The Department is still responsible for unemployment benefit, this often being dealt with in separate offices.

A sub-programme of the Employment Service Agency is 'to aid disabled people to find and keep the jobs best suited to their aptitudes and capacities and to help them to settle into work as quickly and smoothly as possible . . . The Agency has a specialist service, whose central figure is the Disablement Resettlement Officer, the D.R.O.*, who is specially trained to identify and help with the resettlement problems resulting from disablement . . . physical or mental' [15]. The training and functions of these officers are to be extended.

The National Advisory Council on the Employment of the Disabled [16] is the national body advising and assisting in matters relating to the employment, undertaking of work on their own account, or training of disabled persons generally. Its work is implemented through disablement advisory committees, linked, through the D.R.O.*, with the main employment exchanges.

Where prolonged illness or unemployment has resulted in loss of work habits and/or adjustment to industrial conditions, the department provides Industrial Rehabilitation Units*. 'The units have two main functions. Firstly, to provide individually designed courses to help people to build up confidence and accustom themselves to the routines and disciplines of work in a simulated industrial atmosphere. Secondly, to assess individual aptitude and potential and give vocational guidance' [17]. 'An increasing number of people seeking help from I.R.U.s* suffer from mental illness, congenital disabilities or organic nervous complaints, and many have social and personal difficulties' [18]. Others with various degrees of physical disabilities may be recommended to attend these Units. The employment problem of each person at an I.R.U.* is discussed regularly by a team of specialists in charge, a doctor, vocational and/or rehabilitation officer (often an occupational psychologist), a social worker, a D.R.O.* and a chief occupational supervisor. The purpose is 'not so much . . . restoring people to fitness but . . . helping to modify attitudes or help solve personal problems which may be the main barrier to employment' [19]. If an aptitude is discovered and calls for training in a skilled trade, arrangements for this can be made at a Skill Centre [20]. Help is also given in finding a job at the end of the course. If the person is considered fit for work, but not to compete in open industry, he may be referred for sheltered work, in a Remploy* factory or other centre.

For those whose mental or physical disability requires prolonged industrial rehabilitation and who, for this reason, are not suitable for an industrial rehabilitation unit, the department gives support to certain industrial organisations (i.e. at Hanwell, Epsom and Bristol) and special centres such as that for spastics at Welwyn Garden City.

Skill centres. Government instructional factories were established in 1917 by the Ministry of Pensions to meet the problems of training disabled ex-servicemen. They were transferred to the Ministry of Labour in 1919 and have become the skill centres of today.

Skill centres provide training in a variety of different skills. These trainings are often an intensive version of the normal apprenticeship and they are recognised by the unions as being of a comparable standard. This creates an age gap for patients who are too old for apprenticeship but too young for government training, as they would complete the government training at an earlier age than the apprentices. All training is for a skill and as such demands some educational standard, varying according to the course.

An applicant is only accepted for training if there is a reasonable hope that he will then qualify for employment and that he will be able to remain in this. The disabled are taught alongside fit workers to accustom them to normal conditions of employment.

A fundamental need is 'to develop closer links with the health services. Garston Manor I.R.U.*, near Watford, is built in the grounds of a medical rehabilitation centre and has provided experience of ways of linking I.R.U.s* and medical services' [21]. A unit has also recently been opened in the grounds of the Queen Elizabeth Hospital, Birmingham. These should 'help co-operation between the National Health Service*, local government and the Agency' [22].

Residential colleges. There are some residential colleges for those too seriously handicapped to travel daily to a training centre, which are directed to the needs of the disabled, in that all their clients are disabled, whereas, in a Skill Centre, a number of able-bodied trainees are being retrained for alternative employment. The courses offered at a Residential Centre may be different, and perhaps more sedentary. Some residential courses have been provided by voluntary organisations but are financially assisted by the Department of Employment, e.g.:

The Derwen Cripples Training College, Gobowen, Shropshire.
Finchale Abbey Training Centre, Durham.
Queen Elizabeth's College, Leatherhead, Surrey.
Portland Training College, Mansfield, Notts.
St. Loye's College, Exeter, Devon.

Training courses for skilled occupations take anything from six months. The curriculum and length of course can be adjusted for the disabled if necessary.

The Disabled Persons (Employment) Acts 1944, 1958. The acts are administered by the Department of Employment. Their purpose is 'to make further and better provision for enabling persons handicapped by disablement to secure employment or work on their own account'. The acts define a disabled person and require:

(1) The maintenance of a register of employable disabled persons who are otherwise unable to work under normal conditions.
(2) That concerns with a large number of employees should also employ a certain number of disabled (the quota).
(3) The reservation for the disabled of certain kinds of work (designated employment), i.e. lift attendants and car park attendants.
(4) That sheltered employment shall be provided.
(5) The setting up of a national advisory council and of local disablement advisory committees for the purpose of implementing the acts.
(6) The provision of courses of industrial rehabilitation and for vocational training if required.

In order to be seen by the D.R.O.*, if the patient is still undergoing treatment, form DPI* has to be completed by the doctor, and the occupational therapist can contribute to the information required. Form DP17* has to be filled in for registration as a disabled person, and form DP32*, a confidential medical report, may be necessary for the D.R.O.* and the Disablement Advisory Committee.

The acts also enable the department to assist voluntary undertakings which have developed schemes for sheltered employment and to make grants to local authorities who provide employment facilities.

Under the acts, a special company exists to provide sheltered employment. *Remploy Ltd.* runs factories on business lines in which a percentage of severely disabled workers are employed with the help of a small number of non-disabled. Employees are paid at a standard rate and in almost all cases work not less than 38 hours per week. The company also caters for the supply of out-work to disabled persons in their homes, provided they are able to undertake a given amount each week.

The preceding provisions do not apply only to the physically disabled but also to the mentally ill and handicapped.

Patients who have recovered from psychoses or neuroses, and mentally subnormal patients who have been socially trained and are employable, need the same kind of help as others in resettlement, after health care and social services. There is a special need here for close cooperation between the different services, and for obtaining the understanding of employers. The rehabilitation of the mentally ill is helped by the increasing number of psychiatric clinics in general hospitals, which offer early assessment and treatment, and by the externalising of many of the mental hospitals themselves. The facilities listed above can also be used for the mentally handicapped.

The Youth Employment Service also comes under the direction of the Department of Employment, and may need to be consulted in the resettlement of patients up to the age of 18. Some centres specialise in educating and training younger disabled persons, e.g. Banstead Place, St. Loye's College, Exeter, which has a junior intake and provides 2 years of normal school education, Hereward College of Further Education, Coventry (for the physically handicapped), and the Star Centre, Cheltenham (for the physically handicapped school leaver).

The Department of Education and Science and Other Educational Groups

This took the place of the Ministry of Education (for England and Wales) in 1964. Scotland has its Scottish Education Department, Northern Ireland its Ministry of Education. Provision is made for education for long-term patients in certain hospitals, and where hospital schools are run. Special schools, residential and non-residential are provided for the physically or mentally handicapped, for the blind, deaf, maladjusted, etc. An occupational therapist is sometimes called upon to augment the educational services by treatment aid, as is the physiotherapist. Further education is also catered for in making classes available in hospital if there are sufficient numbers.

Correspondence courses are available through the Preparatory Training Bureau* of the British Council for the Rehabilitation of the Disabled* and grants for these may be obtained from local education authorities. Courses are also available in universities, polytechnics, colleges of technology or further education, or in special vocational training centres run by statutory or voluntary bodies.

Voluntary Organisations

There is a large list of voluntary organisations concerned with the disabled in the Consumers' Association booklet *Coping with Disablement* [23]. It is unnecessary, therefore, to amplify this here, except to mention that there is usually close cooperation between local authorities and voluntary organisations. Voluntary organisations, such as the Red Cross and the Royal Women's Voluntary Services frequently act as agents for the local authority in providing residential accommodation, clubs and social activities and certain other welfare services for the elderly or disabled. Where cooperation is lacking, however, there may be overlapping of services to the detriment of the overall scheme and to the confusion of those who should benefit. There are many exclusive associations for special categories of the disabled. They undoubtedly help their members in distinctive ways but more administrative amalgamation is indicated and is taking place.

A knowledge of these voluntary organisations and particulars of those concerned with the training and rehabilitation of the disabled is of particular value to the occupational therapist.

Some well-known and important advisory groups with which the occupational therapist should be in touch, are:

The Central Council for the Disabled*, which, like the others, helps to implement the Chronically Sick and Disabled Persons Act (1970), by dealing with holidays, housing, building and access for the disabled, running the Hesley Hall School for very disabled children, etc.

The Disabled Living Foundation* (with many occupational therapists on the staff), which provides an information service for the disabled, has an *Aids Display Centre*, and involves itself in projects on housing, design of furniture and equipment, incontinence, employment, gardening, physical recreation, music, educational facilities, visual handicap, etc.

The British Council for Rehabilitation*, which arranges conferences on rehabilitation, and on the problems of disease and disablement, with particular reference to their bearing on industry, collects and disseminates information on a wide range of subjects to individuals, government departments and many other organisations. It also arranges, through its *Preparatory Training Bureau**, courses of correspondence for long-stay patients in hospitals.

The Handcrafts Advisory Association*, set up to provide expert advice on design, saleable standards, markets, and business methods for those who need to earn by means of handcraft production.

Voluntary help is being increasingly used within the hospitals. *Leagues of Friends* are established, who may help in a number of ways, from preparing and serving ward teas to equipping and staffing patients' canteens and social clubs. Members of adult and youth organisations visit the patients and join in their activities. Careful 'orientation' of these helpers is necessary but the bringing of the community into the hospital, and vice-versa can only result in better understanding and easier social and industrial resettlement.

The Resettlement of Patients in Work [24]

Taking it that the physical and psychological considerations put forward in preceding chapters are of primary importance, the occupational therapist cannot plan realistic and progressive rehabilitation and resettlement unless she also takes the economic conditions of the patient into account. This is, in the main, the business of the social worker, and the whole resettlement team will share the responsibility of decisions made with and for the patient. It is important for her to study the physical and mental claims of certain types of employment, so that she may contribute usefully to correct placing and re-establishment. Although no undue pressure should be put on any patient, it is the responsibility of the occupational therapist, as well as other members of the team, to ensure that time and money are not wasted and that progression is as continuous as it should be.

To acquaint herself with different aspects and requirements of different jobs the occupational therapist may have to visit industrial and other work centres in her district. She would be helped in her assessment if she had been able to attend even a brief course in *work study* [25], which would give an introduction to work measurement in industry. This includes information on job breakdown, rating scales, bonus schemes, and of stresses and pressures. This, in its turn, leads on to improved planning and layout and new methods of training to achieve skilled performance in the minimum time. Not only can the occupational therapist apply this in her own work in the department, she can also use it as a basis for observation and analysis of occupations for which she may be rehabilitating her patients. The main essential is that the occupational therapist shall be a *trained* observer and shall use the results of her observations to improve the selection and presentation of a therapeutic activity and to gear this to the ultimate re-establishment of the patient.

Industrial work can be used as a rehabilitative measure, within or without the hospital. This is discussed in chapter 22.

The future of patients will be decided with them in the *Resettlement Clinic*, customarily held at regular intervals and attended by the doctor, disablement resettlement officer, social worker, occupational therapist and others treating the patient. The assessment and reports of the occupational therapist, if succinct, explicit and realistic can make an important contribution to decisions to be made. (Presentation of appropriate observations and records of well-planned and graded treatment can indicate to the team the important part that occupational therapy can play in rehabilitation and resettlement.)

Patients for whom occupational therapy is prescribed and for whose future, therefore, the occupational therapist will concern herself in the process of her treatment fall into five main categories:

(1) Those who can Return to their Former Work

The majority of patients can return to their former occupations after discharge from hospital either immediately or after a short period of convalescence. These will mostly fall into class 1 of the insurance categories, but even if in others, they may hope for a satisfactory re-establishment of their former income resources.

Physically disabled patients may have travelling problems. *The Travel Concessions Act 1964* offers solutions for these in appropriate circumstances. The provision of wheel-chairs and motorised invalid vehicles or grants for car conversion can be applied for [26], although there are certain conditions attached to the supply of these and often considerable delay.

A further problem for this and the other groups may be that of accessibility, or mobility, at home or at work. A move or even a change of job (but not occupation) may be necessary, unless alterations and adaptations can be made. For those in the home an application should be made to the social services department of the local authority for information on grants available. The domiciliary or hospital occupational therapist may be called on for advice here.

The patient still able to follow his former occupation may need some help with activities of daily living (see chapter 7).

For psychiatric patients the first three months after discharge from hospital are critical. Success in adjusting to former domestic or work routines will depend on the patient feeling confident to seek advice when difficulties occur, as psychiatric problems are not usually as obvious as physical ones. As most patients will attend an out-patient clinic, or evening follow-up group during the period, the occupational therapist should be available to give advice and encouragement concerning specific occupational problems. Housewives may need to be 'weaned' gradually from a day centre. Those returning to paid employment may benefit from attending part time at first. Some contact with the employer may be necessary through the social worker or direct. A patient may have to go to work, first, from a hospital or hostel, as an intermediate step to return home or living independently. Certain allowances are available for hostel board and lodging.

(2) Those Able to Undertake Alternative Work

The patient may be fit for alternative work within his capacities. This may be obtained with his former employer, or through the employment exchange, and there would be no need for special retraining. He might, or might not, be registered as disabled. The physical and psychological factors referred to above would also apply here.

(3) Those for Work in Sheltered Conditions

These, probably registered as disabled, would be unfit for open employment and might be settled in Remploy* workshops (although there are long waiting lists for vacancies) or in special centres such as the El Alamein Village. They would be unlikely to be sent to industrial rehabilitation units* or skill centres.

(4) Those who would be Sent for Retraining

Patients could be sent to:

(1) *Colleges of further education* for specialised courses.
(2) *Industrial rehabilitation units* for assessment as registered disabled. Here, after assessment, the alternatives would be:
   (*a*) Referral back to employment exchanges for direct placement.
   (*b*) Referral to sheltered work, Remploy,* etc. (see 3 above).
   (*c*) Referral for training within industry at a skill centre or other similarly relevant place.

For these patients there can also be problems of accessibility and mobility and in carrying out activities of daily living. They should be dealt with in the same way as for the former group.

Psychiatric cases fall into three categories:

(1) Patients who have had psychotic or neurotic breakdowns and were previously employed in certain professions, e.g. medical professions, research scientists, etc., who may be advised to discontinue and to seek alternative work with less responsibility but using their experience and knowledge.
(2) Long-term patients who because of age and length of time since they were previously employed usually require new and less demanding work than originally undertaken.
(3) Mentally handicapped patients starting work for the first time after some but not complete training in hospital.

3

For (2) and (3) a carefully planned gradual rehabilitation programme, graded in hospital and progressing to work outside hospital before discharge, is needed. Follow-up for two years is usually essential.

(5) Those who have to be Settled in Sheltered Work in Day or Residential Centres or in their Homes

Some patients will be deemed unemployable in open industry. Factors influencing the decision include the type and degree of disability, the type of local industry, the economic state of the country and the specific knowledge and advice of the disablement resettlement officer. Sheltered employment may be the answer. This offers security although with a small wage packet, and slowness and other limitations imposed by disability are accepted.

For patients likely to show improvement over a period of time, better openings may present themselves in local industry. The patient's work future should be reconsidered at regular intervals. The assessment report compiled at the time of his discharge from hospital, including the psychologist's findings and recommendations, will be of value if he is referred back for reappraisal.

These patients may have to be transferred to the care of the community occupational therapist, but some may have to be resettled in residential homes or in permanent nursing care as an extension of hospital care. Some, who may have been treated as out-patients, but who have increasing disablement due to progressive illness or old age, may first be admitted to hospital or medical rehabilitation centres for a brief period to be helped with activities of daily living, and taught how to make the most of residual ability. For economic reasons, and pressure on beds, these courses may have to be intensive and staff allocation and concentration should be planned carefully. In chapters 7 and 21 of this book full accounts are given of training in activities of daily living and the application of this type of occupational therapy for the aged. Whether in- or out-patients, some should come up to the resettlement clinic (see above) for consideration. They may be capable of contract work under the shelter of a day centre or in the home (see chapter 21 on community work).

Patients may, however, be capable of spasmodic occupation in the home only, and here the occupational therapist needs to be ingenious and realistic. She may set a pattern for diversional occupation within clinical considerations and arrange for patients to be visited by paid or voluntary craft or other helpers [27], supporting this by regular but less frequent visits herself.

For physical cases in this group, who can travel to day centres, there may be problems of transport and accessibility, which should be dealt with as suggested for the two former groups.

Wherever possible psychiatric cases, unable to work in open employment, should attend a sheltered workshop or day centre. Transport might be needed here too, as such patients are often unable to travel on public transport or attend regularly on their own initiative. Those who have to be settled in geriatric or psychogeriatric units, or in homes for the more permanently or progressively disabled may be able to make some contribution to the running of these if helped to do so under careful direction. Others will, perhaps, only be able to share, in varying degreees, in simple recreations. All will need to be helped to maintain their abilities and mobility as long and well as possible.

Suitable housing for handicapped people is considered to be vital and no programme of rehabilitation and resettlement is complete unless this is given careful attention. This is discussed more fully in chapter 21 on community occupational therapy.

Resettlement of the cerebral palsied has its special problems. This is discussed in the chapter under that heading, as are the implications of industrial work in rehabilitation in chapter 22.

Social Resettlement

While the aim of all resettlement is the re-establishment of the patient in his home and the community with maximum independence, circumstances can make this difficult and often something less than satisfactory must be accepted.

What is hoped for *for* the patient is a family with capacity to understand the patient's needs, both for help and independence, with good health, adaptability and tolerance, and a home in which he can make full use of his abilities, to which he can contribute; one in which he can have some degree of privacy when he wants it, and in which his friends will be welcome.

He must also have opportunity to get out to local shops, church, library, pub, friends' homes and clubs, i.e. to the places he used to go to, and to day centres and entertainments run by the community or local authorities.

What is hoped for *of* the patient is that he will make maximum use of his residual ability and that, having understanding of the demands and restrictions his disability will impose on his family, he will be considerate to them.

When return home is not possible it may be for any of the following reasons: architectural or environmental problems; inability of the family to take responsibility on physical or on psychological grounds; the physical needs of the patient being too great to be met even with maximum domiciliary services; the patient's presence being a source of disruption in the home.

Hope of satisfactory rehousing is almost nil in many areas in spite of a system of priorities. There are other difficulties, chief amongst them being an understandable reluctance to move away from the district where relatives and friends are within reach. This is as important to the patient's family as to himself especially if relationships within the home are strained. When alternative accommodation is offered the occupational therapist from the hospital or from the community service can be helpful in assessing its suitability and in advising on any necessary alterations or fittings, etc.

Although suitable housing can make the difference between being able or unable to live at home, a severely disabled person may be wholly without resources when it comes to passing the time. Many people have no hobbies and no interest in reading. Friends call in occasionally but less frequently as time goes by. Local authority day centres and old people's clubs offer opportunity for social contacts, and attendance even once a week breaks the monotony for those who are otherwise housebound. Unfortunately most centres only take people within a certain area and individuals with special needs cannot always be accommodated locally. With financial agreement between local authorities exceptions are sometimes made and this is invaluable especially for those with dual disability whose needs are great. Unfortunately lack of transport for the centres can limit attendance to once a week.

In theory it might seem that the occupational therapy department should be able to supply patients with an interest and occupation for home. Except in rare cases this is not practicable. When a handover to a community occupational therapist can be made the position is better [28].

Statutory provision of accommodation for those unable to live at home falls into two main categories, hospital or Part III* accommodation. Disabled people are allocated according to their need for care and to some extent to their age. It is not easy to ensure that 'a home' will have any provision for activity—making cups of tea, writing letters or following hobby interests. There are exceptions. More local authorities are building special accommodation for different categories of disabled—for old people in particular—where some supervision is provided but where there is also freedom of activity. Clearly any assessment of suitability on physical and personality grounds must be related to the possibilities available. Once the patient has reached his maximum functional ability, discussion with the appropriate social worker is helpful. She contributes by knowing the individual homes in her area, the physical demands which must be met in them, and their atmosphere. In return she is helped by being told of the patient's physical abilities, personality and interests, in addition to the medical prognosis. Everyone who has known the patient contributes to a picture of the individual.

More purpose built accommodation is urgently needed for the young, unemployable, severely disabled. Imaginative yet realistic planning will be wanted to ensure that physical activity and stimulation of interest are maintained, and that the varying intellectual abilities of individuals are catered for. Occupational therapists could contribute usefully in such schemes at the stage of structural planning and later to the choice and fixing of aids such as rails, choice of beds, chairs, work-tables and, if necessary, individual electronic aids [29]. Much of the day to day running of activities could be carried out by trained aides, under the overall supervision of the occupational therapist, and in cooperation with nursing staff. Specialist help may also be available locally.

REFERENCES AND RECOMMENDED FURTHER READING

1. See *Department of Health and Social Security Index of Leaflets* N.1.146, Feb. 1973 (Very comprehensive). Also *Attendance Allowance for Adults and Children*, N.1.205, Dec. 1973, and *Help for Handicapped People*, H.B.1, July 1972.
2. See ref. 1 above, and *The Reorganisation of the Health Service, 1974*, N.E. Metropolitan Reg. Hosp. Board, November 1973. (47 Whitehall Lane, Buckhurst Hill, Essex).
3. See *A Report from the Working Party on Collaboration between the N.H.S. and Local Government*. H.M.S.O.* 1973; *Coping with Disablement*, Consumers' Association*, 1974; chapter 21; and Telephone aids for the disabled. *Occ. Ther.*, 36, no. 9, 1973.
4. *Disabled Persons (Employment) Act*, 1944–1958.
5. Warden-assisted accommodation comes in 2 kinds: (*a*) where the Warden's task is supervisory and (*b*) where active assistance is given to residents (rare).
6. See ref. 1 above.
7. 8. 9. 10. 11. See ref. 1 above, H.B.1.
12. See D.H.S.S.* leaflet N.1. 6, *Industrial Injuries: Disablement Benefit*, June 1973.
13. See ref. 1 above, H.B.1.
14. See *The Employment Service, Plans and Programmes*. H.M.S.O.*, Oct. 1974.
15. See *The Employment Service, Plans and Programmes*, pp. 16, 17. H.M.S.O.*, Oct. 1974.
16. See *Employment and Training: Government Proposals*, p. 6. H.M.S.O.*, March 1973.
17. See *The Employment Service, Plans and Programmes*, p. 30. H.M.S.O.*, Oct. 1974.
18. See *The Employment Service, Plans and Programmes*, p. 32, H.M.S.O.*, Oct. 1974. And see: Worker's Group. *Occ. Ther.*, 36, no. 7, 1973.
19. See *The Employment Services: Plans and Programmes*, p. 32.
20. See *The Employment Services: Plans and Programmes*, p. 22.
21. See *The Employment Services: Plans and Programmes*, p. 33.
22. See *The Employment Services: Plans and Programmes*, p. 33.
23. See ref. 3 above.
24. See chapter 6.
25. As ref. 21 above.
26. As ref. 24 above.
27. See *Handcrafts Advisory Association*, p. 47.
28. See chapter 2.
29. See *Possum** and *P.I.L.O.T.** and *Zambette System 7**.
* See *Glossary*, pp. 454–6.

Part Two

CHAPTER 5

Basic Principles of Physical Treatment

Introduction [1]

Many patients recover from injury or illness without physical treatment of any kind. Some regain fitness with physiotherapy or with occupational therapy, while others need both forms of treatment. Each has a distinctive part to play and each is complementary to the other. While the practitioners share many basic concepts they must accept and respect differences too; differences in approach, in interpretation of treatment aims and in techniques. Each has something to offer which is wholly outside the scope of the other. Some patients prefer one form of treatment to another and this preference should be respected unless it affects progress. The basic tenet must be that the patient's treatment programme must be broad in concept yet realistic in its aims and that it must be right for him. For one patient the best progression might be to step up treatment in both departments, another might benefit more by increasing one while decreasing the other. For example, some jobs and some recreations demand maximal physical effort and in many centres this may be attained best by physiotherapy or remedial gymnastics. Even when occupational therapy includes outdoor work this rarely serves the same purpose for it seldom demands maximal effort. On the other hand stamina in its physical and mental aspects is best built up by occupational therapy and stamina in some form is needed in most peoples' jobs. In occupational therapy there is great opportunity for purposeful activity in a wide choice of treatment media for patients with similar disabilities. There should never be a rule of thumb treatment programme for a particular condition. Physiotherapy for a cellarman and a pharmacist with severe and comparable hand injuries might be similar but their occupational therapy could be wholly dissimilar although the patients' basic problems of use of the hand are the same: both may have difficulty in doing up fastenings on clothes and in using a knife or fork, and will avoid using the hand for picking up a newspaper or for opening a door. At work the demands on their hands are very different and it is the occupational therapist who will ask about this in detail for she has the greater scope for 'tailoring' treatment for individual needs.

Even a good referral from a doctor is unlikely to specify all the patient's needs. The responsibility lies with the therapist. First she must be able to identify dysfunction of movement, then to analyse its cause. Having done this she can plan treatment. For example, a referral for a patient newly weight-bearing after a fracture of the femur may specify quadriceps strengthening and knee mobilising. Less often will the glutei or calf muscles be mentioned and rarely the intrinsic muscles of the foot. Yet all are antigravity groups and will have deteriorated equally during the period of non-weight bearing. Until they can take the weight of the body the patient will be unable to walk without a limp, to climb stairs normally or to hurry, and attempts at crouching, shovelling or Scottish dancing will show up the weaknesses even more clearly.

Treatment starts from the moment a patient walks into the department and takes off his jacket for work. Occupational therapists should be observant of the spontaneous and incidental actions occasioned by the workshop environment for these can form a basis for treatment quite as valuable as the exercise provided by a carefully chosen activity. The best criteria of the success of treatment is the extent to which everyday actions show signs of spontaneity and the extent to which there is a return of confidence and efficiency in carrying out actions requiring special skill.

Demands on the occupational therapy department vary from centre to centre. This depends partly on the overall administrative and medical policy but also on the individual interests of doctors. Treatment for a special group of patients gives opportunity for depth of study and development of special techniques and equipment. It also calls for accurate forms of recording of methods and results. It is hoped that if the occupational therapist has a special interest she, too, will have opportunity to investigate its treatment implications, always bearing in mind that few departments can treat all the patients who might benefit and that priority must be given to those whose needs cannot be met elsewhere.

Planning the Patient's Programme [2]

When planning the patient's programme, the type of occupational therapy will depend upon:

The doctor's prescription. This may vary with the individual consultant's theories of treatment. For example, when a patient has rheumatoid arthritis he may ask for any or all of the following.

(1) Build-up strength in the affected parts.
(2) Assess the need for hand splintage.
(3) Check activities of daily living.
(4) Assess for work.

The treatment given by other departments. An aphasic patient who is receiving regular speech therapy will require speech and writing practice but not the intensive help he would need if there were no speech therapist available. If a patient with a hand injury is attending physiotherapy for specific exercises daily, the occupational therapist can concentrate on the more generalised functional use of the hand.

The length of time the patient attends for treatment. A housewife with family responsibilities will appreciate a short period of treatment with increasing activity. A docker with an industrial injury will benefit from longer periods of treatment incorporating specific activities interspaced with more generalised activities.

The facilities of the department. A small department with mainly light work cannot recondition a man who hopes to return to heavy work. When a department has only one bicycle fretsaw it may be necessary to progress the patient by making him work more quickly, completing 50 circuits in the time it previously took him to do 25, rather than increasing the time he spends on the activity.

The case load of the occupational therapist. The ability of the occupational therapist to give a patient with a head injury the individual treatment he needs, to make hand splints or to carry out clerical assessment will be partly dependent on the number of patients she is treating. (See chapters 3, 23.)

Posture and Working Positions [3]

The points made in this section are best understood by practical personal experiments.

The term 'good posture' implies an upright position of the body in which balance is maintained, without effort, in spite of the pull of gravity. This results in efficiency of movement with minimal effort and indicates a state of physical and mental well being. Posture quickly reacts to fatigue or a change of mood, and after a debilitating or depressive illness or a long period of immobilisation good posture will be at risk.

Working Heights

Chairs, stools, tables and benches of various heights are needed in treatment departments. Simple means of adjusting their height and the angle of their surfaces are invaluable, but no amount of care over these points alone can safeguard the patient's posture. The work must be correctly positioned and the patient closely supervised to see that it remains so.

Choice of working heights. A table of standard height is designed for use when sitting and it is often wrong for standing work. There are exceptions. When strong downward pressure is needed, as for cutting leather or card with a knife and ruler, or when the work itself raises the working level as, for example, packing cartons, a standard height of table is right for workers who are standing. Those sitting for these types of work need especially low tables, with comfortable clearance for the knees. It is a useful guide to think of the optimum normal height for work as being that of the elbow when the arm is by the side. Lengths of arm vary so the work height must be considered for each individual. A patient with short legs may need a low work bench when standing but he may be surprisingly tall when sitting and able to work comfortably at a normal height of table. There may be occasions when adjustments are made to standard working positions and work heights, for clearly defined therapeutic ends. This is acceptable only if the movements obtained follow normal patterns and are carried out without fatigue.

Posture when Sitting

When propped up in a bed or chair none of the antigravity muscle groups responsible for good posture are brought into play. The weight is more often taken on the sacrum and the dorsal spine than, correctly, on the ischial tuberosities. The spinal and abdominal muscles, which together control the tilt of the pelvis and the relationship between the different regions of the spine, are relaxed. The anterior chest wall is depressed and narrowed by abnormal flexion in the dorsal region and by relaxation of the retractors of the scapulae. Movements of the thorax are restricted and breathing is shallow. All the muscles stretched by such a position are weakened. In time their antagonists adapt to a shortened position and later may restrict full range of movement.

In bed the task of sitting well is made more difficult by the pull of the hamstring muscles. Even the relatively young may find it difficult to sit erect when their legs are horizontal and their knees are straight. The same problem faces a patient who has to keep his lower limb elevated while it is in a full-length plaster. If work is too far away the patient will unavoidably flex his spine and round his shoulders to increase his reach. Instead he should be allowed to lean back slightly concentrating on a flat back, and to have his work within reach from that position. With work which is lightweight, mobile and easily handled it is easier to safeguard good posture than with work requiring rigid equipment. The more accustomed a patient becomes to the feeling of any position, good or bad, the more normal it feels. The longer a bad posture is accepted the harder it will be to correct.

Detection of Postural Faults

Some defects are obvious both in standing and sitting, for example a long round back, narrow chest and poking head. Others may only be detected in one or other position; for example, it is in sitting that an arthrodesed hip is easily apparent. The pelvis is tilted backward and rotated, and the lumbar spine is flexed, to compensate for the lack of hip flexion. The body weight will be taken at two points only; by the rounded dorsal spine at a point high up the chair back and by the back of the thigh on the front edge of the seat. The knee on the side of the arthrodesed hip will be straight. To avoid discomfort it is instinctive to sit upright on the front of the seat and to bend the knee of the affected leg so that the foot is underneath the chair. This position relieves the flexion strain on the hip and spine but there is no back support. Patients with this disability often need advice and practical help in adapting an armchair for their comfort at home. Those in sedentary jobs need special consideration to ensure a comfortable working position. Deformity of the knee joints, whether in extension or flexion, is no bar to normal comfortable sitting, provided that there is a foot rest if the feet do not reach the floor. On the other hand severe flexion deformity is at once noticeable in standing. To bring the weight forward over the feet the hips are flexed and then to bring the head and shoulders erect the lumbar spine must be hyperextended. Back pain is a common sequel.

As far as it is compatible with treatment aims, patients with preference for sitting or standing should be given activities which can be done in the position of their choice.

Sitting Balance

Good sitting balance is a prerequisite for standing balance. All patients but the frail elderly or those with irreversible disturbance of the balance mechanisms can be trained to sit erect without back support. This training will usually be initiated by the physiotherapist and supplemented by the occupational therapist. Maintenance of sitting balance, while concentration is partly diverted to accomplish something else at the same time, is obviously a progression on sitting and doing nothing.

Demonstration is the best and quickest way of teaching sitting balance, stressing the following points:

Feet—fully supported, pointing straight forward, slightly apart and directly under the knees.

Weight—on ischial tuberosities, heels and forepart of feet.

Abdominal wall—flattened.

Lumbar region—slightly hollow.

Sternum—raised.

Dorsal spine—flat.

Shoulder blades—held down and together without limiting freedom of arm movement.

Head—erect.

Neck—stretched at the back and chin held slightly down, without tension.

Once this position can be held work is provided to build up stamina in holding it. At first the work must be close to the patient, for instance, using a rubber stamp or peeling potatoes. Gradually it should become possible to reach to one side to pick up the unstamped form and to the other to make a pile of those stamped. Similarly the 'cook' can progress to something in which reach and body movements are needed, such as washing up.

A further progression in the sitting position is to create a less static base by treadling or bicycling. Then the main responsibility for balance is thrown on the trunk muscles. Care must be taken not to restore stability by giving work which has to be held down firmly to the work top. Instead the choice should be something that must be handled lightly and inspected closely while in the hands, preferably while still working the machine; for example accurate shaping of wood on a bicycle or treadle sander. (For methods of strengthening muscles of the trunk and shoulder girdle see chapter 11.)

Standing Balance

Standing balance is a prerequisite for walking. In standing the centre of gravity is raised and the base is smaller than in sitting. More joints must be controlled and more muscle groups are involved, particularly the glutei, quadriceps and all muscles of the lower leg and feet. Able-bodied people stand and sit many times a day without thinking how it is done, but both are acts of skill and of extreme difficulty to many patients. After initial instruction by a physiotherapist, only practice can overcome the difficulty. This practice should be provided in occupational therapy departments as an essential part of treatment. With ingenuity the need to stand and sit can easily be integrated with the chosen activity.

Standing for Work

Patients should be instructed how to stand for maximum efficiency and avoidance of fatigue. The feet must be comfortably apart to give balance and approximately in the same plane as any strong or large movements likely to be made by the arms or trunk. Knees should be 'easy' to give pliability and to help to avoid back strain. To meet unpredictable hazards, and this applies to every patient whose balance is precarious, a diagonal stance is safest. The best way in which to appreciate this is in an underground train, standing but not strap hanging.

Applied Kinesiology [4]

Group Action of Muscles

Any movement brings into play groups of muscles, acting in different roles, and so coordinated that there is skilled performance with minimal effort.

In everyday life much of this is without conscious thought, for the movement patterns become established in the cerebral cortex as a result of repetition.

The arms and legs are accustomed to move in certain patterns with the limb of the opposite side and with those of the other extremity. The best example is walking. The arms swing in opposition to each other, the legs move forward alternately and coordination between the arm and leg of the same side of the body is also movement in opposition. The need to maintain balance is basic. The window cleaner reaching out to the side will lift his opposite arm or, if up a ladder, his opposite leg sideways without thinking about it.

Application in treatment

(1) Muscles are accustomed to work with each other and can only be maximally efficient when doing so.

(2) The limbs are accustomed to move simultaneously or to give stability for movement elsewhere.

(3) The intrinsic muscles of the trunk and those of the shoulder and pelvic girdles are accustomed to maintain posture, to initiate movement and to coordinate in movements of the extremities.

Types of Muscle Work

Concentric muscle work. The origin and insertion are approximated by the muscle contracting against resistance. This is an easy concept for patients. There is purpose in the action and the movement can be seen and felt.

Eccentric muscle work. The muscle 'pays' out by controlled relaxation. This allows the distance between the origin and insertion to be increased by a stronger force, e.g. gravity or an antagonistic muscle. This concept is difficult. The average person is unaware that a muscle works in this capacity.

Static muscle work. The muscle contracts to maintain a position and the relationship between the origin and insertion remains unchanged. This concept of holding is an easy one to appreciate.

Both concentric and eccentric muscle work may be referred to as *isotonic* and static muscle work as *isometric*.

Application in treatment

(1) If mobilising is the aim concentric work is most effective alternating with relaxation or eccentric work.

(2) If there is special need for improvement in circulation, static work is contra-indicated and movement should be stressed.

(3) If there is need to work the muscles maximally in a given time, static work is best, although this is not always practicable.

(4) If the primary aim is strengthening, and joint movement causes pain or is otherwise contra-indicated, static work is best.

(5) If coordination is to be improved the muscles must be trained both in concentric and eccentric work, e.g. quadriceps must control the upward movement of the lathe footplate by eccentric work after the concentric downward thrust. Similarly lowering of the hand to replace a tea cup must be controlled eccentrically by the elbow flexors. Playing draughts could prepare for this.

The Role of Muscle Groups During Activity

Prime movers are muscles working concentrically or eccentrically to promote movement, e.g. elbow flexors working to raise a cup for drinking, elbow flexors controlling extension of the elbow to put the cup down.

Antagonists are muscles which normally produce the opposite movement to that of the prime movers. They reciprocate with the prime movers by adapting in length.

Fixators work statically to stabilise the origin or insertion of the prime movers, e.g. unless the abdominals can control the lumbar spine, contraction of psoas will produce lordosis and will be inefficient as a hip flexor.

Synergists are muscles which contract and relax in conjunction with prime movers crossing more than one joint. By controlling the proximal joint a fulcrum is provided for the prime movers and their antagonists are protected against overstretching, e.g. as the long flexors of the fingers contract they act successively on the interphalangeal joints, the metacarpo-phalangeal joints and the wrist joint. Simultaneous flexion of these joints stretches the long extensors of the fingers and thus exerts a mechanical pull on the interphalangeal joints. These are prevented from flexing fully and gripping power would be ineffectual but for the synergist action of the wrist extensors.

Application in treatment. Some muscles work as often in one role as another and so there is no need to consider which to emphasise. Spinal muscles can most easily be strengthened in their fixator role, working statically to stabilise the spine for efficient movement of the shoulder girdle and arms. Wrist extensors work eccentrically to control flexion as the fingers open out preparatory to grasping. Then as synergists they work concentrically as the fingers flex to grip. They rarely work concentrically in conjunction with the long extensors of the fingers and should not, without good reason, be expected to do so as treatment.

Range of Muscle Work

This can be concentric or eccentric work:

> *Full range*—the muscle works between the fully stretched position and full contraction.
>
> *Outer range*—the muscle works between the fully stretched position and the mid-point of contraction.

Middle range—the muscle works in the middle section of its full range. For most muscles this is the most usual range and it is the one in which they work to the best mechanical advantage.

Inner range—the muscle works between the mid-point of contraction and full contraction.

Application in treatment. Weak muscles are able to work in mid range while still unable to overcome the mechanical disadvantages of outer or inner range. In the case of deltoid or the elbow flexors, sedentary work at a normal table which supports the forearm at rest can provide mid-range activity for both. An activity with varied free movement such as simple jewellery can require the forearm and elbow to be raised from the table while the hands move freely for short periods.

Types of Movement

Passive movement is brought about by some force other than the muscles which normally produce it. Being inactive, the muscles are therefore not strengthened. Existing range can be maintained by passive movement, but cannot be increased by it. When stretching occurs the movement is no longer strictly passive.

When there is loss of muscle power the physiotherapist will normally take the appropriate joints through their full passive range daily in order to prevent contractures, but at some stage of treatment this may become the occupational therapist's responsibility.

Active movements are of three types. In all of them the muscle is working either concentrically, eccentrically or statically and therefore its condition can be improved.

(1) *Assisted movement.* The muscle power can be augmented in various ways. (See pp. 67, 68.)

(2) *Free movement.* There is no attempt to assist, restrict or resist movement. For example, a patient with a newly united fractured humerus would not require assistance but should not work against resistance. Restriction of movement which might jar the fracture would be contra-indicated. Painting or sewing are suitable activities.

(3) *Resisted movement.* A technique used to strengthen muscle. (See p. 68.)

Applied Mechanics [5]

Mechanical advantage can be achieved by using *levers*, *pulley blocks*, *gears* and *flywheels*. Range of movement and speed of action are affected by their use. In many machines more than one of these work in combination and with understanding of their effects the treatment requirements can be met with reasonable accuracy. Everyone makes use of leverage in some form, daily.

The housewife uses the handle of a spoon to lever up the lid of a syrup tin. Pulley blocks are used mainly at loading bays and docks. These have limited use in occupational therapy.

Levers

Two opposing forces, *power* and *weight*, operate on a rigid bar moving at a fixed point, the *fulcrum*. *Power arm* and *weight arm* are the names given respectively to the distance between each and the fulcrum. In a state of equilibrium the power multiplied by the power arm equals the weight multiplied by the weight arm.

In the *first order of levers* the fulcrum is between the power and weight, e.g. a see-saw, pliers, scissors. Tools are designed to give their users mechanical advantage, so the handles are longer than the gripping or cutting jaws, i.e. the *power arm* is longer than the *weight arm*. Theoretically, the longer the handles the greater the advantage, but in practice undue lengthening makes one-handed grip and control difficult. In the *second order* the weight is between the power and the fulcrum, e.g. a wheelbarrow. Power has the advantage and a gardener can push a heavy load with comparative ease. Similarly, the *calf muscle* lifts the body's weight as its contraction pulls the heel up in walking or running. Power is exerted on the *os calcis* by the *Achilles tendon*, the weight falls through the middle of the foot and the fulcrum is the line of the *metatarsophalangeal joints*. Most muscles are examples of the *third order*. The power is between the weight and the fulcrum. Mechanically it is always at a disadvantage but there are compensations. A small contraction produces a relatively large movement, quickly, e.g. if the hand touches a hot surface it is withdrawn instantly by reflex contraction of *biceps* with a power arm only about 2 in long, from the *radial tuberosity* to the *elbow joint*. The joint is the fulcrum. The weight arm is the full length of the forearm and hand. Anyone with muscles below par, i.e. a woman with rheumatoid arthritis, is often in difficulty and, because of this poor leverage, she may be unable to lift a saucepan, however light it is, unless she uses both hands.

The therapist who is considering ways of making things easier for her patient must appreciate the full effects of increasing leverage. Range and speed of movement will be affected too, and the results might counteract the hoped-for benefits. An elderly patient who finds work on a bicycle-saw too tiring with the pedal shanks short, may not have enough movement in his hips or knees to have them lengthened. A lower gear might be the answer but he would have to pedal faster and, medically, this might be contraindicated. Plans for his treatment would have to be reconsidered.

Compromise is sometimes possible. Wood being turned on a lathe should rotate at speed. High gear is indicated, but a patient with spasticity would not have a strong enough leg thrust to use it. Nor would he have the movement and speed needed to gain better leverage by working with his foot further from the fulcrum of the footplate. The compromise might be to use the high gear, to stabilize his foot to give him maximum leverage within his limitations (see p. 190) and to supply the extra power needed by sharing the treadling with him.

Gears

These are a means of regulating speed and effort. Some of the problems related to leverage can be offset by their use. For example, a patient working on the bicycle with short cranks because of limited knee flexion, may need to be in low gear to reduce the power required to pedal. As range of movement improves, the cranks must be extended, but it would be contrary to treatment aims for the strength of his muscle work to be decreased. A change to high gear could offset this.

Momentum

A weighted flywheel is incorporated in some machines. Initially it resists the movement but once this is started the flywheel ensures a steady rhythm and its momentum gives assistance. Therefore a patient pushing a garden roller to improve strength in his leg muscles must push it slowly. Otherwise momentum does the work for him.

Pulleys

These can be used to change direction of pull without friction. If the change involves movement in a different plane the pulley must be of the swivel type. The normal down-pressure exerted by the pectoral muscles, when working a printing press, can be changed by running a strong cord vertically down from the horizontal bar handle of the press and through a swivel pulley at the level of the patient's waist to work the deltoid muscle. The pulley will adjust to variations in the line of pull as the patient abducts his arm with the elbow bent or straight.

Pulleys can be used to increase range of movement, resistance being constant throughout. This is the principle of the pulley block. Each pulley doubles the former range and simultaneously the power required is halved.

Muscle Re-education [6]

Dysfunction in muscle may show itself in several ways: slow reaction, weak contraction, lack of stamina, lack of reciprocal action between muscle groups, abnormal tone, inability to relax.

Muscles which continually take the weight of the body against gravity must be stronger than their antagonists on which everyday demands are less. For example, the calf muscles take full body weight while the dorsiflexors of the ankle normally lift only the weight of the foot: the exception is the acrobat who hangs by his feet.

The most common causes of local muscle weakness are disuse from immobilisation following trauma, and disuse as a natural reaction to movement causing pain, as with joint disease. There may, therefore, be several factors influencing the techniques of local treatment.

There are two aspects of muscle strengthening, building up power and building up stamina. Patients who need more muscle power will also need more stamina, but the converse is not necessarily true. It may be left to the therapist to plan the priorities according to the individual's needs. As the muscle becomes stronger its response to stimuli will be quicker, too.

Work within capacity, however regular, will not increase muscle power. There is only one way to do this, by working the muscle to capacity and trying to work it harder still. Maximal effort will produce local fatigue but this is deliberate and although it may result in temporary loss of efficiency it is not detrimental.

Building up stamina is achieved by working the muscles for increasing periods within their capacity. Circulatory and respiratory function will improve and this will again improve muscle function. In the gymnasium this can be done by working a muscle against light resistance many times, as opposed to working it fewer times, against maximal resistance, when the aim is to increase power. In contrast, a choice of activity should be available as occupational therapy, something that entails changes of position, a variety of actions and a moderate degree of exertion. If by continued effort some degree of skill can be gained with a particular tool, or with certain materials, there will be incentive to work for longer periods. For her own benefit the therapist may measure muscle bulk or draw the contours of, for example, the forearm to show it, but to the doctor, progress should be reported in practical terms relating to performance. The criteria are: how far can the patient walk, and how long can he stand, working, without fatigue, and what is his working speed and efficiency?

When the condition is one of spasticity the whole limb is affected and the balanced interplay between muscle groups no longer occurs. Attempts at re-education begin by trying to gain some measure of relaxation. The patient must be comfortable and in a good position. The limb must be adequately supported. The movement to be attempted is demonstrated slowly and carefully, and the patient is then helped to copy it. For example, he may be helped to grasp a spoon with a thick handle, to do the pick-up movement and then to raise the spoon to his mouth. The therapist must 'feel' the movement herself and coordinate her action with that of the patient. Any improvement will follow the normal pattern of the development of skills from infancy. Gross movements at proximal joints will be possible before any of the more intricate ones at the distal joints. If, after a reasonable period of concentrating on re-education of local function, the muscle cannot work efficiently, an all out drive for functional achievement by any means should be made. This change of emphasis may seem unreasonable to the patient, and the therapist must help him to understand and accept the reasons.

Functional competence may be achieved by trick movements. A patient with weak elbow flexors can compensate by lifting the forearm up on the thigh or by using body swing. He can keep it up by resting it on his iliac crest. Slipping his thumb through a loop of string tied through a front button-hole gives stability and the hand can then be used for lifting and carrying.

When there is serious muscle weakness, function may be improved by arthrodesis, muscle transplants or tendon grafts. The occupational therapist will then be required to re-educate function.

Assistance

Assistance is needed in a variety of circumstances when there is muscle weakness.

(1) Muscles may lack power to overcome gravity or the resistance offered by apparatus, or to control materials.
(2) A muscle may be rendered ineffectual by deficiency in its associates.
(3) Weak muscles are ineffectual in stretching tight structures.

There are various methods of giving assistance:

Choice of working position

(a) To give the muscles optimum advantage. For example, a patient with a weak deltoid trying to abduct his arm from his side may achieve nothing more than a rigidly elevated shoulder girdle and a strongly flexed elbow. If the arm were supported in 45° of forward abduction, further active abduction might be possible.
(b) To eliminate gravity. This is seldom practicable in a natural working position. There are exceptions, for example positioning wood on a sawing horse rather than in a vice allows gravity to assist the downward cutting action of the saw.

Sling suspension will serve in either of the above situations although it brings its own attendant problems (see p. 69).

Reduce resistance by applying basic mechanics

(a) To tools, as lengthening the handles of wire cutters or taking a shorter grip on a wooden spoon.
(b) To machines, as using longer pedal cranks on a bicycle or a lower gear on the lathe.
(c) To work, as in turning wood of smaller diameter.

Choice of materials: using mahogany rather than oak and stitching dress material rather than shopping bag canvas.

Self assistance

(a) By use of the other limb, using both feet side by side on an ankle treadle when one foot would not be strong enough alone, or both hands, one over the other on a leather punch; the reciprocal action of the bicycle as a means of re-educating a weak or incoordinated leg.

(b) By use of body weight and counter pressure to stretch tight structures, using a sanding or polishing block to overcome temporarily spasticity in a hand; kneading shortbread with the heel of the hand to increase extension of the wrist.

Application of resistance can be helpful when the patient is apprehensive of pain or is unable to initiate contraction of the prime movers. It gives a feeling of stability and direction of effort and the muscles react to the incentive to contract. For example, hamstrings which fail to contract when a patient tries to increase his knee flexion with gravity assisting, will automatically come into play if given adequate resistance.

Resistance

This is often an essential part of progressive treatment:

(1) To ensure maximal local muscular effort towards a target fractionally ahead of present performance.

(2) To ensure stronger muscle work in associates —fixators or synergists of a given muscle group.

(3) To build up power in a muscle which is inadequate for its task of mobilising a joint on which it acts.

(4) To offset the effects of mechanical adjustment to apparatus, e.g. with improvement in range of hip movements a patient treated on the bicycle will have the pedal cranks lengthened. The automatic decrease in the amount of power needed is undesirable.

There are various methods of giving resistance.

Reduction of assistance.
Mechanical means.
Use of springs or weights.
Choice of materials.
Use of heavier tools and handling heavier equipment.

Springs

These can be used with the purpose of giving assistance or resistance. The opposite movement to that for which the spring is used will in its turn be resisted or assisted. This could be detrimental to treatment. For example spring assistance could benefit a patient with a weak deltoid but if his pectoral muscles were already disproportionately strong and perhaps tight, self assistance in some form might be a better choice of method.

The resistance offered by extending a spring and the assistance given by its recoil, are strictly proportionate to its full length. While cumulative strength is needed to extend a spring, the assistance given by its recoil is diminishing, i.e. 30 lb and 15 lb will extend a 30 lb spring to its full length and half its length respectively; strength of recoil at full length will be 30 lb, at half length only 15 lb. A patient is therefore not working against the stated power of a spring unless his action extends it fully, i.e. to the length of the inner cord. A spring may already be incorporated in the machine to which an additional one is added and this makes accurate assessment difficult. It does not discount the usefulness of springs. The importance of understanding the effects of using them and of recording this clearly on treatment reports cannot be over-estimated.

When using overhead sling suspension to give assistance, two requirements must be met:

(1) Support for the relaxed limb in the optimum position. For the arm it is usual for the shoulder to be in 45° of forward abduction and externally rotated to bring the hand slightly higher than the elbow, the elbow being flexed through approximately 80°.

(2) Freedom to move as prescribed for treatment, and with appropriate assistance. Only with a high suspension fixing, i.e. approximately 8 ft, can freedom for a wide range of movement and assisted elevation be ensured.

For maximum buoyancy a low-powered spring is essential. Buoyancy may be contra-indicated when there is pain or fear of pain or, exceptionally, when freedom of movement is to be discouraged.

A variety of springs should be stocked, in duplicate, 5, 10, 15, 20, 25 and 30 lb provide a good range.

Weights

Weights offer a predetermined and consistent amount of assistance or resistance regardless of the range of movement. They can therefore be used with greater accuracy than springs but it is more difficult to apply them safely and unobtrusively in treatment.

PROPRIOCEPTIVE NEUROMUSCULAR FACILITATION*[7]

These techniques are now widely accepted and increasingly used in muscle re-education, most particularly with neuromuscular disorders such as cerebral palsy, hemiplegia and disseminated sclerosis. While they can only be fully used by the physiotherapists, the occupational therapists should know how to adapt those which are suitable for occupational therapy. In this way patients can receive stimulation in the same pattern in both departments.

Such techniques can be defined as 'methods of promoting or hastening the response of the neuromuscular mechanism through stimulation of the proprioceptors'. They aim to combine simultaneously known facilitatory factors. The bigger the sensory demand the better the motor response. They depend upon:

(1) *Demand* to raise the central excitatory state and lower the threshold of the dormant anterior horn cells.

(2) *Repetition* to lower the synaptic resistance and to improve the conductivity of nervous pathways.

Basic Principles and Techniques

Patterns of movement. 'Nervous centres know nothing of muscles, they only know of movements' [7†]. Mass movement patterns are spiral and diagonal in character and closely allied to functional movements, for example hand to mouth. Re-education in patterns of movement follows the normal sequence of child development, for example, withdrawal is learned before thrust. While an athetoid will need to learn the whole sequence, a hemiplegic who has an overstimulated withdrawal pattern will start with extensor thrust.

Woodwork provides good patterns of movement; sawing, planing, and hammering are done diagonally across the body. Extensor thrust is needed in dart throwing or treadling a lathe.

Maximal resistance. This demands activity of all motor units available, to stimulate the spindles and increase muscle tension to provide overflow to weaker groups.

Methods of giving resistance are described on p. 68.

Manual contacts. Exteroceptive and proprioceptive stimuli from touch and pressure are important facilitatory factors. Some contactual stimulation is present in most activities of the upper limb. Built up cone-shaped handles increase the area for contact and provide additional pressure. Strapping a paralysed hand to a tool ensures contact.

Traction and approximation stimulate the proprioceptors within the joint structures. Traction is more often applied to antigravity, flexion movements and approximation to extensor movements as these most nearly simulate weight bearing. Traction occurs each time an object is lifted and this can be graded. Approximation occurs on pushing, as in treadling or sawing.

Stretch. All muscles contract more strongly when they have been stretched. Therefore placing the muscle first in the stretched position will facilitate its contraction. A muscle is put on stretch when all the joints over which it passes are at the appropriate end of their range. Work components can be placed to necessitate stretching out to reach them. Children can thread beads on to long lengths of string, or draw on large pieces of paper.

Reinforcement is an automatic response proportional to the demands placed before the body. In picking up a typewriter reinforcement spreads from the arms to the trunk and lower limbs. This overflow of excitation into other muscle groups can be utilised by performing an already strong movement and thereby reinforcing other weak groups of muscles. Bilateral work, as when a hemiplegic uses a double handled saw, is an example of reinforcement.

Slow reversal is based on Sherrington's principle of successive induction that after a strong contraction through the range of the agonist there is an increase in the excitability of the antagonist. Maximal resistance is given to the stronger muscle group followed immediately by isotonic contraction of the weaker antagonist group. Activities requiring movement in both directions such as swinging a golf club, sawing and hammering provide this.

Rhythmic stabilisation is based on the same principle. Alternative isometric contractions of agonists and antagonists are used to stimulate contraction of muscles on all sides of the joint, so giving stability. This is not easy in occupational therapy. It occurs at the wrist when resistance in opposing directions is given by using a coping saw or file.

Training Coordination [8]

Causes of Incoordination

Incoordination may be the result of motor or of sensory defect. It is manifested by an imbalance of the group action of muscles; the fixators, prime movers, antagonists and synergists no longer working in harmony. The cause may be lesion in the brain, in the spinal cord or in the periphery. Voluntary control of movement is diminished or lost according to the site and the extent of the lesion. Prognosis for improvement depends on the aetiology. There may be spontaneous recovery of function without treatment; there may be improvement with treatment, although with some residual disability, and sometimes there will be irreversible deterioration. Even so periodic treatment can slow down the rate of loss of function by building up residual abilities. Personality changes and impairment of mental function reduce prospects of good results. Either may occur in association with a cerebral lesion.

Lesion of the upper motor neurone can lead to some loss of voluntary movements and slowness of residual movements. There is spasticity, as seen in hemiplegia, cerebral palsy or spastic paraplegia. All the muscles in the limb or limbs are hypertonic and the most powerful groups may pull the joints into positions of deformity. In the upper limb these are the muscles concerned with grasping and holding to the body. In the lower limb they are, in the first instance, those accustomed to take the weight of the body against gravity. The typical hemiplegic patient is a good example, with his tight fist and adducted shoulder, his straight knee and spastic drop foot. Gross movements are possible but usually not those requiring fine coordination.

Lesion in the cerebellum produces ataxia. This may affect one limb or the whole body. The gait is unsteady and the whole arm will come into play when any attempt is made to use the hand. This is 'intention tremor'. Speech is slurred and visual acuity is impaired.

Lesion in the basal ganglia produces rigidity or tremor. Both initiation and cessation of movement is inhibited, as seen in the typical Parkinsonian gait. This defect, together with tremor, is a serious discouragement to any active effort, including speech. Hand function is ineffectual, due equally to inability to place the hand for use and to coordinate its movements.

Interruption of sensory pathways. Deficit of tactile sense, kinaesthetic sense or spatial perception impairs coordination. Simple movements can no longer be performed with accuracy or speed even with conscious effort. Transferring a canister from a table to a high shelf can illustrate this. With tactile loss the canister could only be picked up after fumbling with it. Kinaesthetic loss would make it necessary to watch the arm movement while lifting the canister. Loss of spatial perception would make it hard to judge the exact position of the shelf. Related to functional use, therefore, the effects of sensory deficit would be evident through poor motor performance.

Re-education

This is based on an understanding of good posture and good movement, and of the components on which they depend. Interference with function of any one component will interfere with the total function and it may therefore be necessary to improve function of the components first.

Aims of treatment can be broken down:

(1) *To improve local muscle function* by remedial measures as required, e.g. strengthening, training in quicker response, training in rhythm.

(2) *To retrain sensory function*, compensating for loss as necessary. This is needed as it affects posture, i.e. static relationships of one part of the body to another; and as it affects movement, i.e. changing relationships involving balance. It is also needed when tactile discrimination is faulty.

(3) *To make optimum use of function*, planning to conserve energy for the individual's priority needs. For example, a patient might be able to continue at his job provided his writing could be improved. It deteriorates markedly with fatigue. It would, therefore, be sensible to accept help from his wife for dressing and for being driven to work. Treatment should concentrate on his needs at work.

(4) *To help the patient to become maximally confident* in compensatory methods when improvement is inadequate for normal ones, e.g. perching on a stool at the kitchen sink.

(5) *To help the patient to adjust* to the limitations imposed, to allow more

time to concentrate and to do things, and to avoid taking unnecessary risks. This is especially difficult for the patient who has been quick and efficient.

Treatment for the Upper Limb

Useful function depends on ability to pick up and to release objects of varying sizes, shape and weight, to manipulate, and to place the hand for use. Gross action pick-up is possible before precision pick-up and approximate placement before accurate placement. Manipulative skill is only possible after precision pick-up. Conditions resulting in poor coordination commonly affect both handling and placement. The dominant and non-dominant hands should be retrained for their former roles if practicable, i.e. actions needing strength or precision, and the secondary role of stabilisation, respectively. Progression should vary according to needs: use a less stable starting position, e.g. sitting with back unsupported after being supported; use a longer lever, e.g. with the arm unsupported when before, the forearm rested on the table; aim to work faster or with greater precision; include more complex movements; use both hands simultaneously; make less use of eyesight; keep up more sustained effort.

The following examples illustrate some of the principles described.

Example I. Simple assembly of bottles and bottle tops for the hospital dispensary. Repacking in cartons.

> *Starting position.* Sitting up to a table, back fully supported, forearms resting on the table.
> *Placement of work.* Tops and bottles within reach of dominant and non-dominant hands respectively.
> *Action.* (1) Gross pick-up of bottle. (2) Pick up top. (3) Screw together. (4) Replace on table.
> *Progression.* (1) Perching on a stool, arms unsupported: same action.
> (2) As 1, but pick-ups simultaneously.
> (3) Standing with wide base at same table, leaning thighs against it. Bottles and tops in cartons. Reach into cartons, assemble with elbows held into sides. Place bottles on table in rows.
> (4) Work against the clock, assemble smaller bottles and tops, etc. etc.

Example II. Drawing, sitting at a table, paper fixed, following repetitive writing patterns with thick felt pen.

> *Progression.* (1) Writing letters, then words, then using a biro.
> (2) Painting, dipping the brush in a paint pot, then using a paint box.

(3) Sitting at an easel, using a longer brush, holding a
palette, standing at an easel, etc.

Improved control achieved by treatment should be noticeable in general
activities such as feeding and writing. These too can be broken down into
simple forms which should be practised with planned progression.

Treatment for the Lower Limb

Intrinsic strength and control is not enough for useful function. The pelvis
must be balanced on the lower limbs, often on one only. The spinal column
must be balanced on the pelvis. Adjustments of balance are frequently
needed. Hip muscles, abdominal muscles, lateral muscles of the trunk and
the spinal extensors are all involved.

Demands on coordination vary little from individual to individual except
in a minority of cases, e.g. ballet dancers. Safe everyday mobility is the aim,
i.e. ability to change positions and to get from one place to another. Such
differences as there are, are demands on strength or speed of fundamental
movements rather than on increasing complexity. Here again the ballet
dancer and the footballer, are exceptions. Both need perfection of accuracy
in complex sequences of movement, often one leg at a time moving at speed
without body weight. In contrast, normal demands are greatest when weight
bearing. It is not so much control of the leg which is difficult but control of
the body on the leg, although the primary dysfunction is in the leg. This will
of course also show in movement of the leg, e.g. the ataxic patient's problem
in placing his foot correctly when walking.

Specific re-education is the physiotherapist's responsibility, by Frenkel
type exercises and progressive balance retraining. The occupational therapist
can contribute by giving work which will improve strength and rhythm of
leg movements and which builds up an awareness of good posture. The
rhythmic reciprocal movement of bicycling is good local treatment. The
range, speed and strength can be regulated and the action involves muscle
groups in coordination, as in walking. The starting position is not wholly
stable although the pelvis is partially controlled by taking weight on the
saddle and it would not be possible to have freedom of hip movement from
any other form of seat. The patient may need to hold on firmly with both
hands for further stabilisation and this must be accepted until he can
continue an even leg action while simultaneously using his hands. This
ability indicates more than physical progression. Habit must be formed so
that conscious effort is no longer needed for the leg action and can be transferred to the work being done by hand. Until this can be done, another
patient or the therapist must handle the material. A patient with incoordination of his legs is likely to be similarly handicapped with his hands and
the activity must be appropriate. If the machine can provide for work

needing only one hand so much the better, buffing, for example. The other can still stabilise.

The patient must be safeguarded against injury to his ankles if poor control jeopardises the position of his feet on the pedals. Control of the hip joint is responsible for this and correct alignment of hip, knee and foot is important. The therapist may have to apply pressure on the outer side of the knee until the patient is able to control its position for himself. Getting on and off the machine is an integral part of treatment and the therapist should think out the best method for the individual patient.

It is a progression to work on the lathe. The supporting leg is weight bearing, the centre of gravity is higher and the pelvis must be stabilised by the hip muscles. The control needed for this is as important as that for the moving leg. First there is the downward extension thrust through the knee and forepart of the foot to the footplate. Then its recoil must be actively controlled by eccentric muscle work to ensure a continuous smooth action. The weighted flywheel is helpful, giving a feeling of balance and rhythm. Low gear should not be used for incoordinated patients. A treadle sewing machine gives good possibilities of continuous rhythm and the newer models with a slow gear are best. Darning technique is good, first to cover a given area freely, such as coloured felt for a kettle holder; later progressing to embroidery, still in bold blocks of colour but calling for greater control. This technique ensures continuous treadling. A foot power loom makes demands on foot placement not provided by bicycle or lathe as proprioceptive accuracy is required by the pedals being out of sight.

Part of treatment should consist of any activity of interest which will involve part sitting, part standing, part moving from one place to another, handling and carrying. Kitchen work provides this, or sorting and rearranging the contents of a workshop cupboard. Patients who are not fully confident in walking tend to stop short of their objective, not realising that balance and hand control will both be more difficult if picking up is done at arms' length. Training in positioning for reaching and in lifting and carrying will be needed. The feet should be pointed in the direction in which they will be moving, close to the object to be picked up. The knees should be pliable, bracing them will not give added stability. Any article should be held close to the body with the elbows well in. If possible one or both hands should be underneath, for example carrying a tray with one hand forward, one at the back. When walking, concentration should be on this, not on what is being carried. Excellent opportunities for practice offer themselves during the routine tidying up in the department.

Mobilisation of Joints [9]

Before planning treatment to mobilise a joint the cause of stiffness must be known. This will indicate, and may also contra-indicate, certain treatment techniques and will predetermine to some extent improvement to be expected. The patient's tolerance of pain may also influence the treatment content.

Causes of Joint Stiffness

(1) Contracture of the joint capsule, surrounding muscles or interstitial fascia following prolonged immobilisation.

(2) Damage to the articular cartilage by arthritic changes, or by a fracture into the joint.

(3) Tethering of muscle or skin by callus formation or scar tissue.

Aims of Treatment

(1) To improve the circulation through the part.

(2) Progressive stretching of the tight structures.

(3) Re-education of the related muscle groups. In the upper limb the emphasis will be on mobility and in the lower limb on stability.

Stiffness Within the Joint

When this is due solely to disuse it is treated according to general aims. Rate of progress depends on age, the younger the patient the quicker full function is restored, and on any limitations put on activity by the original injury.

Damage Within the Joint

Transmission of pressure through the joint drives the adjacent articular surfaces together, causing pain. Muscle spasm may result and with it inhibition of movement. If the articular surfaces can be separated by traction during movement pain is less likely. Although this technique is not always possible in occupational therapy, transmission of force can and should be avoided.

If the upper limb, pulling against resistance, applies traction to the wrist joint and if the grip is a hook grip as distinct from a palm grip there will also be traction of the metacarpo-phalangeal joints. Work on a bench drill is good for this. The stronger the spring resistance to pulling down the lever the more traction there is. Holding the drill and pushing forward to drill horizontally against resistance would be contra-indicated when pain is a dominant symptom.

For the lower limb a continuous rhythmical movement such as bicycling is good. Although traction is not inherent in this, transmission of force can be avoided by ensuring that resistance to the pedalling action is minimal. Indirectly the work itself gives resistance, so it must be light. Over estimation of the joint range can bring the pedalling to a halt, always at the position in which maximal strain is on the joint. This indicates the need for shorter pedal cranks but these in turn impose a mechanical disadvantage. A weighted flywheel will help to counteract this. Ideally this should be within reach so that manual self assistance can be given to start the movement. Strong work on a foot-power lathe is contra-indicated in the early stages. It is also important to identify the patient who thinks that if treatment is painful it must be doing good; here the opposite is true. It is important to 'run in' the joint surfaces in the same way as running in the engine of a car after a rebore.

Contracted Tissues and Tethering of Muscle or Skin

Treatment must be gentle but persistent, for strong action could tear the soft tissues and so produce further scarring. Muscle held down in callus formation or scar tissue loses its ability both to stretch and to contract fully throughout its length. The former will limit the outer range of movement and the latter will result in lack of stability in the inner range. In weight-bearing joints this is a serious disability. Increase of joint range is contra-indicated unless there can be a corresponding increase in muscle power to control it.

Skin adhering to underlying bone or tendon may limit movement permanently. Local treatment for the skin and passive stretching of the joints by physiotherapy is followed by occupational therapy. Ideally both treatments should be given at least twice daily. Splints to maintain improved range may be prescribed, to be worn between treatments. These must be altered as often as there is change. As a rule they are made of plaster of paris by the physiotherapist.

Assessment of Range

This is frequently gauged by eye by the doctor during his clinical examination. The physiotherapist more often uses a goniometer. Often the patient will have been to both before coming to the occupational therapist. She, too, must record her findings but it is important to avoid unnecessary duplication. Different people measure differently and conflicting readings are confusing. The same person should always measure the same patient. Any alteration in range less than 5° should be disregarded. Short-term cases may show worthwhile improvement in one week whereas long-term patients should be recorded at the most every fortnight. The effects of treatment are constantly assessed: for example, after working on a bicycle the patient will be expected to show by his walk that he has benefited from his treatment.

Doctors often prefer reports from the occupational therapist in terms of everyday function. For example, of a bricklayer 'He can now grip and use a 4 lb hammer for short periods', or of a home help 'She is using public transport and can now kneel'. The method of assessment is immaterial provided it is simple and provides reliable evidence of maximum function. This last is not as easy as it sounds. The therapist must decide exactly what she wants the patient to do and must know what she will look for as he attempts to do it. With knowledge of anatomy and kinesiology she knows how each digit normally functions as a hand closes to make a fist and how their movements are coordinated. Few patients have consciously thought about either. She must discriminate between true loss of function and poor performance. With the latter appropriate encouragement can produce an improved final effort bearing little resemblance to his first attempt.

Special Problems of Mobilisation

Few everyday actions call for the ultimate degrees of joint range but they will be performed more easily and efficiently if full range is possible. Physiotherapy may be more efficient in achieving the ultimate range; occupational therapy is often more efficient as a means of restoring skill and endurance. It is difficult to mobilise certain joints by occupational therapy, e.g. inversion and eversion of the foot, extension and rotation of the hip, and internal rotation of the shoulder. Most of these movements are incidental, occurring in the course of complex sequences. They are not therefore used as primary movements in any purposeful activity. Once range has been increased, muscular control for the movements can usefully be built up by occupational therapy, and activities making use of the regained mobility in its subsidiary role will be beneficial.

It is harder to mobilise a joint than to strengthen a muscle because:

The muscles acting on the joint will have lost power and be ineffectual as a force to stretch the tight structures. They must be strengthened within the existing range before they can be expected to increase range.

Some discomfort is unavoidable, and there may be pain at extremes of movement. It is unreasonable to expect such a position to be held. Incorporating the point of maximal stretch in a continuous rhythmical movement will avoid this, for example, exercising a stiff knee on a bicycle adjusted for maximal range or working a stiff shoulder by polishing a table top on an inclined plane positioned to need maximal elevation to reach the far edge.

Recollection of the 'feeling' of the movement may be lost. Careful re-education is needed. Movement of the limb of the other side can be both a visual and a practical aid in re-establishing joint and muscle sense by reciprocal or simultaneous movement.

Compensatory action in adjacent mobile joints may be substituted for movement in the one with limitation. This is inevitable if more is expected of the joint than it can achieve. Important factors in preventing this include the following: accuracy in assessment of the dysfunction and in gauging the amount of resistance which should be given to the prime movers; choice of an activity within which there is scope for an increasing range of movement as improvement occurs; and careful teaching. For example, a patient with limited ankle movement using a treadle machine accurately adjusted will be instructed in the following order:

(1) Shown the correct working position and be told the importance of keeping still on the seat, not 'shunting' backwards and forwards, and keeping the feet and knees in sagittal alignment.

(2) Practise the movement with the normal weight-bearing areas of the foot in contact with the footplate throughout, emphasising toe-heel action.

(3) Taught how to handle the materials.

It is when concentration is directed to the work that compensatory movements occur. In an effort to bring more power to bear on the treadle and to avoid ankle movement which is difficult, the patient will turn on his seat and the knee of the affected leg will be alternately thrust forward and retracted. This may happen even when the patient has been well taught until it is pointed out to him. If not well taught compensatory action can make nonsense of treatment.

Over-anxiety may make a patient try too hard. Antagonists and prime movers will contract simultaneously and muscle groups unrelated to the stiff joint may also be brought into action, the whole limb becoming tense and all movements inhibited. Both the manner and the voice of the therapist can influence such a patient. He must be helped to try 'easily', to feel the rhythm of the treadle and to work with it.

Progression

This may be made as follows:

By increasing the duration of treatment. The aim must be clear. Either a longer period must be spent on the same activity or there must be additional activity. Time spent is of itself no guarantee of progression.

By working more quickly in a given time the structures restricting movement can be stretched more often. Fifty circuits on a bicycle will have twice the benefit of 25 circuits. In addition the effect on the circulation will be greater.

Application of more force can be effected either by stronger muscle work or by using body weight.

The working position can be changed. A patient with a stiff elbow may progress from sitting on a high stool to reach the lever of an overhead drill, to sitting lower doing the same work, as his range of extension improves.

Placement of work can be adjusted. A similar patient assembling industrial work from boxes immediately in front of him may have these boxes placed progressively further away in order to increase elbow extension.

Adjustment of tools. A patient with limitation of metacarpo-phalangeal joint flexion will require padded tools, including those for A.D.L.* As a progression this padding will be reduced gradually. Care must be taken not to upset the balance of the tool with such padding.

Adjustment of apparatus. Range, speed and strength required to work apparatus such as pedal looms, bicycles and treadles can be regulated to meet changing demands. (See p. 63.)

REFERENCES AND RECOMMENDED FURTHER READING

1. Introduction
   Chapman, H., *The Physiology of Muscular Exercise*. U.S.A., 1967.
   De Vries, H. A., *Physiology of Exercise*. London, 1968.
   Gardiner, N. D., *Principles of Exercise Therapy*. London, 1973.
   Grant, R. W., *Prinicples of Rehabilitation*. London, 1963.
   Willard, H. S. & Spackman, C. S., *Occupational Therapy*. U.S.A., 1971.
   See also: Electromyography—Investigating muscle activity. *Occ. Ther.*, **35**, no. 8, 1972.
2. Planning the Patient's Programme
   See chapters 3 and 23, this book.
3. Posture and Working Positions
   Bramwell, Jones. S., *Selection of Household Furniture and Equipment*. D.L.F.*
      Part I ; *Easy Chairs for the Semi-Ambulant*. London, 1968.
      Part II ; *Tables and Chairs for the Semi-Ambulant*. London, 1969.
   Eklundh, M., *Spare Your Back*. London, 1965.
   Hollinshead, W. H., *Functional Anatomy of the Limbs and Back*. London and Philadelphia, 1969.
   Turner, M., *Faulty Posture, Its Effects and Treatment*. London, 1965.
      And see:
   Ergonomics Pamphlet No. 7. *Posture for Industry*.
   Lifting Patients in the Home. Chartered Society of Physiotherapy*.
   Lifting Patients in the Hospital. Chartered Society of Physiotherapy*.
   Lifting in Industry. Chartered Society of Physiotherapy*.
   How to lift and carry patients correctly. *Occ. Ther.*, **35**, no. 8, 1972.
4. Applied Kinesiology
   Bowen, W. P., *Applied Kinesiology*. London, 1953.
   Brunstrom, S., *Clinical Kinesiology*. U.S.A., 1972.
   Kranz, L. G., *Kinesiology Manual*. London, 1961.
   Wells, K. F., *Kinesiology*. London, 1971.
5. Applied Mechanics
   Hollis, M. & Roper, M., *Suspension Therapy in Rehabilitation*. London, 1965.
6. Muscle Strengthening
   Aids to the Investigation of Peripheral Nerve Injuries. H.M.S.O.*, 1965.
   Daniels, L. et al., *Muscle Testing*. U.S.A., 1972.
7. P.N.F.*
   Knott, M. & Voss, D. E., *Proprioceptive Neuromuscular Facilitation (Patterns and Techniques)*. London, 1969.
      And see:
   Approaches to the Treatment of Patients with Neuromuscular Dysfunction. Study Course, W.F.O.T.*, 3rd Int. Congress, 1962.
   Physiotherapy. 53/1. 1967.

Physiotherapy. 55/1. 1969.
† Rasch, P. J. & Burke, R. K., *Kinesiology and Applied Anatomy* (p. 9). U.S.A., 1971. (Hughlings Jackson, 1834–1911.)
8. Training in Coordination
Sandifer, P. H., *Neurology in Orthopaedics.* London, 1967.
Walshe, F., *Diseases of the Nervous System.* Edinburgh and London, 1970.
9. Mobilisation of Joints
Joint Motion: Method of Measuring and Recording. American Assoc. of Orthopaedic Surgeons. London, 1966.

And see:
Cash, J. E., *Medical Conditions for Physiotherapists.* London, 1971.
Cash, J. E., *Physiotherapy in some Surgical Conditions.* London, 1971.
Cash, J. E., *Neurology for Physiotherapists,* London, 1974
Cash, J. E., *Chest, Heart and Vascular Diseases for Physiotherapists,* London, 1974.
Clark Kennedy, A. E. and Bartley, C. W., *Clinical Medicine.* London, 1960.
Davidson, L. S. P. and MacLeod, C. S., *Principles and Practice of Medicine,* London, 1974.
Sears, W. G. and Winwood, R. S., *Medicine for Nurses.* London, 1970.
* See *Glossary,* pp. 454–6.

Introduction to Physical Occupational Therapy: Part 1

Assessment of the Patient: Reporting and Recording [1]

The *initial assessment* of the patient is made to clarify his status and condition when presented for treatment. This will include a social, medical, physical, functional and where necessary, psychological assessment. It is important that this should be made without delay in order to plan the patient's initial treatment programme and to establish a base line against which progress can be checked. *Continuous assessment* is essential in order to plan each succeeding stage of treatment. A *final assessment* prior to discharge will provide a summary of the patient's condition and suggestions for his future. This report will be sent, as appropriate, to his General Practitioner, Consultant, Disablement Resettlement Officer, Employer, and Health or Social Services Departments.

Assessment may be defined as informed and organised observation, leading to a decision as to the action to be taken. The means used will vary according to the circumstances and to the particular discipline making the assessment; for example, a doctor makes a clinical assessment of the systems of the body in an organised sequence. His knowledge and experience give him the appropriate information to interpret his findings and so make an accurate estimate of the patient's medical condition and prognosis, and to initiate the plan of treatment. The occupational therapist's contribution is in the field of functional ability, and she will be less concerned with range or strength of movement, than with the applied range, strength and coordination in terms of the patient's competence in essential activities. His performance must be assessed in relation to his family responsibilities, his home, his neighbourhood and work situation; or to the institution in which he will be living.

The patient's physical disability must be considered in relation to his particular body and age and to the rate of restoration of his tissues. It is also influenced by his personality and attitude of mind. The occupational therapist, like the other members of the treatment and after-care team, must record her findings in such a way that they will be pliable enough both to meet the doctor's request and to fit in with other colleagues' findings so that a picture of the patient's whole life with its various problems is built up. All reports should be available readily to everyone concerned with the patient and verbal discussion is also important.

Occupational Therapy Assessment

The doctor may require a general assessment of the patient's independence or an assessment of his functional ability to return to work or a more specific assessment of local function before and after reconstructive surgery. The occupational therapist, having read the medical notes, uses an organised pattern of questioning and observation for one or more of the following:

> *A preliminary assessment*, to highlight the patient's overall problems and to identify the main ones.
> *Check lists*, to act as reminders, in detail, and to serve as records of progress.
> *Tasks in context*, to involve both physical ability and initiative.
> *Clearly defined and graded tests*, to give, as far as possible, a measure of a particular ability.

These formal means of assessment are augmented by the therapist's continual observation of the patient's function and attitudes in non-structured situations throughout the day.

Preliminary assessment. This covers:

(1) *Home conditions:*

    (*a*) Type of house, flat, bungalow, residential home.

    (*b*) Main problems; access steps, stairs, upstairs bathroom, W.C.*, etc.

    (*c*) Family at home: relatives or friends near.

(2) *Mobility:*

    (*a*) General: Lying, sitting, standing, walking.
                 Walking with aids or appliances.
                 Wheelchair type, method of transfer, and propulsion.
                 Dealing with ramps, steps, curbs, distances.

    (*b*) Outdoor transport: private, public.

(3) *Upper limb function:*

Handling, reaching, lifting, carrying.

These three sections will give a simple overall picture of the patient's capability in his environment. This is then followed by detailed observation under the following headings:

(1) *Personal care:* washing, bathing, toiletting, washing hair, cutting nails, shaving, making up, dressing, eating and drinking.
(2) *Communication:* by speech, telephone, writing, typing, reading, listening to radio and watching T.V., going out for shopping and social functions by public or private transport.
(3) *Domestic activities:* for both men and women; general housework and preparation of basic meals.
(4) *Work/Education/Training:* problems related to the patient's particular job including the running of a home, and in places of work or education/training.
(5) *Leisure activities.*
(6) *Personality and mental attitudes:* positive or negative attitudes, quick or slow reaction, anxiety or relaxation, cooperative or resentful, dependent or independent.

Much information can be obtained by questioning but this must be substantiated by careful observation. For example, a patient may state that she can undress independently but when asked to do so it may be found that she has taken a certain amount of help for granted.

In some cases it is enough to note that a certain activity can be carried out, even though the method is abnormal and much adapted to the patient's disability. It may be necessary, however, to describe exactly how the task was achieved. This calls for knowledge of the normal method and close observation of the trick movement used or attempted.

Check lists. If preliminary assessment indicates housing and domestic problems, check list (1) can be used when a home visit is made by the occupational therapist. If the home is at a distance but the patient's problems are being dealt with at the Assessment or Treatment Centre the check list may be sent to the Community Occupational Therapist or Social Worker in the home area, with a request for further information.

If the main problem is in activities of daily living a check list such as (2) may be used. A run through of the list at regular intervals will indicate the patient's progress.

Where a group of patients have similar and limited problems, a short, selected list may be sufficient, for example for those with lesions of the hip joint. (See check list (3).)

CHECK LIST I

REPORT ON HOUSING AND DOMESTIC PROBLEMS

Patient's name: Diagnosis:
Address: Age:
                                                      Equipment:

Neighbourhood—Rural/suburban/urban
                       Distance from shops
                       Transport available

Housing—House/flat/bungalow
                     Owned/rented/tied
                     Council/private ownership
                     Pre/post-war

State of repair

Who lives in house?

Who gives care?

Access—From street to house
               To front door (if used)
               To back door (if used)

Garden—Cultivated/otherwise used (e.g. children, washing)
             Approx. size
             Necessary paths—level/steep; smooth/rough; firm/soft; wide/narrow
             Is there fuel store; garage; shed?

Circulation in house—adequate space/narrow passage; easy turn into room/
                 awkward corners

Flooring—Types: Carpet/lino/polished surfaces
             Condition
             Levels

Doors—Widths
           Thresholds

Stairs—Straight/turned. State tread. Rise
           Rails: one side/both sides
           Are they adequate?

Lighting—Dark corners
              Passages

Details of rooms:

    Kitchen—Surface heights—Table
                                 Cooker
                                 Sink

[continued

CHECK LIST 1

REPORT ON HOUSING AND DOMESTIC PROBLEMS—*continued*

Storage—Larder
         Refrigerator
         Cupboards—Doors
                Shelves

    Are facilities adequate? e.g. iron? board?

Bathroom—Up/downstairs   Height of bath

Lavatory—Up/downstairs/outside   Height of seat

Patient's bedroom—Height of bed

Potential for alteration
    House structure
    Furniture—Heavy/light
    Attitude of family—Flexible, understanding, cooperative, over-protective

Patient's activities
    Responsibilities, e.g. children, dependent relatives, business

Occupational needs

Hobby needs

Main problems   Being dealt with by:

CHECK LIST 2

ACTIVITIES OF DAILY LIVING

Bed activities
Ring bell
Roll on to right side
Roll on to left side
Roll from back to stomach and back
Sit up from lying
Sit erect in bed
Sit erect with feet over edge of bed
Use B/P or get out of bed to commode

Personal care
Blow nose
Wash face
Wash trunk and arms
Wash below the waist
Clean teeth
Brush or comb hair

Clean nails
Shave or make up
Turn on taps
Manage bottle
Manage toilet
Use paper
Flush toilet
Get in and out of bath
Cut toenails

Eating
Use fork or spoon
Use both together
Cut own food
Drink with straw
Drink from cup
Reach and pick up plate

[*continued*

CHECK LIST 2

ACTIVITIES OF DAILY LIVING—*continued*

Dressing
Fastening velcro
    zips
    buttons
    fasteners or hooks
Put on clothes over head
    trousers or slacks
    bra
    roll-on corset
    stocking or socks
    shoes
    jacket or cardigan
    tie
    orthopaedic appliances

Mobility and wheelchair activities
Propel forward
    backward
    turn
    use brake
    mount kerb
Propel chair on uneven ground
    up slope
    down slope
Cross street at traffic lights
Wheelchair to bed
Bed to wheelchair
Wheelchair to toilet
Toilet to wheelchair
Wheelchair to bath or shower
Bath or shower to wheelchair
Open and close door
Reach floor
Wheelchair to car
Car to wheelchair
Standing and walking
Bed to standing position
Standing position to bed
Wheelchair to standing
Standing to wheelchair
Chair to standing (state height of seat)
Standing to chair
Toilet to standing
Standing to toilet

Bath or shower to standing
In and out of car
Walk on uneven ground
Walk up slope
Walk down slope

General activities
Turn pages of book
Write name and address
Fold letter and seal envelope
Open envelope and remove letter
Type
Strike match and light cigarette
Switch light on and off
Use telephone
Wind watch
Handle money

Laundry
Wash small clothes in sink
Rub clothes
Wring clothes
Use washing machine
Use spin dryer
Peg clothes on to line
Carry laundry basket

Kitchen
Turn on gas/electric taps
Open oven door and move shelves
Lift cake trays in and out of oven
Lift kettle of water
Turn on tap
Fill saucepan/kettle at tap
Open tins
Cream fat and sugar
Rub in fat and flour
Roll out pastry
Cut loaf of bread
Cut meat
Spread butter
Peel vegetables
Wash up/wipe up
Open/close fridge door

ASSESSMENT FOR HIP DISABILITIES

Patient's number:

Consultant:

Name: Age: Date of admission:

Address: Diagnosis:

Lives at home-House   Domiciliary care authority:

           Flat

           Bungalow   Nursing care needed:

Housing difficulties: Home Help needed:

Family consists of:

Occupation: Outdoor transport:

A.D.L. CHECK LIST AND PROGRESS RECORD

Activity	Admission	Discharge	Remarks
Transfers			
On/off bed			
Domestic chair to standing			
Walking			
Independent			
With aid			
sticks			
crutches			
calipers			
Walking distance in yards			
Stairs			
Steps			
Self care			
Wash lower extremities			
Toilet on/off			
clean self			
Bathing in/out			
Dressing			
Stockings/socks			
Shoes			
Pants/trousers			
Caliper			
Household			
Clean floors			
Pick up from floor			
Clean grate			
Lift from oven			
Carry tray			
saucepan			
Other difficulties and summary			

Signature................................ Date...............

Tasks in context. Having found the patient's main areas of difficulty, suitable tasks in context are chosen. The process of getting up in the morning —sitting up in bed, getting out, going to the toilet, washing, dressing and grooming—repeats many of the functions observed in the preliminary assessment. But as a related sequence of events to be performed in reasonable time this requires perseverance and may uncover factors such as fatigue, pain or spasm not apparent when the activities are performed separately. As well as observing the physical function involved, step by step, points such as the following would be noted:

How much of this sequence could the patient manage safely without help? Could any accident risk be reduced by the provision of aids such as grab rails? Would adjustment in heights of his bed, chair, or toilet help him? Would simple adaptation to his clothes help him? Was any pain, fatigue or spasm noticeable, and if so, was this due to any particular task in the sequence, or was it due to the sustained effort? Could the routine be simplified to make it less tiring or to reduce the time required? What was the patient's attitude, did he give up easily or did he persevere? Was he distressed by failure, was he angered by it or did he accept his limitations?

Household tasks such as planning and cooking a family meal, or washing, hanging out clothes and doing the ironing can be used in a similar way.

It is seldom possible to simulate the patient's job realistically in an occupational therapy department, except, perhaps, for home-making. Nevertheless, it is important to examine his work situation and his functional ability to return to that work, and to assess this in general terms. To do this it is necessary to go through his general routine, checking the following:

What is his occupation? When was he last at work?

Getting up in the morning: can this be done in reasonable time, with or without help, and what are the main difficulties here?

Mobility: can he walk with or without aids or has he to use a wheel-chair —independently or with help? Can he negotiate kerbs, cross the street, etc. In leaving the house, are there steps, slopes, rough ground, and does this apply to place of work? Or has he to travel by public transport: if so, what is the distance to bus stop or trains, what about mounting or sitting in bus or train? What is the distance from transport to place of work? Or—if transport is private, what is the method? Car? Invalid tricycle? Wheel-chair into vehicle or on own. Problems of transfer, getting in and out, getting chair into vehicle, driving, etc. Are adaptations needed for this? Are there parking problems; is there sufficient space to get in and out and to off load a wheel-chair if necessary?

Access to place of work; circulation, steps, slopes; narrow doors and passages, heavy swing doors, awkward corners, circulation in working area. Atmosphere—heat, cold, damp, exposure to weather arriving leaving or at work.

Personal problems: distance and access to toilet, walking or in wheel chair; independent or needing help; difficulties with protective or special clothing, etc.

Meals: distance and access to canteen. Difficulties in eating; confidence in eating in public; facilities for eating packed meals.

The more specific details of the patient's job must then be discussed, such as standing for long periods, carrying heavy loads, the need for manual dexterity, the pressures of piecework, working in a gang or on the assembly line. It is essential to think right round the job. For example, office work does not mean simple sitting at a desk typing or writing. It involves opening filing cabinet drawers, punching and filing letters, handling small cards, telephoning and taking down messages, lifting down and handling heavy directories, running errands and even making tea. The patient may never before have had to consider and analyse his work and may find it difficult to describe or demonstrate it without the help of the occupational therapist's systematic enquiry.

Some occupational therapists may have limited opportunity to assess tasks in context as thoroughly as is recommended here. A residential centre provides environmental facilities often lacking in an out-patient setting; and also offers the advantage of close team work, for round the clock observation.

Once the need for such assessment is accepted, however, it should be possible to a considerable degree in any setting and with team work, to carry out selected sequences of tasks, such as outdoor mobility, walking stamina for specified distances, use of public or private transport, ability to deal with the architectural hazards corresponding to those at the patient's place of work, etc. Facilities for this can be found in most hospitals. Even so there will be cases who cannot be adequately assessed on an out-patient basis: the occupational therapist should therefore identify those who would benefit from residence in a centre which is specially staffed and equipped to tackle the problems of the heavily handicapped and their families.

Defined tests. These must be reproducible, defined in environment and components, and measurable in time. The procedure should be very simple, such as recording with a stopwatch the time taken by lower limb amputees to walk 50 yards on a given flat surface. Several tests may be combined to indicate degrees of competence in a given area, such as mobility.

The occupational therapist's tests should always be related to useful function, and defined tests are most frequently used to compare a patient's ability in different circumstances, for example before and after chemo-therapy, or to compare patient's performance within a diagnostic or functional group. For example, a hand function test may be designed to record patient's ability in cases of rheumatoid arthritis, before and after reconstructive surgery and at intervals during post-operative treatment. The components used such as screw-top jars must be kept specially for the testing and must be used in the same way on each occasion, so that variables in environment are kept to a minimum.

Reporting and Recording

Assessment forms, check lists and tests are of no value unless the occupational therapist draws conclusions from them and presents her findings in a clear, concise way. The information may be presented verbally, by written reports, or charted.

Much relevant information may have been gathered which will be of great use to the occupational therapist later, but initially it is her job to sift from it the points relevant to the referral and interpret them in the terms of the doctor's request.

Compiling a report. Summaries should be based on a simple format with which all other staff can easily be familiar. It is the main difficulties of the case which must now be pinpointed and these can be listed under a few broad headings and possible solutions suggested. Only the brief summary should be put into the patient's hospital notes, a copy also being kept in the occupational therapy files. The report should be signed to indicate to other staff which occupational therapist is dealing with the case. It is as well to look back to the doctor's referral to make sure that an attempt has been made to answer the problem implied. The following example illustrates the summarising of data for reporting.

OCCUPATIONAL THERAPISTS REPORT

                                        Number:
                                        Consultant:

Preliminary assessment: 25th September 1974

Name: Mr Brown.   Ward: G   Diagnosis: Rheumatoid arthritis.

Home conditions—lives in an old cottage with his wife, who works as a secretary, and 16 year old son, studying for O levels. Three steps at front door, patient can no longer manage these. Outside toilet, approach slippery and uneven. Mr Brown sleeps downstairs. Neighbours bring him his midday meal.

Mobility—patient is virtually chairbound and only stands and shuffles three or four steps to transfer from bed to wheelchair and wheelchair to toilet. Has 8G wheelchair and Invacar.

Upper limb function—generalised loss of power and loss of precision function of both hands. Loss of joint range in shoulder and elbows limits his reach to mid-range.

Personal care—can wash face and hands only—shaves himself. Bathroom upstairs, wife washes him. Cannot get off toilet. Has difficulty cleaning himself.

Dressing—dependent on his wife, who dresses him before she goes to work every morning.

Communications—has to be helped into Invacar, but goes out to friends. No other problems.

Work—was an electrician, and was still working part-time until 15 months ago.

Mental attitude —Mr Brown resents being dependent on others and is worried that his wife is the wage earner. He is friendly, easy in manner and appears eager to get some work.

Suggestions—occupational therapist to meet domiciliary O.T.* or social worker at cottage re roughened concrete path to toilet and ? sloped concrete path from gate to back door. To try out toilet heights and grab rails. To look into dressing and clothing problems. Possibility of some part-time work discussed with medico-social worker. O.T.* to test his aptitude for figures—(his writing is clear although slow) and ? adding machine and typing.

Signed..

Date..............

Presenting a report. To fulfil its purpose the report must be presented in good time to be considered in the planning of the patient's treatment. A written report may be handed to the doctor, or put into the case notes before the round or case conference. More often a verbal report is required, given formally to the consultant on the round, or informally in day-to-day contacts. Formal reporting needs practice and experience, preceded by careful thought and thorough investigation. (Written notes must be kept of this.)

Before making further interim reports, it is necessary to check with the notes taken on rounds or clinics to see that any adjustments in plans or requests have been taken into account. Progress should be defined and reported objectively. An accurate report of unsuccessful therapy is as valuable as one which records a good response to treatment.

Finally the doctor should be given relevant data before he writes his discharge letter to the general practitioner. Other people may also need information from the occupational therapist before the patient leaves, for example the medical-social worker in contact with the local education authority may need particulars of the typewriter recommended for a disabled child. A domiciliary occupational therapist who is to follow up the patient will appreciate a full report from her hospital colleague.

The disablement resettlement officer may need a detailed report to augment or take the place of the D.P.1.* The employer may need a report showing whether the patient should manage his former job or is needing alternative work.

In this chapter assessment in context has been discussed in relation to the patient. It is equally vital that occupational therapists assess and reassess their own competence in the context of the hospital or service in which they work. Medicine is an ever-changing and progressive concept and the occupational therapist can only give her contribution to this complex by a continually questioning approach to her own attitudes and techniques.

Visual representation. There are various methods of using graphs to give a visual record of progress. Ideas for adapting these can be gained from the literature on work study. In presenting a statistical analysis it is essential that the sample be large enough to be relevant and that the axes and scale of the graph are so proportioned as to present a correct picture. Visual records have the advantages that they can show fact more clearly than a written report; the doctor may find a visual record quicker to assimilate in a busy clinic; the patient may benefit by keeping his own programme charted. Charts save space in the filing system and can be usefully adapted as visual aids when lecturing. An occupational therapist may use them for example:

(1) To record increase in finger flexion, by *contour* drawings.

(2) To record the length of time each day the patient was standing continuously at a given job, by a simple graph, a *frequency polygon*.

(3) To show the daily or weekly output from an industrial outwork section, by blacked-in pillars on a graph, a *histogram*.

(4) To show comparison by '*profiles*', for example a series of assessment records considered in relation to job placement can build up a knowledge of the degree of capacity needed for a particular trade or job.

(5) To show a patient's personal attributes in relation to resettlement with a *five* or *seven point scale*. Great care must be taken to assess the 'average' realistically and not be over optimistic about the patient.

(6) To show the proportion or percentage of different disabilities among patients attending the department, with a '*pie*' *diagram*.

Factors which may Complicate Treatment

Breathlessness

There are many causes for this, amongst them intrinsic pulmonary pathology, inadequacy of respiratory musculature, cardiac disease, overweight, fatigue or emotion. A healthy individual can also become breathless, but his respiration rate returns to normal in approximately two minutes, even after strenuous exercise. The onset of breathlessness for no apparent reason, especially if accompanied by distress, is a danger sign. Medical advice is needed at once and meanwhile the patient must be kept at rest in a comfortable sitting position.

It is not unusual to find that a patient sent for treatment for other reasons becomes breathless with only moderate activity. In the majority of cases chronic bronchitis is the cause. This and its sequel, emphysema, are common in men of middle age especially those who have done heavy work, and are heavy smokers. Every bronchitic patient knows his limitations, and these are the basis for planning the effort content of his treatment. Sudden exertion in any form, hurrying, stooping and lifting should be avoided. Work involving the large muscles of the chest wall may be contra-indicated as this interferes with respiratory rhythm. Anxiety can also have this effect: the physical or psychological demands made on the patient should be within his capacity. Contrary to common belief the dirt and dust in an occupational therapy workshop is rarely an irritant to the bronchitic. He is infinitely more breathless out of doors on a windy day.

The asthmatic patient, who may also be emphysematous, is affected by windy weather too, but his breathlessness commonly springs initially from an allergy individual to him. This may or may not have been isolated, and his treatment must be given wherever there is least likelihood of precipitating an attack. Psychological factors are also important. Patients may need to be taught or reminded that the important thing is to breath out well. If the air can be expelled, fresh air will automatically take its place. Most patients with respiratory difficulty sleep better propped up; a firm back rest is more comfortable than a pile of pillows.

Fatigue

Stamina against fatigue is a personal characteristic varying markedly between individuals. When treating patients whose mental or physical conditions contra-indicate their being fatigued, close observation is needed. It is a factor which, once assessed, can be guarded against, but it will in the first instance become apparent during treatment. Such patients include the elderly, the depressed, all those who have been ill or inactive for a long time and those with systemic disease. Physical comfort is a basic essential for these patients.

For some others, fatigue may be an intentional and inescapable part of a graded reconditioning treatment plan. It should then be thought of as healthy tiredness and patients must be helped to accept it. At first it may reasonably persist into the evening but after a few days this should diminish and disinclination to do anything at the end of the day may indicate over-fatigue and the need to adjust the programme. In residential centres this can be observed. Out-patients—especially any who appear or say they are too tired—should be discreetly questioned. Signs of acute over-fatigue must always be watched for—change of colour, sweating, dizziness, shallow breathing, distress. Rest must be given immediately. Possible causes will be sought and the treatment programme altered according to the findings.

Onset may be sudden, for example in children and adolescents, the first being unaware of it and the second reluctant to admit it. It may be gradual and not realised until concentration is broken into. This is a special hazard of occupational therapy and if it occurs the symptoms must be recognised—slump posture, yawning, falling off in performance, drowsiness and irritability. These symptoms may equally indicate boredom and it is often difficult to differentiate. It is easy to bore a patient who must be guarded against fatigue. However 'light' the activity may have to be it must be appropriate to the patient's intellectual capacity, or hold his interest for some other reason. This could be its therapeutic value to himself or its end value to someone else.

Early signs of fatigue which is in itself not contra-indicated can be counteracted by short rest or exercise periods, change of company or perhaps just change of working position. Change of occupation may or may not be appropriate according to the treatment aims.

Hypertension

Patients with hypertension should avoid excessive strain, but those sent for treatment without instructions for 'sedentary work only' are unlikely to be adversely affected by the physical exertion of, for example, sawing or planing. Sudden exertion, such as hurrying for a bus or excessive stooping or lifting should be avoided. A gently graded programme, with prescribed rest periods, which builds up tolerance for activity within safety limits, is therapeutic. Complaints of increased headache or dizziness must be noted and extra rest periods allowed. These symptoms are common and can occur unrelated to the patient's physical activity. The patient's blood pressure is not necessarily known to the therapist unless it is directly associated with his condition. Some degree of hypertension is common in middle age and after, and any sign that such patients are not feeling well should be noted.

Pain

Pain inhibits physical activity and interferes with concentration. Work done with bad pain may be no criterion of true ability. Some people have to live with pain and can accept it, others cannot, although an explanation of its cause sometimes helps. For example, a patient with thalamic pain following a cardiovascular accident may need repeated explanation and reassurance.

While local pain after an injury is expected, it is less easily accepted when it occurs during treatment. Stretching of tight structures round a joint, or breaking down adhesions, will be painful at the time but will lead to greater mobility and less pain. Patients with a low pain threshold must be encouraged to persevere in spite of discomfort. Pain is noticeable in facial expression. Unobserved observation is important: there are some whose forbearance is unusually low and who therefore manifest their discomfort, but there are others who show no evidence of it unless asked. Most important are those who will not admit to pain but may show it in unguarded moments. If pain persists after treatment or if there is sudden acute pain during treatment the doctor should be consulted. Patients with irreversible pain, as following a brachial plexus lesion, may be referred specifically for diversional therapy, which can be most valuable. Pain lowers resistance to fatigue, both physical and mental, and this should be realised when helping the patients to choose an activity. It is important to find something that will hold his interest, and yet can be done for short periods. Individual treatment at agreed regular times, preferably shortly after medication, is indicated.

Phantom pains must be expected after amputation, their duration being proportionate to that of pain prior to operation. Patients can be assured that this will decrease progressively once a prosthesis is used.

Oedema and Effusion

Oedema is an abnormal accumulation of serous fluid in the body tissues. In its acute form it is a common local symptom after injury, both at the site and distal to it. Immobilising the part in plaster makes its dispersal more difficult but there is usually improvement if the limb is kept elevated. It is unusual for occupational therapy to be given while there is gross oedema, but patients may still have some degree of local swelling when treatment starts. If so, the limb should be kept elevated when not in use. For an oedematous hand a sling is worn to support both forearm and hand, the hand resting higher than the elbow. For the lower limb a chair seat with a cushion will keep the leg horizontal.

Treatment for a patient with an oedematous hand must first improve the circulation. Use of gravity to assist venous return will be further helped by muscle activity and the larger the muscle groups involved the greater the effect. Grip and release action of the hand can be combined with elbow and shoulder movements as in wall draughts. Alternatively, by placing the components suitably, continuous change of position and variety of movements can be involved in doing simple assembly work. Movements which include the inner range of elbow flexion are best. Pressure on the walls of the vessels crossing the joint and in the substance of the muscles of the forearm and upper arm will further stimulate the venous return. When continuous elevation is needed during treatment support must be given. Without this the shoulder and shoulder girdle muscles must maintain the position, working statically. This is contra-indicated for the circulation will be impaired. Either the elbow can rest on the work table or bench while the hands are working on a higher level or a Guthrie Smith type of sling can be used. The patient must be taught to exercise his limb between treatments. The initial instruction is given by the physiotherapist but the importance of exercising regularly and purposefully should be stressed in both departments.

It is more difficult to treat the lower limb in elevation. When oedema is present, for example, after a Pott's fracture, the patient should elevate his foot during rest periods in his treatment session. Between treatments full range movements should be carried out at regular intervals with the leg in elevation: toe movements fully down and fully up; maximal foot and ankle movements by describing the biggest possible imaginary circle with the big toe; and static quadriceps contractions.

The oedema can persist especially in the lower leg, gradually consolidating to produce a permanent thickening of the part. This can restrict movement and is often a distressing symptom especially to women patients. Other forms of chronic oedema also occur in the lower leg. Following widespread spastic or flaccid paralysis, or joint destruction, there will be insufficient muscle and joint activity to counteract the effects of gravity on the venous circulation, as in advanced disseminated sclerosis or rheumatoid arthritis. It is common, too, in cardiac and renal illness. Severe chronic oedema is characterised by 'pitting'. It is an intractable condition. Blocks to raise the foot of the bed may effect temporary improvement by promoting postural drainage. Should such a patient come to the department, prolonged standing is contra-indicated. Some walking followed by elevation is allowable. Healing properties are diminished when circulation is bad so knocks should be avoided. Such patients should have routine chiropody.

Effusion is excess of synovial fluid within the joint. The swelling is fluctuent and there is no pitting. Pressure may push the fluid from one place to another within the capsule of the joint but unlike oedema it returns immediately pressure is removed. Heat, pain and muscle inhibition are the symptoms. Two common causes of effusion are rheumatoid arthritis and trauma, as in internal derangement of the knee. Postural draining can do nothing to disperse the fluid because it is contained, but elevation, especially of the leg, may give comfort. Treatment is rest, sometimes with temporary splinting or with supportive or compression bandaging. If treatment is prescribed while the symptom persists this aims to improve circulation through the part and to build up the adjacent muscles by static contraction and relaxation.

Defective Cutaneous Sensation

This is one aspect of perceptual dysfunction indicated by anaesthesia, as in paraplegia or leprosy, and by hypersensitivity, as in a median nerve lesion. Dressing and other personal care activities, especially those requiring precision outside the range of vision, may be made impossible by defects affecting the hands and although treatment referrals may not indicate the need, help should be offered. A patient with sensory loss in his hands or in weight bearing areas is at risk wherever he is. Help may be needed in minimising potential hazards in the patient's home and there must be strict observance of precautions during treatment. Patients must be trained to use their eyes and their commonsense in compensation for loss of sensation.

The main dangers come from excessive heat, from friction and from accidental knocks. Many of the risks from excessive heat are obvious: holding a cigarette until it burns down to the fingers, holding a hot mug between the palms of the hands or sleeping in contact with a hot-water bottle. Other less obvious ones are picking up metal from a bench where brazing or soldering is done, picking up a plate from the rack over a hot cooker, or, when straining vegetables touching the pan lid while holding its handle. Protective gloves are not always the answer. Although the fingers and thumb are more likely to get burnt than other parts, if they are covered the hand will be clumsy. A 'mitt' made of leather or crepe bandage either covering only the palm and ball of the thumb or coming halfway up the fingers, gives partial protection. Plastic tumbler holders, insulated mugs and a variety of kitchen tongs are available commercially.

Friction can be caused by contact with a rough surface or equally by repeated rubbing against a smooth one. Any tool handle, however smooth, will quickly raise a blister if it is not held securely and most patients with sensory defects also have some degree of muscle weakness. A skin graft may be puffy and soft, further predisposing it to damage. Certain areas of the hand are more prone to injury in this way than others and the patient must be taught to look regularly for any signs of pressure or friction, particularly in the web between the thumb and index finger and along the palmar aspect of the metacarpo-phalangeal joints. String should never be wrapped round the fingers to get a better grip. This can cut into the little finger at the joint line and not be noticed. Similarly a splinter may not be noticed and if it festers healing will be slow.

Wheelchair driving wheels can cause damage, especially to patients who must compensate for poor grip by using the 'heel' of the hand. Although the skin thickens and becomes harder with continual use the hand can be bruised. Damage can also be caused by friction as the wheel runs through the hand. Leather mitts help to prevent this and car steering wheel gloves fitted on the wheels of the chair give extra protection.

For paraplegics special care is needed during treatment on a bicycle. Rubber padding on the pedal crank and foot straps on the pedals will prevent damage to the internal malleoli. Similarly, padding is essential on the saddle. In spite of this the patient can become saddle sore although unaware of it and the risk is greater when there is adductor spasm. Treatment should be for short periods only.

By its very nature an occupational therapy department is not a place in which a patient can be safeguarded against knocking himself or occasionally being knocked, but there are hazards in every home and the patient must be trained to take responsibility for himself.

A patient with local hypersensitivity needs protection against pain caused by movement or physical contact, a common symptom where there is scarring, otherwise he cannot be expected to use his hand normally during treatment or at home. Sponge rubber padding can be put onto tools or he can be given the soft pliable mitt already described. When a finger tip is affected Tubigrip is satisfactory. The overall treatment plan must be built up gradually as tolerance and function improve, working with soft light materials at first and progressing, if appropriate, to tougher and heavier ones.

Muscle Spasm

Cramp. Special circumstances can produce temporary muscle spasm in a healthy individual, for example an athlete or a swimmer whose activities make exceptional demands on the circulatory system. Cramp with acute pain in the calf muscles after walking only 100 yards is abnormal and constitutes a severe handicap. This intermittent claudication, according to the demands of work or the travel involved, may constitute a resettlement problem.

Clonus. This is an involuntary reaction to overstretching a muscle or to stretching it too suddenly. It occurs in patients with hypertonic muscles and precautionary measures should be observed during their treatment. Clonus will occur in the calf muscles if the foot is inadequately supported, for example when the heel drops down from the back of the footrest of a wheelchair. A calf strap will help to prevent this. It can also occur when the patient is treated on the bicycle. The cause may be lack of support for the foot, particularly the heel, or excessive dorsi-flexion while working the machine. A foot piece should be fixed to the pedal so that the fulcrum of the patient's ankle will not be behind that of the pedal. The foot must be securely held in the right position. Two factors dictate the range of dorsi-flexion; first the relationship between the pedals and the saddle. The hub of the pedals must be further forward than vertically below the saddle and the saddle should be high rather than low. Secondly the range of dorsi-flexion is related to that of knee flexion; the longer the pedal cranks the larger the range of movement. The cranks therefore should not be too long.

Protective spasm. Acute spasm as a reaction to pain is not uncommon, as for instance with back injury. The contracted muscles, by acting as a splint, prevent movement at the site of injury. The spasm in itself is painful and a vicious circle is set up. If this happens in the department the patient should be allowed to adopt any position which may give relief and a doctor should be informed.

Spasticity resulting from lesion of the upper motor neurone cannot be cured. In certain conditions medication can provide prolonged relief. Short-term relief by physical methods is also of value. By overcoming spasticity of the knee flexors a chairbound patient, who might otherwise develop contractures which would prevent him from straightening his knee, will be able to do so. It is important for such patients to be able to get onto their feet for transfer independence. Physiotherapists use a variety of techniques to overcome spasticity, among them manual stretching and positioning. Prolonged passive stretching can also help, for example night splinting to overcome spasticity and prevent contractures in the hand of a hemiplegic patient. Occupational therapists, too, should know the techniques of manual stretching. The hands are used with relaxation, placed immediately above and well below the joint affected by the spasticity. So as to gain maximum mechanical advantage while applying counter pressure, body weight can be used. To break spasm in the hamstrings of a patient in a wheelchair the therapist stands facing and level with the patient's knee, with a wide base, hips and knees bent, and back flat. Manual pressure is exerted *downwards* above the patella to stabilise the thigh and simultaneously *upwards* from behind the patient's ankle to extend the lower leg. The position of the lower hand is maintained by static contraction of the wrist flexors. As the spasm yields the body weight is transferred from one foot to the other until the knee is maximally extended. It may be necessary to break spasm in quadriceps before a patient can be moved into a comfortable working position or even before he can be wheeled through a doorway into a passage. A comparable technique is used. One hand hooked under the inside of the knee pulls up to flex and maintain flexion of the hip. The other hand exerts downward pressure from above the ankle, assisted by body weight.

To break spasm in a patient's right hand the therapist hooks the fingers of her right hand under the tips of the patient's fingers. Allowing his wrist to flex, she straightens first the distal and then the proximal interphalangeal joints by exerting counter pressure across the back of his fingers with the ball of her thumb. Then with her other hand she grasps round the patient's thumb while pressing on the back of his forearm with the front of her forearm. Using both hands and maintaining extension of the interphalangeal joints she abducts his thumb and extends the metacarpo-phalangeal joints of his fingers. Finally with counter pressure on the back of his forearm and upward pull on his extended hand, she extends his wrist. This stretching may be necessary as a preliminary to placing the patient's hand round a tool or onto a hand 'block' in order to exercise his elbow and shoulder.

Many patients know the circumstances most likely to induce their spasm and with this information the therapist can hope to prevent its incidence. The precipitating cause may be loud noise, being touched unexpectedly from behind, inexpert handling when changing positions, sudden or jerky movements, for example coughing, or strong emotion. The severity of the attack also varies from patient to patient, in one individual merely causing a temporary interruption of treatment, in another causing loss of balance while sitting or standing. Precautions may be needed to prevent accidents which might occur in the home or elsewhere. In particular the housewife must be encouraged to find methods of working which will minimise potential risks in her kitchen.

Loss of movement and the deformity which can result from muscle spasm create problems in self care activities. Management of clothing below the waist is especially difficult. If hand function is also impaired methods must be worked out by which someone else can give the required help most easily. Clearly this someone should if possible be party to the planning and must always be offered practical instruction. Spasm is not always to the patient's disadvantage however. In spastic paraplegia it is the presence of spasm in the antigravity muscles of the lower limbs which enables him to stand and walk.

Defective Vision

The occupational therapist may be the first person to notice defective vision as it can show in poor standards of work and inaccuracy in performing tests. Her first responsibility is to take any necessary precautions to avoid accidents with tools, machines, etc., and secondly to report the defect to the doctor if there is no reference to it in the medical notes. Defective vision which cannot be corrected by glasses, for example, cataract, can be a problem in resettlement, since most types of light work require some degree of accuracy. Severe impairment of sight makes rapport difficult. Watching facial expressions is an important factor in communication. This may be a particular problem with head injury patients.

A further problem arises when defective vision occurs with a physical disability affecting balance and locomotion. When walking, the proximity of people and objects such as table legs is not apparent. This is a real hazard. Special supervision is needed for those unable to appreciate the risks who move heedlessly. The frail, elderly, short-sighted patient is more likely to trip and fall. The hemiplegic with sensory loss on the paralysed side must learn to use sight in compensation. When there is the additional complication of *hemianopia* he must be trained to turn his head to the affected side to offset the 50 per cent restriction of his visual field. *Diplopic* patients will need opportunity to adjust to this. An eye patch may be of help. But monocular vision also presents problems, for example working on a lathe, playing ball games.

Newly *blind* patients are rarely referred for occupational therapy. Special facilities are available through the Royal National Institute for the Blind* for those who would benefit from an intensive course of rehabilitation. Treatment may be prescribed when blindness occurs together with locomotor dysfunction. It is unlikely that the patient will know his prognosis and nothing must be said or done to indicate this. Practical help should be offered to overcome some of the problems which the patient meets even before his discharge and 'while he is not able to see'.

This is achieved by teaching him to judge distance by recognising the effect of sound on different environments such as corridors and rooms, by listening for the approach of voices and footsteps, encouraging him to participate in everyday activities and fostering a sense of achievement by making something (basketry is contra-indicated because of its association with the blind disabled), giving him practice in recognising coins and supplying any necessary aids, such as a writing board, which are available from the R.N.I.B.* [2]

In a strange environment even the patient accustomed to his blindness will need special consideration. The other patients are liable to be over helpful. A blind person will instinctively take the arm of his helper when walking, and this is right. The instinct of the helper to take the patient's arm is wrong, for in this relationship the patient will be leading.

Precipitancy

The therapist should know which patients are troubled by precipitancy so that she can anticipate their needs. This is a usual problem for old people and those with kidney disease, bladder dysfunction or spasticity. Getting up from or being lifted from a chair can cause it and this is a problem when an active programme is planned. Anxiety which can aggravate the condition, is understandably common. Accidents may happen due to strange surroundings or any emotional factors. Where there is improvement in the patient's general medical condition the problem may be resolved.

The aphasic patient, particularly if he is not independent in walking, has special reason for anxiety and this will seriously interfere with concentration. The therapist must agree a sign with him which will substitute for speech and he must be assured that he will be given the help he needs.

Patients with precipitancy are worried and distracted by it. Every new patient should be shown 'where to go' and some may need to be shown more than once. Staff of other departments are likely to be involved and a routine must be agreed between them, for example the patient to go at regular hourly or two-hourly intervals even if he feels no need, but not more often. Valuable staff time is saved if the patient can be independent in walking or propelling a chair and managing clothes. If he can be trained to take responsibility for carrying out the routine at the hospital he is more likely to continue it at home. The importance of doing this must be stressed both to him and to his family.

Incontinence [3]

Patients whose incontinence is the immediate result of spinal injury or colostomy are taught at an early stage to deal with its associated problems. An appliance is necessary. In the case of a patient with impairment of hand function a member of the family may need to give assistance. Later the patient may be helped to become independent and this is an important part of A.D.L.* training. Nursing staff are always ready to demonstrate the basic practical techniques that the patient would normally carry out himself and the occupational therapist may be able to adapt the method so that he can manage despite his manual handicap. Some patients are wrongly labelled as incontinent by hospital staff. It may be difficult to discriminate between genuine calls for help from those who are unable to reach the W.C.* in time, or to control a bottle, or to handle their clothing adequately, and the false alarm cries of confused and perseverating patients. Patients with progressive neurological disease present a different problem, being reluctant to admit to incontinence and to accept the help they really need.

The Disabled Living Foundation* has made an extensive study of the problems of incontinence and of the practical ways in which those who are incontinent can be helped. Therapists should refer to their publications before trying to think out solutions themselves. There is a considerable choice of specially designed clothing available commercially, and there should seldom be the need to devise adaptations. Alterations to garments already in use can be tried out, to test different styles, before buying new ones.

Damp clothing increases the risk of damage by pressure or friction especially if sensation is defective. Patients should, if possible, be taught to turn onto their sides in bed [4] and, in order to relieve pressure when sitting, to push up on their hands. Commodes are usually obtainable from Social Services Departments, the British Red Cross Society or St John's Ambulance Brigade. Wheelchairs of most types are available with commode seats through Artificial Limb and Appliance Centres.

Treatment on a bicycle may be indicated for a patient whose incontinence is only one symptom of a syndrome, but risk of friction on the saddle may be a stronger contra-indication, as will be the wearing of an appliance.

General Problems

While some people like the feeling of movement and get positive pleasure from it, others get none at all and dislike physical activity. Physique may be one factor contributing to this. Awkward proportions, clumsiness, lack of rhythm or obesity may create difficulties of themselves and self-consciousness greatly adds to these. The therapist must be considerate of genuine distaste for certain forms of treatment which might show up ineptitude and indeed she may have experienced such feelings herself and understand them well. By making a good relationship with the patient, and with expert teaching, slowly and with much encouragement, lack of confidence can often be overcome. Once there are signs of success, these together with interest in what is being done or made will provide further incentive.

Another problem is unsuitable clothing. In some centres regulation garments are provided and there is much to commend them. They are comfortable and movements are unrestricted. Certainly a tight skirt for

bicycle or lathe work is unsuitable, for it restricts the hip and knee movements of both legs. For men on treatment for improvement of leg function
shorts are preferable to trousers but 'uniform' is unpopular with many
people. The occupational therapist must set a good example by wearing the
right type of shoes and she can then both explain and demonstrate the
importance of a broad heel, good support round the instep and adequate
breadth across the toes. Ill-fitting shoes are detrimental to footwork during
treatment and in walking.

Illiteracy

Patients who are illiterate or semi-literate may pass through occupational
therapy departments more frequently than realised. Unless something
disturbs the pattern of life at home or at work they may be content and the
status quo should not be disturbed.

Difficulties arise when a change of work is medically indicated. Most of
the men who are illiterate are labourers, doing highly paid heavy work. They
have no skills to offer an employer and even if offered lighter work they
might be unable to accept because of poor pay. Often this would fall below
the weekly income considered minimally adequate for their family needs
while living on contributory and/or Supplementary Benefits. Acceptance at
an I.R.U.* or Skill Training Centre is unlikely and so is Government
Training (see chapter 4). Reports from the department on personality,
willingness, reliability and standard of work at simple tasks may help the
disablement resettlement officer in his efforts at placement. Occasionally a
patient expresses regrets at his lack of learning and admits to a feeling of
inadequacy. Perhaps at home he has been unable to give his children help
with their homework. Anyone who shows himself willing to work and wants
to learn to read should be given individual tuition for a trial period. The
occupational therapist will see how the patient reacts to a learning situation
and he himself will gain some idea of what will be involved. It is important
not to raise his hopes too high, however promising the initial progress may
be. If the trial period is successful, plans should be made for tuition to be
continued outside the hospital and after working hours. It is often best for
the medical-social worker to make these for in most cases there will be
related family matters to discuss and such tuition will do nothing to change
the current resettlement problem.

Psychological and Psychiatric Problems [5]

A patient who is referred for physical treatment may also be mentally ill.
The occupational therapist should concentrate on the physical aspects of
treatment and refrain from uncovering the psychological problems, but

should use her experience of these to guide her in her approach and in a supportive way. If they are proving an insuperable barrier to successful treatment the referring doctor should be consulted. The patient's general practitioner may be aware of the situation so there can be joint consultation.

Euphoria. This condition, in which awareness of reality is blunted, may create problems for the therapist but it is often a merciful dispensation to the patient, occurring as it does in circumstances which would seem more likely to cause depression. For example, some patients with head injury are euphoric, and those with advanced disseminated sclerosis frequently are. Acceptance of the situation as it is, provides no stimulus towards improving it and application to treatment is often inadequate to effect worthwhile change. If so it should be stopped. On the other hand it has been known for a severely disabled patient to be helped by his euphoria to get back to work. Difficult to assess, unrealistic in general outlook, he went out full of optimism and confidence and got himself a job.

Anxiety. Anxiety is the normal reaction to stress in some people and therefore not uncommon with illness or injury, especially if the patient does not understand his condition. It is not a symptom which the patient will talk about but it often prevents him from giving his best effort to his treatment. Sometimes he may have been given no explanation by his doctor; often his anxiety has come between him and his ability to understand or accept what he has been told. In either case the therapist can help. A straightforward explanation—even including a little anatomy or physiology—may be enough although repetition and reassurance is often needed. Any improvement should be pointed out. It is essential for the same explanation to be given by whosoever may be asked and it is helpful to be present when the doctor is giving his.

An anxious patient may also be distracted from treatment and made more anxious by watching others with obvious disability. His placement in the department in relation to others must therefore be planned carefully.

Hysteria and functional overlay. While a patient with hysterical illness may be referred for physical treatment, these labels are also ascribed to the manifestation of symptoms in physical conditions which appear out of proportion to their cause, or to the continuation of symptoms after treatment which normally relieves them. Patients with such hysterical features are frequently lacking in self esteem. Minor trauma may provide an excuse for not returning to an over demanding job or may serve as an excuse for gaining attention from an inattentive family, for example, a menopausal woman whose children are now grown up. This seems to occur particularly with back injuries where it is difficult for the doctor to assess the precise degree of physical trauma. But there is a danger here in assuming too easily that this is the case when there may be in reality an undiagnosed physical cause. The occupational therapist can often help the doctor to differentiate here. Achievement, especially that acknowledged by others, helps to re-establish self esteem. This can be used as part of a programme of treatment which will indirectly demand of the patient the actions that he finds difficult. When the hysteria is manifest in, for example, a stiff hand or knee, physical treatment is particularly vital since a functional stiffness can all too soon become a permanent one.

Hopes of final compensation following an accident may be a cause of hysteria. Although intended to be fair to the claimant, the present legal procedure for settlement of claims is, in practice, often against his best interests and delays his rehabilitation. It is important to assure the patient that his symptoms are recognised as real to him but important, too, to encourage him to be active in spite of them, hoping that his pain tolerance and his confidence may be built up gradually. This is 'easier said than done', especially if return to work will expose him to risk of further trauma, and settlement of the claim is often the only solution.

Reactive depression. Reactive depression is common in patients with physical illness; for example the hemiplegic who is suddenly incapacitated, or the rheumatoid arthritic with continuing pain. Injury, and again that in which pain is a significant symptom, also causes it, for example a brachial plexus lesion. A relatively minor illness or injury is often enough to depress an individual who was only just managing his life previously and therefore has cause to fear for his future. It is as important to deal with the depression as with the physical condition.

Epilepsy. Many epileptics live normal lives, stabilised on drugs, and with no disability. Such individuals, coming to hospital and being sent for treatment for some other reason will present no problem. There are patients however who are liable to have fits—those who have not been stabilised, and those who forget to take their drugs or perhaps forget to bring them when they come for out-patient treatment. It is wise to have a reserve supply in the department for this type of patient.

Patients who have suffered head injury or have had brain surgery may develop epilepsy at a later date and could have a fit during treatment, possibly a first one. In addition to taking the necessary steps for the patient's safety and comfort it is important to observe and later to record in detail the features of the fit—what the patient was doing; whether he fell and if so how and to which side; whether he lost consciousness, if so for how long, and did he complain of headache or other symptoms after regaining it; were there convulsions, if so in which limbs and how severe? A doctor should be asked to come but the same therapist should stay with the patient throughout. He may be frightened and temporarily unable to recognise his surroundings after the attack, and in need of reassurance.

Most epileptics know the warning signs of their fits and take appropriate action in time. Other patients should always be encouraged to continue with their work and the patient himself can usually resume his too, after a short rest. If a patient has repeated attacks occupational therapy is contra-indicated, in consideration for other patients and in view of possible risks in a crowded department. For a patient who may have a fit, correct placement in the department is important, away from machines, and away from anything on which he could hurt himself, or from anybody who could be hurt by him. It is known that the epileptic who is bored is more prone to having a fit than if fully occupied and interested in what he is doing.

Mental subnormality. Many of those who are mentally subnormal but able to live at home, live less physically active lives and are less venturesome than their more independent contemporaries. It follows that they are also less likely to have the sort of accident which is associated with activity. For other reasons however they may be referred for treatment as are other patients. Extra supervision may be needed to stimulate effort and to encourage perseverance. Distractibility is a common problem as, at times, is curiosity. This may lead to the patient wandering to watch others at their work or to join a group of visitors.

Data of the mental condition may be lacking both in the referral and in the medical notes. Until this is available from the appropriate authority, extra precautions must be taken relating to machines and tools. Direct contact with the patient's family is always helpful and is sometimes essential. Behaviour problems, such as occasional outbursts of temper, may arise, but many of these patients will be easy-going and of happy disposition. Messages to the family should be given direct, even if the patient is also asked to deliver them.

Accidents in an Occupational Therapy Department [6]

If a patient falls he should not immediately be helped to his feet or into a chair. He should be given time to recover his composure and to speak before being moved or helped to move. If a fracture is suspected, or if the patient is confused or acutely breathless he should not be moved and a doctor should be called.

An accident form must be filled in after any accident and if possible an adult person who falls should be seen by a doctor the same day. An increase in symptoms or a new symptom, for example a swollen knee, may be attributed to the accident at a subsequent clinic. Accurate information is expected and this presupposes accurate observation.

PROBLEMS OF COMMUNICATION

The following deals with problems other than those arising from confusion, amentia or mental illness. There may be mechanical defect, for example, deafness or inability to control a pen. There may be dysfunction of the speech centre in the brain resulting in faulty interpretation or inability to 'find' the words for speech. For normal communication it is necessary to have both receptive and expressive powers.

Defective Hearing

This is the most common cause of poor reception. A hearing aid helps some forms of deafness and some people, but certainly not all. Many old people simply 'can't be bothered' with it. Others find the noise physically intolerable, and many find the mental effort of listening too tiring. The therapist must respect these attitudes. She must also be able to help the patient who uses an aid to get the most out of it. She must understand and be able to repeat the instructions given initially by the technician and she should also check periodically that the patient is using the aid correctly. Misuse is the commonest cause of poor performance.

There are also rules for the speaker, especially relating to the very deaf listener:

(1) She must be seen before speaking, say something, e.g. the patient's name, and then allow time for him to 'switch on' mentally and perhaps also to switch on the aid before continuing to speak.

(2) Watch the patient's expression. It will usually show whether or not he is understanding.

(3) Notice if he is fingering the aid while you talk. This will prevent it from functioning well or indicates that it is not functioning.

(4) Speak towards, but not too close to, the receiver and at a speed suited to the individual's powers of reception and interpretation, remembering that one word missed can destroy the sense. As a rule a voice pitched in middle range is the best. Gesticulation distracts from listening and turning of the head adversely affects the volume of sound to the receiver. It also interferes with lip reading.

(5) Avoid saying too much at a time, a part of it may have been missed.

The main value of an aid is for person to person conversation. Background noise interferes with this and often the volume of sound in a group makes interpretation impossible. A deaf patient should therefore be placed where he can see what is going on round him. Otherwise, with his aid switched off, he will frequently interrupt his work by turning round to avoid missing something or will be isolated, both detrimental to treatment. In practical aspects of treatment, demonstration is the best form of teaching.

Receptive Aphasia

This is the result of brain damage, as in a patient who has had a stroke. There is lack of understanding of the spoken or written word and responses to speech may be bizarre. This in itself does not prove lack of intelligence. Commonly the patient will also have speech loss. Interchange of ideas is impossible and for practical things, demonstration is the only means of communication. The patient is frustrated and may become anxious and depressed.

Language Difficulty

Language difficulties create the dual problem of understanding and expression. It is not confined to foreigners but is equally a problem for 'English-speaking' immigrants who have different intonation, pronounciation and colloquialisms. The therapist who has difficulty in understanding her patient is probably herself not understood.

Dysarthria

Dysarthria is a problem of expression. There is difficulty in articulation due to a motor defect in the muscles of lips, tongue, palate or throat. Some hemiplegic patients are dysarthric. It is also a problem in neurological conditions such as motor neurone disease. When there is simultaneous impairment of hand function and writing is impossible it is difficult to find a substitute means of communicating. A spelling board may be the answer.

Expressive Aphasia

This is the result of brain damage as in a patient who has had a stroke. There is inability to find words or to formulate sentences either for speech or for writing. Reading aloud is also difficult. The patient may have receptive loss. He is usually aware of the defect but if not speech may be voluble although incomprehensible. There is no substitute means of expressing thought for the patient with aphasia. The dysphasic patient has a lesser degree of the same disability. Speech is hesitant and the vocabulary restricted.

Inevitably the occupational therapist becomes involved in the speech problems of her patients, for speech is an integral part of the everyday activities which are treatment media in her department. Diagnosis and specialist treatment are in the province of the speech therapist but in many treatment centres speech therapy may be available infrequently or not at all. There should be consultation to decide how best the treatment given by the speech therapist can be supplemented during occupational therapy. In addition to encouraging spontaneous speech, short periods devoted to articulation, improvement of vocabulary, formation of sentences and writing are valuable. Patients with a speech defect must on no account be treated as unintelligent.

In some department the new Bell and Howell language master* [7] has been tried out in consultation with a speech therapist. This has a headphone device and when used in conjunction with a text, it provides two sensory input channels. The text, on cards, may be represented in pictures, words, or both together. The patient can run the card through the machine as many times as he wishes. He can then repeat the word or sentence 'spoken' by the machine, or write it down as required. At a certain stage of recovery of speech an aphasic patient can benefit from this training method but it must also be the right patient. For anyone with anxiety it is contra-indicated.

Inability to Write

Some patients who are unable to write are illiterate. Others have a manipulative problem and must learn to use the non-dominant hand or to overcome dysfunction in the dominant one. Those with expressive aphasia often have lost the use of the dominant hand and are at a loss for words too. Subjectively the severity of the 'handicap' depends on the patient's former writing habits. An unskilled worker may want only to sign his name, a student must be able to write.

Some solutions to the problem:

Educating the non-dominant hand. The first step is to get used to the feeling of the pen as a tool—picking it up, adjusting its position until it is comfortable in the hand, settling into an easy position for writing, with the forearm fully supported and the weight of the hand taken on the ulnar border and little finger. If possible the other arm should be supported on the table from the elbow too. This gives general balance to the position. Next there should be practice in shading-in shapes with lines at different angles, preferably, too, in different colours. Naughts and crosses are also good, putting the pen down after each turn. Until familiarity with the tool is established it is a waste of time to attempt writing as such. In the case of an aphasic patient the decision as to the right time to begin making words is unquestionably the speech therapist's. Close liaison is obviously essential.

Compensating for dysfunction in the dominant hand. First the deficit must be identified from the following: grip on the pen, pressure on the paper, control in forming the letters, movement of the hand across the paper. The cause may be motor or sensory or both. If function cannot be improved by treatment, alternative methods, possibly with aids, must be sought. A thick pen is the easiest to grip, a felt-tipped pen needs least pressure. A rubber band round the pen may prevent the fingers from slipping, and applied jointly round the pen and the fingers it adds pressure and stability to the grip. A splint may bring the fingers and thumb into an improved position for holding the pen or an individually designed aid may substitute for grip. Whatever change from former habit may be necessary, it is only by arduous practice that competence and familiarity will be achieved. Patients need help to persevere. When able to practice reliably without supervision they should do so at home where more time may be available.

Alternatives to writing. Typing is sometimes a possibility. Learning is time consuming and the final speed achieved may be only a fraction of the normal. Many disabled people have, however, time to spare so this is no problem. Electric typewriters are helpful for those with uneven pressure; they are less good than standard machines in cases of ataxia. For anyone too ataxic to write or type a spelling board with the letters widely spaced will help.

The medium of tape-recording can be used with great satisfaction by some patients too disabled to write or type for answering letters, for study or for original work. Electronically operated equipment is also being developed [8]. This covers a wide range of activities until now beyond the achievement of the most severely handicapped and the field of communications is one of them.

REFERENCES AND RECOMMENDED FURTHER READING

1. **Assessment of the Patient: Reporting and Recording**
   Cooper, B. M., *Writing Technical Reports*. Pelican, 1964.
   Reichman, W. J., *Uses and Abuses of Statistics*. Pelican, 1961.
   Shearring & Christian, *Reports and How to Write Them*. London, 1965.
2. *R.N.I.B. = The Royal National Institute for the Blind*. London*.
3. *Incontinence: Some Problems, Suggestions and Conclusions*. Disabled Living Foundation*, 1970.
   Management of Incontinence in the Home: A Survey. Disabled Living Foundation*.
   A Guide to Disposable Incontinence Pads and Draw Sheets. Disabled Living Foundation*.
   And see: The challenge of incontinence. *Occ. Ther.*, 37, no. 6, 1974.
4. Wareham, T., *Return to Independence*, London, 1965.
5. See this book, chapters 12 and 16.
6. See this book, chapter 23.
7. See this book, chapter 7 (p. 112) and references under Collins, D. W. & Maling, R. C.
8. See P.I.L.O.T.*, P.O.S.S.U.M.* and Zambette*.
* See *Glossary*, pp. 454-6.

CHAPTER 7

Introduction to Physical Occupational Therapy: Part 2

Activities of Daily Living [1]

Activities of daily living include the personal care activities, to which most patients attach great importance, and general activities. The personal ones include getting in and out of bed, bathroom activities, dressing and feeding. The general ones include opening doors, turning on switches, handling money, telephoning, writing, picking up and carrying. When relevant, the minimal basic kitchen activities are also included. In practice there can be no firm dividing line, for the environment in which a patient carries out his personal activities will involve him with the general ones. For example, the patient may need to put his shoes on, perhaps a leg iron too, before he can walk, and this will be especially difficult during the night unless there is a light switch within reach of the bed.

Functional assessment, i.e. assessment of the patient's ability in these spheres, may be the only form of treatment requested for a patient when he is first allowed out of the ward. In some cases it is satisfactorily completed in one or two days, and no other physical treatment is indicated. Equally, it may be the beginning of a comprehensive progressive treatment plan which will continue when he becomes an out-patient. Short-term or long-term assessment is a form of treatment, not something distinct from it, and it should be recognised and referred to as such.

The therapist must be able to assess the individual patient's total needs, physical and psychological, but in planning a programme to meet these she must take account of his physical and mental capacity to make efforts and to withstand fatigue. In no treatment is this perhaps so crucial as for the patient who has had an acute illness—for example, a stroke. He may present differently day by day, so his programme must be flexible and this automatically affects timetabling in general. The therapist must be adaptable and she must be able to keep relationships good with the many people who will be directly or indirectly affected by changes she may have to make, for example, ward staff, porters, other therapists, and other patients.

She must also be able to identify the causes underlying poor performance, and to initiate measures which will improve the chances of success. There may be need for clarification with the doctor on any of the following: medication to relieve depression or to control spasm; referral to the medical social worker, to the speech therapist for assessment, referral to the physiotherapist for improvement of balance, or to the occupational therapy department to improve motivation. A visit to see the home and to meet the family may be necessary at this early stage. The patient may not yet be well enough physically for the effort that will be involved nor may he be able to see the point of trying until he has recovered further from his disability. Furthermore he may take it for granted that there will always be someone else to do it for him. Sometimes he feels it will be impossible even if he does try. For such a patient it is important that something, however small, such as lighting his own cigarette should be achieved on the first attendance, or, if not achieved, that it should be seen to be a possibility. In contrast to the above types of patients, there are others who are determined to keep their independence, and set themselves seemingly impossible targets and reach them. Both types are met with amongst those who have become disabled recently and amongst those with years of experience of disability, some of whom may not have been assessed comprehensively before. The disability in itself is not the deciding factor. Rather it is the handicap imposed by it which will influence results and this is dependent on the attitude of mind of the patient. It is unrealistic to expect that a husband who was largely dependent on his wife before his stroke will be enthusiastic about independence after it. While the advantages of doing things for himself would seem obvious to the therapist, the outlook of and decisions reached by the family must be respected.

Because attitude of mind and performance vary so much, it is not possible to generalise and to say 'this is the answer for the arthritic patient: this for the hemiplegic'. Although the therapist will think along similar lines for patients with similar diagnoses until she gets to know them as individuals, the treatment plan should be an individual one. Its content must be appropriate for the physical environment of the home and for the way in which the home is run. For example, a woman with severe arthritis and living alone may be able to move about once she is up, and with home help, to provide herself with meals. She may, however, be unable to get out of bed, to wash or dress herself, to undress or get into bed. A district nurse could help with both, but she would be in bed by 5 p.m. Clearly the problems of undressing and of getting into bed should be given priority. If solutions are found, the patient must practise until she is confident and can prove that she has the stamina to accomplish both at the end of a normal day.

Functional Assessment/Activities of Daily Living Units

Many hospitals and rehabilitation centres have purpose-designed units for functional assessment and training, and special staff allotted to them. This is good in that it ensures full facilities for those who need them, but it is bad if staff elsewhere shelve all responsibility related to their patients' problems. A man may temporarily have difficulty in tying his shoe laces with one hand. He hardly needs to be sent to a special unit to learn how to do that. It is easy for therapists of all kinds, not to mention doctors and nurses, to fail to think of the patient's disability as likely to present a problem of daily living at all, or to realise that, if the patient needs help in putting on her shoes and stockings after treatment, she may also be in difficulties with her pants or girdle, with bathing, with getting up from her armchair and with picking things up from the floor. If so, referral to the unit would be the right action. Similarly, the arthritic patient who was managing satisfactorily before a flare up of her disease, may have new problems after it, and should be referred back if the doctor finds her clinical condition has deteriorated.

There are varying views as to whose responsibility it is to cover this aspect of treatment. The best service is probably given by an occupational therapist and a physiotherapist who are really interested, working together, collaborating to find the answers to complex problems, but each being able to cover the total needs of patients with clearly defined difficulties, such as those caused by having a stiff hip or painful knees. The important thing is that the patients who need help should be recognised as needing it and that it should be available to them. Both physiotherapists and occupational therapists should learn the basic techniques, for in some places there are physiotherapists only, and in others, only occupational therapists.

A unit, purpose planned for running by one occupational therapist can take the form of a bed-sitting room with simple cooking facilities, bathroom, and storage space. This can fit into an area of 24 feet by 20 feet.

Physical help with heavily disabled patients must be available easily from another therapist. Ideally the unit should be close enough to the rest of the department for another member of the staff to keep an eye on the patient, who can be left to practise provided such supervision is available. Practice in writing, basic sewing techniques, and ironing, as well as assessment of feeding problems, can be given at a kitchen table. This must have easy access for at least one wheel-chair.

The skills of personal care activities are acquired gradually in childhood, improved by practice, and then taken for granted. Some patients who are sent for assessment need only to be given opportunity to try these out in a suitable environment and it is then clear that they still have them. Others can re-learn them by practice, in spite of a disability, and some must learn new ones. The therapist who guides this learning relies on her ability to break down complex sequences of movement, to analyse their components and to adapt these to meet the needs of each patient in the light of individual loss of function.

Break-down of normal method of standing and sitting

> *Standing.* Move forward on the seat.
>
> Alternative methods:
>
> > (*a*) Pull on the arms and slide forward;
> >
> > (*b*) Transfer weight to one hip and push the other hip forward. Repeat to alternate sides;
> >
> > (*c*) Push up on the chair-arms to raise the hips, then lower them further forward.
>
> Place feet in a good position, slightly apart, with one foot a little in front of the knee and the other a little behind.
>
> Lean forward with hands on the chair-arms. Push up to raise the hips. Continuing to lean forward, transfer the weight to the feet by straightening the arms until the hands can be lifted from the chair-arms.
>
> Gradually straighten the knees and hips to stand erect, raising the eye level simultaneously to look straight ahead.
>
> *Sitting.* Feel the front of the chair with the back of both legs. With weight still over the feet, bend the hips and knees and let the hands reach back to the chair-arms. Gradually transfer the weight from the feet, back on to the hands and then through the hips, on to the chair-seat. Move back so that the base of the spine is against the chair-back (by the reverse action of (*a*), (*b*) or (*c*) above), and straighten the spine to get full support.

Adaptation of the normal method of standing and sitting for the hemiplegic patient. Instructions are to be read in conjunction with the break-down of the normal method.

> *Standing.* Move forward on the seat by (*a*) or (*b*) or by pressing back against the chair-back with the shoulders, if there is ability to sit upright again.
>
> Lift the affected leg, by hand if need be, to place the foot slightly in front of the sound foot.
>
> Look to see that it is correct. Place the other foot correctly.
>
> Put the walking aid in front and to the side of the sound foot. Put the sound hand on the chair-arm, well back, and turn slightly to that side.
>
> Lean forward over the sound foot, pushing with the hand and foot to raise the hip from the seat. Continuing to lean forward, transfer the weight to the sound foot by straightening the arm. Gradually

straighten the knee and hip to stand erect, and that of the affected leg at the same time.

Transfer the hand to the walking aid and check the position of the affected foot before walking.

Sitting. Approach the chair with the sound side towards it. When in front, but towards the far side of the chair and still leaning on the walking aid, turn, back to the chair-seat.

Transfer the hand from the aid to the arm of the chair, preparatory to taking weight on it. Keeping the weight over the foot and hand, and with the head bent forward over the knee, gradually bend the hip and knee of the sound leg until the weight can be transferred slowly back through the hips to the chair-seat.

While still leaning forward, move back on the seat so that the base of the spine is against the chair-back. Move the feet into good position under the knees, lifting the affected leg by hand if need be. Straighten the spine to get full support, having the shoulders in good alignment.

The more ways of accomplishing the various activities that the therapist knows the better. She should try things out for herself and she will learn from the patients, for example, from the little girl with flail shoulders who was unable to reach behind her back to pull up her pants but found it easy to get there by putting her hand on the basin and then turning her back on it. Method as such does not matter. It must be effective for the patient who uses it, and, above all, it must be safe.

The therapist is constantly asking herself 'Why?' Why can he not stand up from his chair? He may not have transferred his weight forward over his feet. Why can he not turn down his collar? If he has shoulder-girdle weakness he should support his elbows on a table. If he has diminished sensation in his fingers his collar and tie should be in position before he puts his shirt on. Why can he not get down the step if he can get up it? The solution can only be found by first working out the reason for his difficulty.

On a check list personal care activities appear as separate items, e.g. mobility, dressing, toilet, feeding, etc. In practice they cannot be isolated, and mobility is essential for them all. Skilful use of hands is almost as important, although it does not appear on check lists in its own right.

There are now several illustrated publications dealing with the techniques of Activities of Daily Living [1]. What follows here is intended only to follow up the principles already expressed under some of the headings which appear on check lists.

MOBILITY

Few people move just for the pleasure of moving, or walk for walking's sake. Movement is a means to an end; stooping to pick something up, walking to get to the bus stop. Difficulties arise because of its purpose; the demands on balance and skill in handling in the first example, and demands on stamina in the second. In the context of self care, mobility is concerned with moving in bed, and from bed to chair; shifting weight from one hip to another while sitting or crossing and uncrossing a leg; standing and sitting down again; walking safely even a few yards. All are skills. *Correct heights of seats and beds* are an important factor in sitting and standing. These should be to the buttock crease for those with stiff hips or weak quadriceps, to the upper border of the patella for those who are severely spastic or ataxic, so that the thigh is at once fully supported when seated. Not everyone gets into bed by sitting on the edge first. Children and old people often kneel and then keel over into lying. This avoids the difficulty of having to move back and turn through 90° after sitting down. The bed must be low enough for the whole lower leg to be on it in the kneeling position. Whatever the height, a firm bed is easier to move in than a soft one. Those who can only turn with difficulty need a wider bed than the standard 2 feet 6 inches single one. This makes no allowance for inability to move back on to the same bit of mattress during the turn. The therapist must be able to teach alternative methods of sitting up in bed, those based on the break-down of normal methods, and also tricks such as pulling up on the legs of pyjama trousers or on stockings worn for the purpose.

Steps. Difficulty with a single step may be overcome by going up and down sideways. Patients find this out for themselves, but when applying the same technique to the much higher *bus step*, there can be risk of losing balance when getting off unless special training is given. The rail is held slightly below shoulder level; the outside foot steps out and back, *out* to leave room for the other foot and so ensure a steady base, *back* to avoid undue strain on the hip or knee joint of the leg still on the bus.

Training in use of buses includes the following 'Don'ts'.

(1) Don't get on if last in the queue. Wait for the next bus.

(2) Don't get on unless the conductor is downstairs and sees you.

(3) Don't get on any bus which is obviously in a hurry.

(4) Don't trust your walking stick to steady you. It is no steadier than its user. Try always to have one hand on a rail or seat back.

(5) Don't hold your stick in your hand and hope to hold the rail with it too. Hook it on to your arm.

(6) Don't get up while the bus is going. Tell the conductor where you want to get off when you buy your ticket, and remind him as you get near to the stop.

(7) Don't spurn help, but don't let it prevent you from moving safely as you have been trained to do.

If at home, a single 8″ step is impossible, it may help to fit a half-step, i.e. a 4 inch high block. This is fixed at the lowest level. If there is not room for the full width, 10 inches is wide enough, fitted to one side. The same method can be used for a flight of stairs. If the disability is limitation of hips or knee movement, each half-step is fixed at the same side of successive steps. Climbing is normal, lifting up alternate feet, foot *A* always onto the original step, foot *B* always onto the half-step.

Often the seemingly less important things can make all the difference. For example, remembering always to grip a stair rail well ahead, so that the hand will be comfortably to the side after stepping up or down, and remembering to slide it forward again before taking the next step. Some nervous patients may become more confident by coming downstairs backwards, some arthritics prefer this too as it puts less strain on the hip and knee joints. They should be taught to stub the toe gently against the raiser at the back of the step before taking weight on the foot, so that it will be fully supported.

Slopes. The steeper the slope, the greater the need to lean forward going up and backwards coming down. Those with no disability make these adjustments without thinking, those with disability may need training and practice in making them.

Wheel-chairs

First it is important that the chair is right for the patient, for the places in which he will use it and for the purpose for which he wants it. He can have two chairs from the Department of Health and Social Security if there is good reason for a second one, e.g. one kept at work, one at home, if the patient is unable to lift a chair in and out of his car. The best way to choose the right chair is to let the patient try the range of possible ones for comfort and for ease of propulsion. Most chairs have adult, junior and child sizes. Small adults are comfortable in junior chairs. There are reasons for differences between models and these are pointed out below.

Types of wheel-chairs

Self-propelling. Back or front-wheel drive; right or left-hand drive. Of these some are rigid, some folding.

Patients with double above knee amputations who use their chairs without their prostheses are in danger of tipping backwards on slopes. Their propelling wheels can be set back $1\frac{1}{2}$-2 inches.

Push-chairs. Folding light-weight chair for indoor/outdoor use; intended as a chair to take in a car; can be foot-propelled. Heavy sprung chair for outdoors only.

Commode chairs. Available rigid or folding.

Standard extras

(1) Extension to back-rest (various sizes).
(2) Domestic arms.
(3) Tray.
(4) 2 inch/3 inch cushion for seat/back, with/without firm base. Some models come complete with cushions.
(5) Extension to brake lever.
(6) Body-retaining strap.
(7) Leg rests, adjustable.
(8) Calf-retaining strap.
(9) Extension to foot rests.
(10) Swinging removable foot rests (becoming standard).
(11) Heel-retaining straps (standard on some models).

Advantages of alternative features

(1) Propulsion
Back-wheel drive. For sideways transfer and easy frontal approach. Can be propelled while patient's back is supported. For ease of tilting, if pushed out of doors.
Front-wheel drive. For ease of propulsion on carpets, and for outdoor use if self-propelled.
(2) Tyres
Pneumatic: A more comfortable 'ride' but need maintenance.
Solid: Less effort needed to propel, e.g. over carpets.
(3) Arms
Standard. Patients with poor sitting balance/weak back muscles can lean forward, taking weight on the arms; easier 'push-off' for standing.
Domestic. Closer access to table/desk.
A patient can have a pair of both types if necessary.
(4) Front castors on light-weight push-chair.
Fixed: for outdoor use.
Swivel: For easy turning indoors.

Points about pushing chairs out of doors

'Pushers' need to be taught:

(*a*) How to tilt the chair.
(*b*) Whether to go up/down kerbs forwards/backwards.
(*c*) That is is *not* safe to tilt on swivel castors.

The heavy model has features which counteract the seeming disadvantage of weight:

It has pram wheels; it has a pram handle which gives a mechanical advantage when tilting; it is sprung and it is comfortable provided the canvas seat and back are kept taut. It also has a waterproof 'apron'.

General points

(1) New chairs are 'stiff-jointed' and need oiling, especially folding chairs.
(2) Few patients or their relatives understand their chairs.
(3) Patients must be encouraged to maintain their chairs by asking their local Appliance Centre to do this for them regularly or as soon as there is need.

Wheel-chair clinics. Technical officers from the Appliance Centre of the Department of Health and Social Security* are able to give advice on individual problems. Where, as at some hospitals and special centres, wheel-chair clinics are held, the technical officer is an essential member of the team together with the doctor, and therapist. The medical needs are considered, the patient's functional ability and his limitations are known, and his and his family's wishes in respect of the chair are taken into account. The technical officer knows the chairs currently available and improvements being made in their design. He also knows about chairs likely to be available in the future. Occupational therapists and physiotherapists should be able equally to contribute at such a clinic.

The patient must be taught how to transfer to and from the chair, how to propel and manoeuvre it. The family must know how the patient has been taught. They both must know about the chair itself: how it folds, how the brakes work, how to lift it, and how to manage it at kerbs, i.e. how to tip it and whether it should be taken down backwards or forwards. If the patient needs help in transferring to the chair, someone must be taught how to do so, e.g. a patient with paralysed legs will often be able to move his body but will be glad of someone to lift his legs. The helper must first think about the placement of her feet, then the placement and use of her hands and how her body weight may be used to advantage. This sequence must then be practised under supervision with the patient, and there is no other way of learning.

Hoists. The therapist must know the model which can be supplied to patients through the local authority so that she can demonstrate it, teach its use and be aware of its advantages and disadvantages. She must know the full range of slings available from the manufacturers of the hoist so that she can recommend different ones if those supplied with the hoist are not satisfactory. Occasionally she may find herself designing slings to meet a special need. She must be prepared to explore alternative possibilities when the hoist available locally is for any reason unsuitable.

DRESSING AND UNDRESSING

Undressing is easier than dressing. It is, therefore, less tiring and should be tackled first with severely handicapped patients. Gravity helps, and results are not so important as in dressing. Thinking ahead, it is best to avoid turning clothing inside out and allowing everything to fall on the floor. With dressing, results are judged on personal appearance. Individual's standards vary. For some people the fact of being in day clothes again is enough to increase morale. For others it may be an embarrassment to be dressed but inadequately groomed. Anyone who was accustomed to an immaculate appearance and unable to achieve this without help, should be given help, and should not be made to feel that he has been wrong in wanting it. Patients should be encouraged to persevere and to try to achieve standards at least minimally acceptable to themselves, unaided, in case help should not be available at home.

Few patients realise the importance of a well-balanced starting position. Sitting implies relaxation, but as a starting position from which to dress there must be good balance to withstand the extra strain of leaning forward, twisting to the side or reaching up. These movements add to the difficulty of standing safely too. It may help to lean against the side of the bed, facing it, with knees slightly bent. Every patient must find his best position for each stage of dressing. Often it is easier to pull up trousers when lying on the bed if balance is poor, either by rolling from side to side or by lifting the hips. Having found the best position he should always use it for practising. This is one of the reasons why liaison with the ward staff or with the family at home is so important.

Methods found by the patient for himself are likely to be the best for him. Any patient willing to try should therefore be encouraged. If he is seen to be struggling unsuccessfully, the therapist can often see the reason for the difficulty and the solution to it. Many now standard methods have been discovered in this way. For example, a hemiplegic patient was convinced that he could not tie his tie. Given a thumb loop on the short end, which could then be held taut by his paralysed hand, he had no difficulty. Later, he found that there was no need for the loop. It had, however, served its purpose by giving encouragement initially. Patients referred early for assessment have had no time to come to terms with their disabilities, and encouragement is much needed.

Relatives may be glad of advice about the right kind of clothing to buy. If there are indications that the patient may put on weight, this should be remembered. Material which has 'give', raglan type sleeves, wide neck openings, minimal trimmings, generous opening when openings are needed, few and large fastenings, slippery linings in sleeves that have to pulled up over others, garments that are light to handle, will all make it easier for the disabled patient to become independent. Garments which open all the way down the front are not always the best; they are difficult to put on, while sitting. Provided there is an opening big enough to slip over the shoulders, it is easier for most patients to put things on over their heads. For a patient who must be dressed by someone else while lying or sitting, full-length back openings are best. Several garments can be put on from the front before the patient must lean forward to have them fastened. Fastenings are best off centre to avoid discomfort.

Shoes should give support to the instep and the heels must be broad. This is more important than the height. For patients with 'difficult' feet, e.g. arthritics, there are shoes now available through surgical appliance firms recognised by the Department of Health and Social Security*, which are moulded over plaster of paris casts of the feet. Imprints of the soles of the feet are also taken and the soles of the shoes conform to these. They are light-weight, seamless, comfortable, and known as 'space' shoes. A home shoe stretcher, with various appropriate attachments, is also available and could be a useful piece of equipment in an A.D.L. Unit.*

Fastenings on surgical appliances need not be difficult if the therapist can be with the patient at his initial appointment with the fitter, so that his preferences for direction of pull, his 'handedness', his preference for positioning of fastenings, and his special problems of gripping can be explained.

BATHROOM ACTIVITIES

It is more difficult to feel confident in the bathroom than anywhere else, yet it is the place in which the patient most dislikes being dependent. Surfaces are shiny and can be wet and slippery: there should be a mop at hand. It may be difficult to get into the bathroom with walking aids, and the patient may be without the support of his shoes or surgical appliances. Rails are advisable, placed to give support from the door to the lavatory, bath and basin.

The lavatory. The same optimum heights for sitting apply as in the bedroom, but because it is usual to supply rails or a frame round the lavatory some patients can manage with the seat slightly lower. Horizontal rails are used for pushing down on, diagonal rails for pulling up. Rails on a wall should be $1\frac{1}{2}$ inches in diameter with a clearance from the wall of 2 inches.

A patient with painful knees must be able to take her weight off these joints while sitting down and standing up by pressing down on rails or arm rests. A frame round the W.C.* or a horizontal rail on each side wall of a separate lavatory or one horizontal rail and a high stool slightly to the front on the other side, will be suitable. These arm rests should be 8 inches above the seat, because it is difficult to get purchase in pressing down if they are higher. They should project forward 1 foot 9 inches from mid thigh, and for safety and comfort they should be 3 inches wide and padded. The patient with painful knees may have painful hands and she will use the full length of her forearm on the arm rest.

A patient with severe limitation of hip flexion will need horizontal rails projecting further forward (as in Plate 1). If a frame is used this must be fixed firmly. He may also require a raised sloping seat, but not more than 2 inches lower at the front than the back. He will need to lean back, and if a low-level cistern can be exchanged for a high one, a sloping back support can be fitted between the seat and the wall. Whether or not his knees are stiff in extension, the method of standing up will be the same. He will press down on both arm rests, reaching gradually further and further forward, simultaneously drawing his feet back with very small steps until his legs are vertical. With the final push-off to take the weight on to his feet he will normally make a quarter turn. A hemiplegic patient, or one with progressive paralysis will need a diagonal rail, or rails. This should start just below shoulder height when sitting and be angled at 30° to the horizontal. As the patient stands up he slides his hand or hands forwards up the rail. A patient, perhaps elderly and confused, who can manage the lavatory but lacks confidence in her balance will be helped by having a chair or stool by her side to hold on to.

A patient who transfers sideways from a wheel-chair will be helped by having an extension flush with the seat and approximately 9 inches wide, on the far side. This must be fixed firmly in order to take the weight through the hand, leaving the seat itself free. Such patients must of course be able to transfer to right or left as required.

The bath. A patient can be taught to sit down in the bath through kneeling or half kneeling instead of sitting directly from standing. Hemiplegic patients who are confident in moving, and patients with painful but mobile knees may prefer this method to one using a seat, for they can then use any bath. A flat-bottomed wide one is best. A non-slip bath mat is indicated for any disabled or elderly person. This may be the sole aid, or it may be used in conjunction with a bath seat. A towelling bath robe is good for drying.

A simple side-to-side board over the end of the bath may be the answer for those who cannot stand on one leg. This will mean sitting down with the back to the bath and then swivelling round through 90° while lifting in the legs. Those who find this turn difficult need a stool of the same height which clips to the over bath seat so that they need only slide along sideways after sitting. Such a stool is also useful to sit on at the washbasin.

A patient who feels unable to get up out of the bath can be helped if the side panel of the bath is set $\frac{3}{4}$ inch in from the top rim of the bath, so as to allow for a firm finger grip, otherwise a slot could be cut in the panel. A damp towel or face cloth on the edge will prevent the grip slipping. He may also need an inside bath seat. This must be fitted to the individual bath and should come a third of the way up from the bottom as the most difficult movement will be getting from there to the seat. An over bath seat and/or a grab rail may also be needed. The latter should be about 3 feet long, 5 inches above the edge of the bath and 1 foot 3 inches from the sitting end. With practice and as confidence increases this inside bath seat may be discarded. It can, of course, be lifted out of the bath during bathing.

It is important for the therapist to arrange for a member of the family to come and see that the patient can manage the bath and is confident in doing so. If she does not, it is unlikely that he will be allowed to bath at home and follow-ups confirm this. It is sometimes discovered that the district nurse has been called in to give a blanket bath.

Home visits in some areas disclose primitive bathroom and lavatory facilities, often out of reach. Commodes of different types can be supplied. If a solid one with a wide base and arms is wanted, it is wise to ask for it. Standard models are often too low.

FEEDING

The only problems which the therapist in an assessment unit should be expected to tackle are those of the one-handed, who can be taught the press-down-and-rock technique of the Nelson knife, and those of patients who need something to thicken a knife handle because of poor grip. Anything more complex should be dealt with in the occupational therapy department itself.

The choice of tableware is one part of the problem and the need for correct positioning of the food in relation to the patient's mouth is the other and more complex aspect.

Cutlery. Knives and forks are normally held as are all small tools. The handles are pressed into the palm by the fourth and fifth fingers, given lateral stability by pressure of the thumb against the middle finger and stabilised from above by the index finger. Extra downward pressure during use comes from flexion of the wrist. Deficit in any of these will reduce efficiency, as will sensory impairment or incoordination. Having identified the deficit there are two possible lines to pursue: to substitute for the deficit, perhaps by providing a splint which will stabilise the thumb in opposition so that the normal grip and action can still be used, or to suggest a grip in which opposition of the thumb plays no part. This example is a simplification, for a patient whose only problem is lack of opposition would find his own answer. But the more complex the problem the greater is the need to be analytical as a first step towards solving it.

Most knives, forks and spoons present difficulty if grip or control is poor. The handles are too thin and too slippery. If pain is a factor, as in arthritis. weight is an added disadvantage. Manufacturers are becoming more aware that there are problems. In addition to certain standard products with a feature which facilitates grip, for example *Nycraft* cutlery has a groove in the handle, *Melaware Manoy* range has been specially designed for the severely disabled. The full range includes *tableware*, two plates and a beaker, and these have proved invaluable for patients who have previously been unable to manage without help.

Positioning. In Plates 3 and 4, an acting patient is seen with a special table which proved satisfactory for a man with severe tremor and muscle weakness. Note the head support, the inclined plane of the forearm support, the relative heights of the hand and the plate, the nearness of the plate to the mouth. Note the adjustable legs of the table and in the companion photograph, the totally different angle of the table top for reading. With such a patient trial and error must play a part and there is better chance of success if the equipment can be built up in the department, basing the design on assessment of the patient's functional abilities and disabilities.

KITCHEN ACTIVITIES [2]

Making tea, washing up and putting away what has been used, will be part of a full A.D.L.* assessment. This tests mobility, ability to remember, for the kitchen will be a strange environment, orientation to the job in hand, attention to safety with gas or electricity, and, to some extent, it tests standards. One attendance may be enough but with a patient whose performance is variable, it is important to assess her both on a good and on a less good day.

Retraining of the housewife to overcome problems brought to light by fullscale kitchen assessment is the province of the occupational therapist and one of her most valuable contributions in rehabilitation. No here else can a substantially disabled housewife re-establish herself with confidence in new techniques and in her ability to plan, and to work to a plan. Preparation of food and cooking to a high standard is possible in spite of disability, with careful choice of what shall be attempted, and the sooner something can be sent or taken home for enjoyment by the family, the better.

The therapist in a kitchen unit will be a much better therapist if she is already a good cook; the kind of cook who knows the difference between boiling and simmering, and understands the reason why a white sauce must be brought to boiling point. She will not, as a rule, be teaching her patients how to cook, but she will often find herself having to remind them, or having to share with them the development of new ideas and methods. She must also have some understanding of appropriate simple diets, and of meals that can be cooked with limited facilities. She should also know the basic principles of cleaning utensils and equipment, e.g. that it is easiest to clean the inside of the oven or the outside of the kettle when they are warm. Patients in their own kitchens will have to do these things and practice may be needed, as it may, too, with general household tasks.

Much has now been published about the need for better planning of kitchens for the disabled [1]. The occupational therapy kitchen should demonstrate good principles of planning and work study methods should be encouraged. At the same time the patient's own kitchen must be in the therapist's mind and any particular hazards to safety must be given attention.

Treatment is planned to be realistic and the best kitchen units have meals cooked and eaten in them. Timetabling is not easy unless in a residential centre, and failures of transport not only deprive the patient of her treatment but can deprive the therapist of her most reliable cook. Sometimes this provides just the incentive needed for another patient to take additional responsibility.

It is good to encourage men who are likely, in the future, to spend most of their time at home, to take an interest in kitchen activities. Good relationships with other members of the patient's family are vitally important to the successful resettlement of a disabled housewife or of a volunteer kitchen helper, and any time spent to achieve this is time well spent. Some patients will only be able to make a minimal contribution but this should be encouraged because it will increase their self respect. There are others who are capable of taking over a major part of the work, but without encouragement and even pressure from their families will be content to do little.

One patient can be a full-time responsibility for the therapist; sometimes she can have three or four at once, for it is hoped that less obvious supervision needs to be given to patients as they improve. Onlookers in the kitchen should be discouraged on grounds of safety.

For a comprehensive scheme of treatment there should be equal emphasis on building up physical stamina and improving physical skill, and on building up confidence and ability to take increasing responsibility. There is much work to be covered: training in sitting balance, in neat finger work and in safe mobility; the need to try different tools, e.g. potato peelers or whisks; the need to try different ways of holding and pouring from a kettle; and the need to practise planning the timing of cooking a full meal. There is scope for practical sessions with a group of patients, discussing such common problems, as storage, handling equipment and materials and of saving energy and compensating for slowness.

The kitchen is also an excellent place in which to treat patients for improvement of local function. A student can learn a lot at the sink, with a saucepan and a Brillo pad, remembering that both the outside and inside need attention. Housewives who have had back strain and are physically unsuited to lifting by the right methods, will benefit from talking to a therapist about ways in which they can save their backs during the course of their work (see p. 229. Back Care). The kitchen is also the obvious place in which to work out possible solutions for patients with feeding difficulties, remembering that these will vary with different foods. It is best to start on something easy like rice pudding or mashed potatoes rather than fried eggs or salad which are difficult.

The kitchen therapist must be well organised, resourceful, observant, and confident in the techniques of her craft, cooking and home management, combined, always, with the application of her use of physical and psychological treatment techniques.

SPECIAL EQUIPMENT

A therapist should make herself familiar with the channels of supply of aids, in her own area, e.g. rails, bath seats, walking aids, wheel-chairs, hoists, commodes, etc., with where she can get information about the range and supply of more specialised equipment, e.g. special beds, alarm systems etc., and about general facilities for the disabled. The Disabled Living Foundation* provides this service. It is largely staffed by occupational therapists, a wide range of equipment is on view and, by arrangement, assessments can be made there. The Central Council for the Disabled* and the National Fund for Research into Crippling Diseases* are also useful. Some aids may be made locally in Occupational Therapy Departments, Day Centres, or Hospital Day Units, the needs of the patients or clients being met in the process. Manufacturers may make equipment or adapt their products for specific needs. Occupational therapists must understand the design of commonly used equipment, to be able to take measurements in patients' homes and to make realistic recommendations [3].

The following is a suggested line of thought for the occasion when seeking an answer to a practical problem. It is in order of priority:

(1) Avoid the difficulty, e.g. a patient who is not confident enough to bend down when she is standing, should not put her handbag on the floor when she sits down unless she will remember to pick it up again before she gets up.

(2) Try another method, e.g. a patient with stiff hips can slip his feet into his shoes if he stands in front of the shoes, and bends his knee back so that his toes point downwards. Approximately $25°$ of knee flexion is enough.

(3) Use an aid; ideally one available in the shops, e.g. the Helping Hand, designed for picking up, or something designed for one purpose which can be used for another, such as a dish mop to wash the back of the neck.

(4) Make a special gadget—only as a last resort. A good example of such a gadget is the *spring wire button hook* for those with 'fingering' difficulty, such as arthritics and those with tremor.

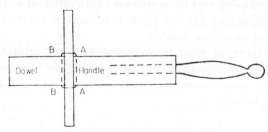

FIG. 2.   Spring wire button hook: ½ size.

Method of use.

Push the wire loop right through the button hole from the outside of the garment to the inside.

Hook the button into the wide part of the wire loop and pull the button hook back so that the button slides into the bulb of the wire loop. Pull on the button hook and ease the button hole towards the bulb so it is over the button.

Keeping the handle flat against the body, and without twisting it, swing it like the hand of a clock through 360°, until the button is through. (N.B. It is easier to keep it close to you and untwisted if you change hands. If you are doing up the top button, you must lift your chin out of the way of the handle.)

To free the button hook, keep the handle close to the body and push until the button slides into the wide part of the wire loop and can be freed.

Note. With a button that is wider than the widest part of the hook, it will be necessary to tilt the hook first to one side and then the other, to get the button in in the first instance, and, later, to free it.

A thin piece of dowel attached to the handle with a rubber band, put on like a square lashing, as in the diagram, helps those with poor grip. The finger should be above the dowel bar for pulling (in position A) and below for pushing (in position B). The user should find out the best position for the dowel bar.

The therapist must be able to demonstrate in slow motion, right-handed or left-handed, any technique which the patient must learn. The ease with which this is done may influence a patient's attitude of mind towards his problems for the better. A bad demonstration can be disastrous. From time to time there will be need for the occupational therapy department to provide a major piece of equipment individually designed for a patient whose needs may not otherwise be met.

Two examples of such projects have already been referred to, the walking trolley described and illustrated in Plate 16, the second, the adjustable table illustrated in Plates 3 and 4. Before undertaking such projects it is essential to list the various aspects upon which decisions must be taken.

The following points relating to designing a chair were listed at the time of planning and making the one illustrated in Plates 1 and 2.

Is a special chair really necessary?

What would it achieve for the patient?

> Comfort/independence in standing and sitting/opportunity to be active while sitting/independence in feeding, etc.

How does the disability affect the patient's method of standing and sitting? How would this method dictate the design of the chair? and what factors relating to the various parts of the chair should be considered?:

> *Seat.* Height. Depth. Width. Angle. Soft/hard. Texture.
>
> *Back.* Height. Angle. Adjustability. Head Support. Wings. Shaping for the spine.
>
> *Arms.* Height above seat. Forward projection. Open/solid sides. Contour and texture of top. Provision for fittings.
>
> *Legs.* Need for extra wide or deep base for stability. Need for brake. Ferrules/domes/wheels/swivel castors. Need to plan without a low front cross-bar.
>
> *Footrest.* Angle to give support for feet. Need for leg support. Size to allow change of position of the feet. Method by which it could be brought into position by the patient. Method by which it could be removed by the patient.

What provision should be made for activities the patient might want to engage in? e.g. typing, painting, sewing, clay modelling.

How would these dictate structure, dimensions, surfaces, etc., of, for example, a work tray?

How would such a work tray be got into position and be removed by the patient?

What special fittings would be necessary on the chair? e.g. reading light, containers, controls for walking aids not in use.

Re-education of Work Habit

Motivation for Work

To increase a patient's motivation it will be necessary to increase his sense of personal endeavour. His attitude of mind is as important as his physical condition. Some people are able to activate themselves while others are not.

The therapist must show an understanding of the psychological implications of disinclination to work, or doubts as to capacity to work. It is essential to explain, sometimes repeatedly, the patient's condition to him and the methods which will be used in treatment. Much encouragement may be needed but, equally, the patient may also need a bracing talk. It is not sufficient for the doctor and the therapist to know that he is progressing. The patient must be made aware of this too.

There are many factors which inhibit motivation. It is important that social problems relating to the home situation, family relationships and finances are being dealt with by the medical social worker. Unless this is done the patient may be unable to concentrate on treatment. Lack of confidence also impedes progress. The doctor and therapist may consider that the patient is fit for his former job while he himself is unconvinced. General improvement should help in restoring self confidence and the opportunity of trying out similar work will help to convince him. A purposeful, stimulating atmosphere in the department is essential and the choice of 'neighbours' is of primary importance. Lack of confidence can also be a problem in resettlement. For example, a bricklayer with rheumatoid arthritis who could not return to his previous job showed aptitude for clerical work but was unable to visualise himself as a white-collar worker. After two months spent on hospital and departmental form filling and accounts in the occupational therapy department he felt confident enough to go for an interview and accepted a clerical job.

The provisions of the welfare state offer a number of positive disincentives to work. A patient may benefit financially by remaining on the sick list or on unemployment benefit rather than undertaking the only work for which he is capable. This is especially true of a man with a large family who may literally not be able to afford to work. Another disincentive arises from the method of settling compensation claims. Many people may be subconsciously reluctant to recover maximally before the amount of their compensation is decided, while the lawyers cannot settle this until the optimum recovery is reached. It is in the patient's best interest to return to work as early as possible. Compensation helps to make up loss of earnings but the lump sum will not vary and the longer he is off work the harder it will be to readjust to it. In some conditions, such as hand injuries, delay in fully cooperating in treatment may lead to a permanent disability which could have been prevented. The occupational therapist is the best person to assess, practically, when the patient is ready for work. For example, a man who cannot flex his spine when asked by the doctor in a clinic may do so readily when he is levelling up a table on the workshop floor. In consultation with his staff the doctor will tell the patient when to return to work and may ask the patient's solicitor to endorse this advice. No solicitor would ethically support a malingerer and when faced with such medical opinion must advise accordingly.

Elderly people who are not returning to work in the commercial sense may have problems of motivation. A housewife with family responsibilities has an incentive to make a maximal effort, but many men, unable to adapt to a workless future, have none. All too many have had little opportunity or inclination for leisure activities. Others may have had to leave a home and garden for a flat in a different neighbourhood. Loneliness and inactivity lead to depression. This should be recognised and patients who are at risk should be referred for help through the appropriate channels. Local authorities are doing much to help in preparation for retirement and provide club activities for able bodied and disabled old age pensioners.

Building up Work Tolerance

The occupational therapy department should provide a choice of activities by which different types of patients can build up tolerance to fatigue and become reacclimatised to a work situation, including noise if appropriate. A nervous patient, after surgery, may be pampered by his wife and fail to take any active steps towards reconditioning himself, even if there is the opportunity at home. A cardiac patient, told after many months that he is now fit to think about work may doubt this and be afraid of his fatigue. Both patients could be helped by occupational therapy carefully planned and graded to improve stamina. The therapist must observe individuals even when supervising a group. A man on a full day's programme may not do a full day's work. He may arrive late and leave early or spend a disproportionate time leaning against the bench. Standards can be set too low; even a good day's work in the department may fall short of the demands the patient will meet at work. This is particularly true of labouring jobs.

Travelling to work is another important factor and a tiring one. Many people could work if only they could get there. Training in the use of public transport may be the physio- or occupational therapist's responsibility, as agreed between them. Some patients only need to be told they may now use a bus, others must have practice with a therapist; taking at first simple trips at quiet periods, advancing, if need be, to rush hour travel. It will be a progression in treatment to come by public transport or to walk instead of coming by ambulance. Refund of fares can be arranged in some cases.

Retraining in Specific Skills

A skill is a facility for doing something and it is achieved only by constant practice during which special movement patterns are laid down in the brain. Interruption of these patterns will result in poor performance; physical incapacity to hold and manipulate the tools will do likewise. Speed may be lost through long-term lack of practice but this can return quickly with use, as for example with typing. While performance is likely to be poor, the skilled craftsman should not be asked to use the tools of his trade unless he wishes to do so. He must be treated through some other medium, until strength, mobility and control have improved enough to assure reasonable results. From then on retraining of the skill will best be achieved by making increasing demands in terms of speed of work, accuracy and endurance. A skill may be temporarily lost by a patient's inability to assume the working position his job will demand. A gas fitter, for instance, must be fully mobile, able to crouch and to reach. Treatment for restoration of function so that he can do both of these is as important to him as is the use of his tools. The occupational therapist should ask about hobby or recreational interests so that treatment can be relevant to them too. The keen amateur footballer will need more lower limb strength and agility than a man who only takes the dog for a walk.

When there is permanent injury, more complex retraining will be needed. A machine operator with sensory defect in the hand must learn to use his eyes to compensate for this. A hemiplegic housewife must compensate for loss of the use of one hand by developing extra skill in the other, skill to separate an egg, skill to write.

For some patients the occupational therapist will have to arrange for the provision of adapted tools. For example, a draughtsman severely paralysed by poliomyelitis was able to do work of his previous standard only after each piece of his equipment had been adapted to his individual method of pick up and use.

Preparing the Patient for Resettlement [4]

In this context resettlement means getting the patient back to some form of work. For the majority of patients who were working prior to attending for treatment this will mean return to their former jobs. A small proportion will need resettling in alternative work, and of these only a minority will be retrained. Some may no longer be employable.

During his initial period of treatment the patient may need help with activities of daily living. When assessing his ability to return to work he may need any of the following:

(1) Improvement of local function and increasing use of it in purposeful activity related to home, travel and work.
(2) Physical and psychological reconditioning.
(3) Assessment of personality.
(4) Positive motivation.
(5) Practice or revision of skills.
(6) Assessment of fitness for a particular job, including means of travel.
(7) Assessment of abilities or potential abilities for alternative work.
(8) Prevocational study.

(9) Refresher course or retraining.

(10) Social resettlement, particularly in relation to housing.

The occupational therapy department can contribute directly or indirectly to all of these, working in conjunction with personnel in other departments in the hospital and, as necessary, outside it.

It is important for someone to identify the patient who would benefit from any such help and to do so early. He himself may be unaware of the facilities available. The apprentice for example, with long hospitalisation ahead of him would benefit from a course of study in theoretical aspects of his training. Facilities for prevocational work, advice, supervised study and in some cases practical work, are available. The adult education authorities can supply such tuition. The occupational therapist will not necessarily be involved.

For a patient in another hospital with less good facilities, the occupational therapist and the medical social worker must take the initiative: enlisting support from the doctor and ward staff and perhaps from a psychologist, arranging for tuition through the education authority or through the Preparatory Training Bureau* of the British Council for the Rehabilitation of the Disabled*. The success of any such scheme depends on there being somewhere to study, perhaps a side room. Much depends on the patient's stamina to persevere. The harder he finds this the more help he will need: a teaching machine with suitable programmes from a library can be most helpful.

An out-patient sent for improvement of local function following an injury may, on interview, appear likely to have difficulty about future work, e.g. the building-site labourer with bilateral fractures of os calcis. General assessment should begin at once. As soon as his need for resettlement in alternative work becomes certain specific assessment can begin concurrently with continuing remedial treatment.

Facilities for Assessment

The occupational therapy department provides facilities which can be utilised in many ways to assess patients. These will vary but the following are some useful examples.

Purposeful mobility: carrying on the level, up slopes, up stairs and outdoors: using a wheel-chair, pushing a trolley, hurrying, climbing ladders, sending a patient round the hospital as a messenger to deliver notes to other staff members and checking the time and method of delivering them: taking the patient out to test ability to use a bus, train or bicycle: sending a patient out shopping, first with staff or student, then with another patient and finally alone: providing a shopping list of increasing variety on succeeding occasions requiring visits to several different shops.

Heavy work: shovelling gravel to different heights, into a wheelbarrow and higher, pushing and tipping a wheelbarrow, digging a pit in the garden, concreting, cross-cut sawing, stacking industrial outwork, doing such work in the boots that will normally be worn.

Assembly work: industrial outwork such as binding cable forms, assembling castors, 'local' i.e. hospital, production lines making rockers for walking plasters, wrapping and packaging items for the central sterilising department, etc. This may be simple repetitive work or something more complex which may be broken down into several processes. It may require neat finger movements or gross grip, similar or dissimilar bilateral hand action.

Housewife equivalent: bed-making, cooking, laundering, cleaning the bath, shopping and checking prices.

Clerical work: typewriting, duplicating, using an adding machine, filing.

Simple job simulation may be used to check whether a patient can manage a specific part of his job, for example a carpenter assembling a mortice lock and making a dovetail joint; an electrician changing a plug or mending a fuse; a draughtsman producing or copying a working drawing; a painter preparing and painting wood. Experiments with very simple tasks may give an idea of the type of work possible for the problem patient with ostensibly nothing to offer an employer, tea making and taking it round the department, making deliveries outside the department, sweeping the carpentry shop at the end of the day, answering the telephone and taking messages.

Miscellaneous projects can be used to check learning ability, for example the use of an adding machine: the therapist will teach the patient how to make sub-totals, totals and correct mistakes. The next day she will check what he can remember. If necessary she will teach and check again, noting how often this is necessary. She will observe how he takes corrections and learns by his mistakes, how persistent he is and what his standards are. Ability to follow written instructions can be assessed by cooking from a recipe, and following diagrammatic instructions by making some item such as a bath seat from a drawing.

Although the facilities of an occupational therapy department provide excellent media for assessment, the therapist will have two major problems:

Standards must be realistic in appraising the results of such experiments. Restacking timber in the department woodstore for an hour, even daily, would not prove fitness for a five-day week of labouring. Similarly a patient who does better than average at clerical tests devised in the department may still be of lower standard than an office clerk. Performance should be compared with recognised standards, not those of fellow patients. Validated tests are best.

Occupational therapists who use locally devised tests should attempt to standardise them. The test must have a clear aim. It must be administered in exactly the same way to each patient and under the same conditions. A method of scoring must be devised which will eventually make it possible to relate individual scores to some well defined reference groups. Records should be kept of patients' achievements so that a body of knowledge is built up about the test. The tests can also be tried out on other groups of people to give further information. The help of a psychologist interested in test development could be used to advantage.

The provision of a true work situation is rarely possible. With ingenuity working conditions can be simulated for short-term trials. A hairdresser recovering from backstrain could spend an afternoon shampooing and setting a succession of volunteer patients. This may be sufficient to restore his confidence and to give him a good indication of what he can manage but it will still not provide the equivalent of a five-day week.

A trial period of work arranged in the appropriate department of the hospital can overcome both of the above difficulties. Tripartite understanding of the purpose of the trial is vital for its success.

(1) It is arranged only if the patient understands the conditions and wishes for it. It is an extension of treatment, therefore unpaid; he must work at times laid down by the department to which he is going and as far as possible do whatever work is asked of him; he must not expect the trial to lead to the offer of a job.

(2) Any aspect of the work which is contra-indicated must be explained to his temporary 'foreman'.

(3) The therapist must have an objective and realistic report of the patient's ability and fitness for the job. 'He is very good' should mean just that, and '. . . considering how much his hand slows him down' should not be withheld if it is true.

Such trials are invaluable for patients who think they are fit enough but have no way of proving it, for example, the school meals helper who, for an hour and a half five days a week, must handle heavy stacks of plates, at speed. Working in the hospital canteen during the lunch hour will prove or disprove it. They are valuable too for the patient who, though considered medically fit by the doctor and assessed as likely to have no problems by the therapist, lacks confidence. Sending a patient insufficiently skilled or motivated, and not yet physically fit or, above all, one who is a troublemaker, can jeopardise the chances of repeating such trials, whereas with a suitable patient it can make for good future relationships with the department concerned. It can even occasionally lead to a job for the patient—a providential by-product.

Occasionally it is possible to arrange for a patient to have a trial period of work in his own firm, with a prospective employer or even at a local government training centre. This can be a great benefit but good relationships with local industry will be necessary to achieve it.

General Assessment

This is built up over a period of time and should be continuous. The patient's general behaviour in a variety of situations is observed: his reaction to other patients, to staff, and to his environment; his attitude to his disability and to the idea of work, also the changes in these attitudes and reactions. There will be opportunity to get to know the patient as a person, what he does at home and his outside interests. There will be assessment of the patient's physical adaptability relating to working positions: standing, sitting, stooping, crouching, and of his ability to lift and carry. His liking for different kinds of work can be tried out: simple repetitive work; work with variety; work with the hands or on machines; solitary work or work with others; creative work or routine work; and preference for certain materials, e.g. wood, metal, bricks, soil, etc. The need for tests of the 3 R's may become apparent and also tests of eyesight. The patient's standards for behaviour and performance will be shown by his personal appearance, his responsibility in organising himself, e.g. being punctual and caring for tools and materials, by his work effort and its results. A Work Assessment Report may be helpful. This should be written in specific terms in order to give guidance to the doctor, D.R.O.* or employer. In the course of such assessment it may be necessary to provide the patient with practice in an area of difficulty shown up by a test, and then to re-test him. It will be important to know after what period of time re-assessment on the same test will be reliable. Usually this will depend on the length and complexity of the test.

Patients on a comprehensive assessment programme should, if possible, be sent at an early stage to a psychologist for assessment, ideally one who understands the occupational therapist's aims and methods. The psychologist will apply and interpret standardised intelligence tests to assess the patient's level of functioning, and will identify his special abilities and optimum channels of learning, and also any special problems—for example, in brain damaged patients. She will also apply tests of personality. The means she uses are in the main beyond the scope of the occupational therapist, but the tests she uses do not take the place of those given by the therapist, nor can the latter take the place of those given by the psychologist. They reinforce one another. Preliminary findings from the occupational therapy department will be a guide to the areas in which standardised testing is most needed, and the psychologist's findings indicate the areas in which practical assessment is most likely to be profitable. The psychologist can also contribute by giving an unbiased opinion of the patient's attitude both to his disability and to his future.

Beginning in 1974, those occupational therapists who have completed specific courses in psychological testing will be able to use some of the 'tools' available to psychologists. Courses to train occupational therapists in psychological testing were begun under the supervision of the British Psychological Society, in conjunction with the British Association of Occupational Therapists [5]. Some of the tests occupational therapists have been trained to use are:

(1) *Raven's Standard Progressive Matrices* (1938), which uses non-verbal items to measure general intelligence.

(2) *The Mill Hill Vocabulary Scale*, which uses vocabulary questions to measure verbal ability.

These two tests are designed to be used together in place of a single test of general intelligence. By doing this it is possible to assess, separately:

(*a*) The present capacity for intellectual activity, largely independent of a person's educational and cultural background.

(*b*) The fund of information acquired, whatever the present capacity for intellectual activity. It will also be possible to gain some insight into the psychological significance of any discrepancies between (*a*) and (*b*).

Although these two tests can be freely purchased and are widely used by occupational therapists, nurses and others, they will be more effective tools in the hands of an occupational therapist who has taken a course in psychological testing. In fact, the indiscriminate use of these tests, or any others, without proper recordings and controls, tends to destroy, eventually, the test's usefulness.

(3) *A.H.4 and A.H.5* [6] intelligence tests.

(4) *The General Clerical Test.* This is a general and differential test for use with all types of clerical personnel. Individual sections test clerical speed and accuracy, numerical ability, and verbal facility. The total score is a measure of general mental ability, weighted in favour of someone who possesses clerical aptitudes or skills.

(5) *Revised Minnesota Paper Form Board.* This is a paper and pencil test measuring spatial perception as indicated by the ability to visualise the assembly of two-dimensional geometric shapes into a whole design. It predicts success in mechanical jobs and in those aspects of engineering which involve design, and is related to art as well as mechanical abilities.

These last three tests are not freely available to the public.

Other tests which may be useful and should be available to occupational therapists include:

(6) *Schonell's Diagnostic and Attainment Testing* [7], containing a number of tests, instructions for their use and norms. It includes a quick and simple measure of word recognition and good arithmetic tests.

(7) J. C. Daniel's and H. Diack's *Standard Reading Test* [8]. This includes a good spelling test and also measures hand–eye co-ordination, picture–word recognition and visual discrimination.

It may also be useful to refer to the standards laid down by the Department of Employment for candidates applying for training. The D.R.O.* may have tests in mathematics or English for some disabled persons referred to him. The Skills Centres ask for certain basic educational requirements, as do the Queen Elizabeth Training College and other residential training centres. These give frames of reference to which the occupational therapist can work.

Methods of Specific Practical Assessment

These will be governed by the patient's physical condition and prognosis, his mental condition and attitude and his previous level of employment. It is helpful to have got to know the patient and to have preliminary findings of general assessment before starting something more specific; but he may have been sent for assessment only, and if so, both forms must be carried out concurrently. It is important to explain to him the object of the programme which will be planned. Some patients, perhaps apprehensive or on the defensive, may first have to be assured that they will not be expected to know anything they have not been taught, that instruction will be given and time allowed to practise what has been learnt. A patient who has ideas about what he might do should be given opportunity to try it if possible. These ideas are often unrealistic, the demands of clerical work or storekeeping being underestimated.

Unless the purpose of the tests is understood and the patient cooperates in doing them the results are valueless. The performance level will be lowered by unfavourable conditions. Physical comfort, lack of distraction and good equipment are necessary, also adequate staff supervision. The patient's reactions to the situation should be noted.

Two forms of test may be given:

Tests with a clearly defined single aim, i.e. assessment of an attribute which would be needed in some types of job but not in others. The aim must be clear in the therapist's mind, i.e. a dexterity test is given to test dexterity only. Results will be valueless if placement of the equipment demands an effort of reach which slows down performance, e.g. a patient with muscular dystrophy may have excellent facility with his hands but be unable to combine this with hand placement. He must be allowed to work in his position of choice, at knee level perhaps, tests of hand placement being given separately. Some patients will know their optimum working position, others may need the therapist's help in finding it. The final choice should be noted.

Examples of single aim tests

(1) *Finger dexterity*, using precision grip and manipulation, one handed or two handed, e.g. assembling nuts and bolts, graded $\frac{3}{8}$ inch to $\frac{1}{16}$ inch against a time clock. Or putting paper clips onto two pieces of paper, folding them and putting them into an envelope.

(2) *Hand eye coordination* with or without a tool, e.g. using tweezers, pick up a brad, insert it into a hole in a block of wood with metal surface drilled at regular intervals, and put a washer over it. Repeat many times. Or drop a marble through a hole to roll down a slope, catching it as it rolls, and repeating.

(3) *Strength of grip*, using a Terry's 'wrist strengthener' which has a spring of known strength incorporated in it.

(4) *Colour discrimination* using a peggotty board and arranging pegs in shades of different colours or copying a design made with such pegs.

(5) *Sensory function*. (*a*) Tactile—picking up articles of varying shapes, using different appropriate grips also identifying textures. (*b*) Stereognosis—recognising objects of different shape held in the hand. These tests must be done without using eyesight and it is better to have a solid panel providing a screen than to ask the patient to shut his eyes.

(6) *Reaction time span*. The interval between a light going on and pushing a bell is recorded. This is of special relevance when consideration is being given to suitability for driving.

(7) *Spatial relationships*. Fitting a variety of widely differing shapes into the relevant spaces on a board, some with only slight differences. The purpose of this type of test must be explained. To adults, especially to those with some brain damage, they seem childish, yet they are relevant to the demands of some kinds of work, e.g. fitting parts into jigs.

(8) *Ability to measure*, using ruler, calipers, compass, protractor, set square.

(9) *Perseverance*. This is an essential quality for the patient with potential abilities but without an educational or work background of value in the context of resettlement. The test could be a mathematical or otherwise academically oriented problem, it could be a constructional puzzle or a long-term "finicky" project as individually suitable.

Each of the preceding tests needs to be standardised to maximise its value. For example, the items used to assess finger dexterity should be kept together for this purpose; the paper, paper-clips and envelopes should be of standard size, design and quality; a scale by which to interpret results should be made available; and the conditions in which the test is to be given should be clearly stated. The environmental conditions in which the candidates have to work may in themselves, be an essential factor to include in the test, i.e. interruptions or noise in office work, etc. But uncontrolled variations in testing conditions can reduce a test's reliability and destroy its validity. The result cannot, then, be meaningfully interpreted. For example, a patient should not be in risk of having his chair bumped, nor should he be expected to work with cold hands. These factors could, respectively, disturb or slow down his work pace and reduce his score.

Occasionally the occupational therapist may be asked for an assessment at short notice. It is then useful to have available a battery of test material, ready for immediate use, from which the most appropriate instruments can be selected for the case in hand.

Reasons for giving tests to assess aptitude or competence in a particular type of work may be any of the following: the patient's wish to try; the psychologist's findings; the occupational therapist's findings; the requirements of the patient's job; the requirements of possible jobs available through the D.R.O.*; or the entry requirements for courses run at Skills Centres or other training establishments.

It is a saving of time if assessment can be made without having to break the work down into its components and it is not even always necessary to strive for maximum performance. If eighteen words per minute will meet the typing requirement of a patient's job and she can maintain accuracy at that speed, this is good enough.

When performance is poor with a cooperative patient working in good conditions, at any type of test, the factors responsible should be identified. Sometimes, the patient himself will know these: fingering difficulty, the result of motor or sensory defect; not seeing well enough, the result of intrinsic defect of vision or poor patient work relationship; lack of facility with the alphabet or lack of concentration. A disabled person may be physically unable to adjust his position to effect a good working relationship with equipment. The equipment must be correctly related to him.

Treatment might improve a function which lowers performance, alternatively the patient might, with practice, learn to function competently in spite of difficulty or disability. When the reason is general lack of aptitude this should not be interpreted as failure on the part of the patient. It is as important to know what sort of work would not be suitable as to know what would.

Examples of tests for competence

(1) *Educational assessment.* Broadly speaking this is assessment of the patient's abilities expressed in words or figures and recorded by pen on paper. The medium of a typewriter may be necessary. Sometimes the level of proficiency in terms of educational standards as such is of value. The occupational therapist should be able to assess the

patient's ability to write English and to spell by giving him standardised examination papers and tests. Such tests for adult patients must not be childish in content, nor should they be marked strictly on school lines. The overall impression of ability and the types of error made are more important than a percentage score. More often the important factor is the patient's ability in relation to known requirements for particular jobs, e.g. fractions, decimals and algebra for radio and television repairs, the 3 R's with emphasis on simple calculations with money for general office routine. Suitable textbooks, simple but adult in content, should be available for the patient who will need further instruction and practice before further testing.

(2) *Clerical assessment* can be broken down into separate items for some of which validated tests are available, i.e. typing, and those who have taken the appropriate training course may use the General Clerical Test (No. 4 above). Standards must be set for routine jobs such as copying lists; adding figures, with or without an adding machine; abstracting information from directories; compiling invoices; filing alphabetically, numerically or by colour, etc. Factors to include in setting such standards should include accuracy, speed and presentation. Where norms for a test are not available, local ones can be established for tentative use, on the basis of the hospital clerical staff performance. Such tests can be graded and the gradings refined and better defined as the test data accumulate.

Additional material which may be useful in assessment.

(1) *Tests for Guidance and Assessment* (GASS tests) published by the National Foundation for Educational Research. These tests were developed for schoolteachers and are also available to occupational therapists.

(2) *A Clerical Assessment* used at the Passmore Edwards Rehabilitation Centre, Clacton.

(3) *Psychological Testing* [9] Anne Anastasi, published by Macmillan. This gives information about the origins of psychological testing, the meaning of standardisation, reliability and validity, norms, and the interpretation of tests.

RELATING ASSESSMENT TO RESETTLEMENT

Successful resettlement is the result of efficient team work, the disablement resettlement officer and the medical social worker discussing the patient with the doctor and the members of his treatment team. The machinery of this will vary. In some hospitals a resettlement clinic is held where the patient and his family are invited to meet the team and together discuss all aspects of the problem. In other centres there are weekly D.R.O.* conferences attended by the occupational therapist where all the patients with resettlement problems are discussed regularly until specific conclusions have been reached. But in all centres informal discussion of the patient should take place as opportunity and need arises. It may fall to the occupational therapist to take the initiative in arranging such discussions where none exist. She may also act as a coordinator in seeing that decisions taken at such a conference are in fact implemented. A comprehensive follow up system is beyond the scope of most hospitals. Some rehabilitation centres and research units have such a system and this is to be applauded. Unless statistical evidence is available it is difficult to establish that the methods employed to assess and resettle patients are efficient. Where no follow up exists the occupational therapist may be the appropriate person to see that the badly disabled patient is given an appointment for review at a clinic, perhaps in six months time, when his medical condition and any problems of social or industrial resettlement can be reconsidered.

Social resettlement is interrelated with industrial resettlement, and an unsuitable home situation may make work impossible. For example, it must be possible to get in and out of the house or flat; it is compulsory for the owner of an electric tricycle to have a garage with charging facilities. Even when these points can be met the distance to travel may be too great. It is unrealistic to expect someone who unavoidably takes a long time getting ready to leave home, to undertake a long journey also. Rehousing which would overcome the relevant problem is rarely possible. For the patient with a family prepared to move or with no family ties, application can be made for accommodation in one of the special centres planned for the disabled where homes or hostels and workshops are in close proximity.

Travelling is an important factor in resettlement. The patient must be able to get to work.

(1) Getting to and from a distant bus stop—this will require stamina.
(2) Negotiating a complicated journey with several changes—this requires both stamina and agility.
(3) Managing the rush hour. If this proves a problem, shift work or night work may be considered.
(4) Where public transport proves impracticable for any of the above reasons, an invalid tricycle may be the answer.
(5) When the patient already has a car, this may need adapting.

Suitable work must be available in the district. There may be nothing the patient could do, for example in a coal-mining area where there is little light work. A patient from a rural area will not be accepted for training as an arc welder if there is no prospect of a job afterwards. In theory moving to a town with a better employment prospect would be advisable, in practice it creates other problems. The salary or wage offered must not only provide for the patient's needs but must be in excess of the benefits drawn while unemployed. Light work is often designated as 'women's work' and paid as such. The ultimate success of holding down a job may be determined by the employer being sympathetic and work colleagues being compatible.

Assessment for Direct Placement

When a patient's physical condition precludes a return to his previous employment, direct placement is the quickest way of resettling him. Whenever possible he should return to alternative employment with his previous employer, who will be more sympathetic to his present and future problems, especially if he has a good work record. Sometimes false hopes are raised at an early stage by the employer's assurance of finding suitable work. When the extent of residual disability becomes apparent this is not possible.

Previous experience or a former skill may be utilised to advantage. For example, a patient with osteoarthritic hips, a bricklayer for thirty years, needs semi-sedentary work, which might be found for him at a builder's merchant, checking materials. His potential for this work could be assessed by the occupational therapist. A patient might have left a job as a switchboard operator to become a travelling representative and many years later have to give that up because he is now wheel-chair bound, although able to drive an invalid tricycle. He might return to switchboard work after a refresher course on modern equipment.

Many patients have no alternative skills to offer and many show no potential for learning. Educational standards are often poor. In addition to such patients who will previously have done labouring or manual jobs, patients who have never worked are referred for assessment. They will all need both general and specific practical assessment. Direct placement will be their only hope of employment for they would qualify for neither an Industrial Rehabilitation Unit nor Skill Centre.

A visit to the patient's firm or to a prospective employer may be helpful. The technician and the medical social worker may be included. The occupational therapist will report on her assessment of the patient verbally, possibly leaving a short report for further consideration. She will list the patient's abilities and personal attributes, his mental and physical limitations. In connection with the latter she may need to check the access to where the patient will be working, the lavatory facilities, canteen facilities and possibly car parking facilities. Should a particular job be available its requirements should be noted in detail so that the patient can be given a practical assessment of his ability to meet them and the problems involved. Such a visit may be particularly valuable when the patient is aphasic or very obviously disabled, for example with a tremor. The occupational therapist will not only speak about the patient's abilities but her enthusiasm may encourage the employer to give the patient a chance. Contacts with local firms over re-settlement of their own employees may lead to help in finding jobs for other patients later.

Resettlement through Special Units

The various facilities offered by the Department of Employment and other bodies for the assessment, training and employment of disabled people are fully described in chapter 4. The assessment undertaken by the occupational therapist will be determined by the resettlement possibilities and her report will vary according to where the patient is being sent and to whom it is written, for example, the disablement resettlement officer or the medical officer of health.

Assessment prior to attending an Industrial Rehabilitation Unit.* In depart-ments where a full assessment is not possible the occupational therapist should identify the patient likely to benefit from an Industrial Rehabilitation Unit.* She will do this by a general assessment, utilising such facilities in her department as are appropriate for the particular patient. The Disablement Resettlement Officer* generally welcomes any information about the patient and will hand this on so that the Industrial Rehabilitation Unit becomes part of a continuous process of resettlement.

Assessment for goverment training or training within industry. Assess-ment for either of the above may be done without going through an industrial rehabilitation unit. Such assessment should be specific to the limited types of training appropriate for the patient. The report should include the reasons for advocating training and how the patient fulfils the basic physical and educational requirements of training indicated by the Department of Employment and Productivity or laid down by the employer.

Referral to sheltered workshops and other centres. The assessment of the patient may show that he is only likely to manage some form of sheltered employment or occupation. A report detailing what he can and cannot manage to do will be of help not only to those planning the next stage, but as a yardstick to measure further improvement.

Job Analysis

This is the counterpart of work assessment but there is no readily available reference book, which meets the needs of occupational therapists. D.R.O.s* have two manuals: (*a*) *Classification of Occupations and Directory of Occupa-tional Titles**, which lists jobs by name and itemizes the processes involved; (*b*) *Job Information Manual** which gives cross references to jobs with different titles but for which skills required are much the same. Neither touches on functional aspects. The occupational therapist needs a breakdown of the physical demands and personality requirements for jobs of different kinds—something to which she can refer when planning an assessment programme for a patient, and refer to again when considering the results of that assessment. With its help she could form an opinion on the patient's work prospects with more assurance.

In the absence of any such material department staff can gradually collect information for their own use. They can talk to patients, whose first-hand experience is invaluable, even if some of them have to be encouraged to give the relevant information. Occupational therapists can make opportunities for watching people at work, and can analyse how the work is done. There are some forms of work which they try out for themselves, and they can also arrange to consult employers and supervisors.

In the early stages it is probably best not to have a structured form, but to record actual findings under general broad headings. The amount of information under any one heading could vary markedly from job to job. This would indicate the relative importance of different aspects in each, e.g. manual skills or personal qualities, etc. Later it might be worth developing different forms for different types of work, more applicable to local requirements, i.e. for work of different types, such as labouring, skilled trades and sedentary occupations, etc. The factor of greatest overall importance is that the material collected should be presented in such a way that any occupational therapist will find it understandable and useful, remembering always that the character of jobs can change and that no home-made reference file on such a topic can be comprehensive.

Headings on a form might include the samples shown below. The findings entered here are relevant to (*a*) a *lorry driver* and (*b*) a *shop assistant*.

(1) *Work Environment.*
   (*a*) Out in all weathers.
   (*b*) Indoors, and generally good.

(2) *Hours of Work.*
   (*a*) Variable, day or night, i.e. anti-social.
   (*b*) Regular. Part-time sometimes available. Rush hour travel.

(3) *Contacts at Work.*
   (*a*) Sometimes alone: sometimes with a mate: at stops en route.
   (*b*) With fellow workers, supervisors, customers, etc. Rarely alone.

(4) *Personality Requirements.*
   (*a*) To be reliable, level-headed and self-reliant.
   (*b*) To be honest, conscientious, equable, friendly, polite and patient. Appreciative of the need for high standards in personal appearance.

(5) *Routine Physical Demands.*

   (*a*) Lifting for loading/unloading: generally physically fit and with good stamina.

   (*b*) Stamina for standing for long hours. Ability to handle goods safely.

(6) *Special Skills Needed.*

   (*a*) Driving (an appropriate licence).

   (*b*) Sometimes lifting, carrying, packing. Dexterity to use cash registers and/or to make quick monetary calculations.

(7) *Prospects for Advancement.*

   (*a*) None.

   (*b*) Good.

(8) *Contra-indications for the job.*

   (*a*) Black-outs, intemperance, history of gastric or duodenal ulcers.

   (*b*) Defective hearing, eyesight or speech, severe enough to cause anxiety or embarrassment.

REFERENCES AND RECOMMENDED FURTHER READING

1. **Activities of Daily Living**
Bramwell Jones, S. (1969) The household needs of the disabled. (A guide to the selection of furniture and equipment). *Br. Hosp. J. soc. Serv. Rev.*
Collins, D. W. (1967) New developments in aids and prostheses. *Rehabilitation.* (Re P.I.L.O.T. aids*.)
Eckhardt, M. E., *Homemaking for the Handicapped*, New York, 1966.
Goldsmith, S., *Designing for the Disabled*, London, 1967.
Hart Wheeler, V., *Planning Kitchens for the Handicapped Homemaker*, monograph XXVII, New York Medical Center for Rehabilitation.
Howie, P. M., *A Pilot Study of Disabled Housewives in Their Kitchens*, London, 1968.
Jay, P., Walker, E. & Ellison, A., *Help Yourselves*, London, 1972.
Jay, P., *Coping with Disablement*, Consumer's Association, London, 1974.
Kamenetz, H. L., *The Wheelchair Book, Mobility for the Disabled*, U.S.A., 1969.
Lawton Buchwald, E., et al., *Physical Rehabilitation for Daily Living*, New York and London, 1952.
Lawton Buchwald, E., *Activities of Daily Living for Physical Rehabilitation*, New York and London, 1963.
Lowman, E. & Rusk, H., *Self Help Devices*, Institute of Physical Medicine and Rehabilitation. Part I, 1962; Part II, 1963.
Maling, R. G. (1968) Control in severe disability. *Rehabilitation.* (Re Possum aids*).
McLurg Anderson, T., *Housework with Ease*. Scottish Council of Physical Recreation.
Nichols, P., *Living with Handicap*, London, 1974.
Nichols, R. J. R., Hollings, E. M. & Wilshere, E. R., *Equipment for the Disabled*, Horsham, 1974.
Rogers, X. & Stevens, B. (1960) Dressmaking for the disabled. *Occ. Ther.*
Rusk, H. A., *Living with a Disability*, New York and London, 1953.
Walter, F., *An Introduction to Domestic Design for the Disabled*, London, 1968.
And see:
Clothing Fastenings for the Handicapped and Disabled. D.L.F.*, London, 1968.
And list of publications on clothing for the disabled, D.L.F.*, London.

Lord Snowdon's Chairmobile. *Occ. Ther.*, 35, no. 6, 1972.
Stand-up wheelchair. *Occ. Ther.*, 35, no. 8, 1972.

General

Belbin, E., *Problems in Adult Training*, London, 1972.
Bradley, W. H., *Proceedings of a Symposium on the Disabled Young Adult.*
National Fund for Research into Crippling Diseases*, 1967.
Nichols, P. J. R. & Bradley, W. H., *Proceedings of a Symposium on the Motivation of the Physically Disabled*, National Fund for Research into Crippling Diseases*, 1968.

2. See *Gas Aids for the Disabled*, issued by British Gas, and *Electric Aids for the Disabled*, issued by the Electricity Council.
3. See this book, chapter 21.
4. See this book, chapter 4.
Vernon, P. E., *Personality Tests and Assessment.* London, 1957.
Rehabilitation of the Injured Workman. Study Course I. Third International Congress W.F.O.T.*, 1962.
Work Adjustment as a Function of Occupational Therapy. Study Course V. Third International Congress W.F.O.T.*, 1962.
5. There may be other courses available to occupational therapists, i.e. those on which personnel officers are trained to use the same tests.
6. A.H.=A.W. Heim, author.
7. Published by the National Foundation for Education Research Publishing Co.*, 2 Jennings Buildings, Slough, Berks SL4 1QS.
8. Granada Publishing, Park Street, St Albans, Herts. Can be purchased from Dillon's University Bookshop, 1 Malet Street, London WC1 or other university bookshops.
9. See General Bibliography, p. 453.
* See *Glossary*, pp. 454-6.

CHAPTER 8

Occupational Therapy for the Upper Limb

The hands are positioned for use by movement of the arms and what the hands do determines the pattern of arm and shoulder girdle movements, their direction, range and strength. For example, when tucking a shirt into the back of trousers or a skirt with an up and down movement of the hand, the shoulder is extended and internally rotated. For choice the hands are used in front of the body and at a comfortable distance from it, where they are easily seen and controlled. Consequently the arms are below shoulder level and the shoulder and elbow joints are moving through a limited range. Although everyone has some regular need to reach up, if only to take off a pullover or open a window, relatively few have to use force or to work overhead for long periods. The arms, as distinct from the hands, develop their appropriate skills too. Shoe cleaning is a good example. Try it using the 'wrong hand': the awkwardness is not in holding the brush.

The dominant hand is used for holding implements of all kinds and for actions that need fine finger movements. The non-dominant hand reaches for materials and acts as a stabiliser. But even when the hand is used for precision work the muscles of the shoulder girdle, upper arm and forearm all come into play, if intermittently, to effect change of position and placement, although the movement may be minimal.

Principles of Assessment

Isolated movements are rare when using the upper limb. Assessment therefore must be of the whole limb. This will include assessment of anatomical function in terms of range, strength and control, and of purposeful use, such as opening a door, handling a newspaper or writing. Findings are recorded and also, if identified, the reasons for poor performance. These can usefully include the patient's contribution. Treatment is planned on these findings.

The therapist must know exactly what she is looking for. Functional achievement and anatomical function are not synonymous. While it is important to know if the patient can reach the back of his neck, ability to do this does not prove that he can abduct and externally rotate his shoulder. Clear instructions must be given if this is the movement to be assessed. The therapist will stand in front of the patient with her back to him and demonstrating on herself, say 'lift your elbow out from your side and reach down between your shoulders as far as you can with your middle finger'. She can then mark the spot on the patient's back with her finger and say 'now try it with your other hand' and note the difference in achievement. If this action is performed easily there will be no need to test elbow flexion, but if it is not, and if limitation of the elbow is thought to be the reason, flexion should be tested. Again, a target gives incentive; 'touch your shoulder with your fingers' rather than 'bend your elbow'.

The therapist can help the patient to make his best effort to supinate and pronate by standing in front of him and carrying out the movements herself as he tries to do them: 'bend your elbows, tuck them into your sides and pull them well back. Now turn your palms *up*. Keep your elbows in and turn your palms *down*.' There should be no need to handle the patient.

Initially hand function is assessed by testing the ability to close and open a fist. The tips of the fingers are hidden on the palmar crease, the knuckles fully flexed, the index at 90° and the little finger at approximately 100°, so giving a markedly arched and sloping line. The thumb, including the ball, is wrapped round the closed fingers with its tip bent against the middle phalanx of the middle finger, the wrist cocked back. Coordination is noted too, the finger tips coming together and bending towards the palm, simultaneously with the thumb moving out from the palm and across it, to enclose the fingers at the moment they are maximally flexed. As with other tests, demonstration may be essential and the therapist must be able to do this in slow motion with either hand, pointing out each special feature. The patient may need reassurance that it is normal for the little finger to bend towards the ball of the thumb. This is because of the mobility of the fifth metacarpal bone which moves forward when the metacarpo-phalangeal joint is flexed, so cupping the palm. Demonstration of opening a fist draws attention to controlled flexion of the wrist as fingers and thumb extend and abduct as widely as possible. If the patient closes and opens his fist well, showing all the above features, there is no need to test the components of the action. If there is deficit it must be followed up, assessed and recorded. He must be shown first to bend the finger tips down towards, or to touch, the base of the fingers while keeping the palm flat and uncreased. Then he must bend the palm and swing the tips of all four fingers towards the ball of the thumb, touching it if possible.

Strength of cylinder grip can be tested by asking the patient to grasp the therapist's wrist. Hand shaking is contra-indicated because the therapist may hurt the patient, or vice versa. Strength of pinch grip can be tested by the patient trying to prevent the therapist's hooked index finger from breaking out of the ring made by pressure of his thumb tip against the tips of his index and middle fingers, also by asking the patient to pinch grip, tripod pinch or key grip a piece of card which the therapist then tries to pull away.

There can be no rigid rules as to the order in which assessment is made, but with some patients it can be completed quickly by direct methods. With others only a part can be covered at the first interview. The patient's reaction to it forms part of the total assessment of him as an individual and this will influence his treatment plan.

Planning Treatment

In deciding on the form and content of the treatment plan most likely to meet the patient's needs it helps to clarify aims if suggestions can be written down with reasons for their choice, for example, low level work to encourage gravity assisted movement of the shoulder, or playing with a yo-yo to encourage normal coordination of hand and wrist.

However local the dysfunction, treatment should, if time permits, include some general use of the whole limb. To ensure that this continues throughout the day the therapist will emphasise the importance of using the hand or arm normally, reaching out to pick things up, reaching up to switch on lights and reaching down to get money out of a pocket, also using it for dressing, washing, feeding, etc. When the hand itself is the injured part the patient can be encouraged to keep his other hand in his pocket, until the habit of using the injured one is re-established. With improvement of function the general activity of the treatment session will be brought more into line with the patient's normal activities of job and home. Sometimes there will be opportunity and incentive for him to take over responsibility for this himself, e.g. by turning out and painting his garden shed.

The Shoulder and Shoulder Girdle

The shoulder girdle comes into action as soon as there is appreciable movement of the shoulder joint, and its muscles lose strength when function of the shoulder joint is impaired. A professional or white-collar worker will not be aware of this unless through his recreational interests. Manual workers will be. Pushing, pulling, 'humping', stacking, pickaxing, scaffold erecting, and bill posting all demand strong hands, arms, and shoulder girdles. To strengthen these muscles, and until such time as the patient is fit to try something more precisely simulating his job, he will be given progressively resisted arm work of any kind, resisted by the materials he must lift or shape, by the weight of tools he must control, or by such measures as springs.

Shoulder movements which are difficult for all patients are antigravity movements, away from the body and above shoulder level, i.e. the ones least used normally. In all of them both the shoulder joint and the shoulder girdle are involved and when the shoulder joint is stiff or its muscles are weak, the shoulder girdle moves excessively to compensate. The patient has real difficulty in preventing this. The therapist must direct the patient's thinking away from his shoulder and towards his hand, towards moving it outwards or sideways and on letting his elbow come away from his side as he does so. These movements are helped by leaning slightly 'into' the movement, i.e. towards the side of the moving arm. This lowers the point of the shoulder and discourages the shrugging movement of the shoulder girdle which raises it. To encourage this 'leaning' action, placement of the patient's work or his placement in relation to apparatus needs to be planned carefully. For elevation, which is the patient's greatest difficulty, it is important to think of the two movements which comprise it, first, abduction through slight flexion and with the elbow extended no more than a right angle. The hand should 'gain' on the elbow so that it is leading at the horizontal level. In doing this, external rotation has been initiated and must be continued as the hand reaches up vertically, the elbow straightens and the upper arm moves towards the side of the head. Full elevation is not an easy target for occupational therapy although it should be tested by the therapist in each patient with a stiff shoulder or hand. Treatment is still valuable although the activity may require less than full range. If the components of the movement, i.e. abduction and external rotation, and strength of the deltoid muscle, can be improved, elevation will improve.

Patients sent for treatment with loss of shoulder function are likely to fall into one of the following categories.

(1) Those with pain following trauma or a frozen shoulder who are unable to abduct the arm beyond 45°. The hemiplegic patient can, for treatment purposes, be included in this group.

(2) Those with full passive range but a painful arc of movement between 60° and 100° of abduction. This is the result of soft tissue injury.

(3) Those with some limitation of movement and some discomfort at the extremes of their range but no acute pain, for example, after capsulitis, dislocation of the shoulder, fracture of the shaft of the humerus.

(4) Those with deltoid weakness. The muscle quickly loses power with disuse of the limb for any reason. It is not uncommonly paralysed in dislocation of the shoulder, together with the external rotators.

Aims of treatment for patients with pain. First, pain must be avoided. Therefore the patient must not be given any activity which could cause him to move into the painful range. This means, too, that he must not be expected to put his tools away on high shelves or to hang up his jacket on a high peg. Second, muscle power in the limb, including the shoulder girdle, must be maintained by any activity wholly within the pain free range.

This is especially important for men who must ultimately go back to heavy work. It is possible to saw and to do routine woodwork jobs entirely without discomfort while being unable to abduct beyond 45°. This is reassuring for the patient and if his job requires no more of him than his treatment does, he may feel confident enough to return to it.

Aims of treatment for patients with limitation of movement but not acute pain are to increase range of movement and to strengthen the limb for its normal role at home and at work. An example of treatment for a housewife with limited elevation following a fracture of the humerus is described below.

Activity. Gentle rhythmical mobilisation in abduction by polishing a table top from a sitting position.

Action. Holding the polishing cloth, she moves her hand in clockwise circles of varying size, covering as large an area as possible from the centre line of her body as far as possible to the right. The therapist will teach her how to emphasise an easy, smooth rhythm with the arm and body moving together.

Treatment points

(1) The table top will be taking part of the weight of her arm.
(2) Emphasis on 'out and round' will encourage her to 'lean into the movement'.
(3) At moments when her elbow is straight she may be achieving abduction approximately to shoulder height.
(4) The pattern of the movement allows for contraction of anterior, middle and posterior fibres of the deltoid.
(5) The circular action ensures that the point of stretch and discomfort will soon be passed.
(6) The patient can do this usefully at home once she has demonstrated an understanding of the treatment aim and how to practise.

Gravity can assist movement of the shoulder joint when range is restricted and muscle power is inadequate to mobilise it. Any activity for which the patient leans forward from his hips will bring it into play, for example working at floor level while kneeling, or at knee level while standing with feet apart and knees pliable. Some housewives still polish their floors by hand, home dressmakers cut out on the floor, painters kneel to paint skirting boards and logs are sawn on sawing horses. Side to side movement is the most beneficial for it encourages abduction, but any movement that can be carried out free from tension, in however small a range and in whatever direction, is helpful. It may be inappropriate to ask a patient to work from such positions when almost the same result is achieved by using a downward sloping work top. The central section of a woodwork bench can be made adjustable for this, with the angle variable and including an upward slope (see Plates 19 and 20). For the initial warming up period of mobilising, sanding on a downward surface is excellent. By trying to reach as far as possible and by rotating the trunk in doing so, flexion becomes abduction, sometimes without the patient realising it. The deck game of shuffleboard is good treatment too. With incentive to push the disc a long way, the player instinctively leans down low and there is a good range of elevation through flexion. Using a broom can give a somewhat similar result and a housewife can be shown how to do this to best advantage.

Aim of treatment when there has been deltoid weakness. The aim is to strengthen the muscle as recovery takes place. To eliminate gravity, the physiotherapist treats her patient lying down. The occupational therapist must use other means of giving assistance, remembering always that the patient will be able to lift his bent arm from his side before he can lift a straight arm, and will be able to hold it in abduction before he can abduct it from his side. When there is also weakness of the external rotators the normal degree of rotation must be assured as the arm is assisted into abduction. This must always be such that flexion of the elbow brings the hand up to the mouth.

The Elbow

All treatment after injury to the joint or near it is undertaken with care. Occupational therapy is rarely prescribed at the stage when activity must be restricted to mid range of elbow movement. If it is, use of the hand involving predominantly rotation of the forearm, as in simple model making, light assembly, solo card games, or painting small articles, is suitable treatment. When resting, the elbow must be flexed and the patient should wear a collar and cuff sling between treatments. Only when this is discarded can treatment be progressed in range or vigour. There must never be increase of extension at the expense of flexion, and regular checks must be made. The patient must be told not to carry heavy loads to try to straighten the arm.

Treatment following immobilisation for injury elsewhere in the arm can be as vigorous as the injury permits. The extremes of flexion and extension are difficult to achieve by occupational therapy with general work, for they rarely occcur in routine daily activities. Flexion brings the hand to the shoulder and only by hand to shoulder movement can full range be achieved. Apparatus can be adapted mechanically so that the movements are isolated, and the range and resistance predetermined. It is a matter of opinion as to which gives the greater benefit, isolated work for extremes of movement or general free activity moving in normal working range with its usual associates.

The Forearm

In turning the palm of the hand up or down in normal use, the rotating action of the forearm is usually supplemented by adduction or abduction of the shoulder. It must therefore be expected that the patient who has limited forearm rotation will compensate by excessive shoulder movement. It is also normal to move the elbow in coordination with the forearm, extension as the hand reaches forward in pronation to pick up a biscuit, and flexion as it supinates to reach the mouth. If there is limitation, lack of supination is the greater disability, for the body obstructs the shoulder adduction which is needed in compensation. To strengthen the supinators or pronators it is not necessary to isolate movement of the forearm. The muscles will be working with any strong effort to twist the hand to right or left whether the forearm rotates or not, and regardless of any movement which occurs elsewhere. In contrast, for mobilisation, it is necessary to help the patient to isolate the movement. The best starting position is the one in which assessment of range will be made, elbow tucked in to the side to discourage abduction of the arm, well bent and pulled back to discourage adduction through flexion. Activities in this position can be used until the patient has the feeling of the movements which are required and as a means of teaching him how to practise at home. Solomon's knotting can be successful if a careful breakdown of the method is made, as is turning over cards from a pack when playing patience. Once there is the feeling, greater freedom can be allowed but it is wise to choose activities in which the elbow is bent.

In many departments, patients who have forearm or full-length arm plasters following injury are not sent for treatment until the plaster is off, if then. With a fracture at the wrist, if the position during immobilisation has been a good functional one and the fingers have been kept fully mobile, there may be no need for occupational therapy. When a patient is sent for treatment while still in plaster it is likely to be because he has stiff fingers. Between treatments the patient should try to bend the fingers so that the tips touch the hand where the plaster ends at the palmar crease and then to swing them over to reach as far down the plaster in the palm as possible. If the fifth metacarpo-phalangeal joint is restricted by the plaster it should be freed. Some surgeons insist on their patients wearing a collar and cuff while in plaster.

A Colles fracture may be immobilised with the wrist in flexion, rendering use of the hand difficult, and both the fingers and the shoulder may be stiff in consequence. Occupational therapy will then be needed when the plaster is removed, especially as this is predominantly a woman's fracture and someone else may have taken over the domestic duties. The first aim of treatment is to re-educate the coordination of extending the wrist as the hand closes to grasp. The feeling of the movement must be re-learned. Initially it will be difficult, and often the joints are painful. The housewife can try to shine up the outside of saucepans, keeping her palm and fingers in contact while moving the hand forward and back rhythmically. She can be given a plastic sponge, 4 inches by 3 inches, or a large face flannel; after soaking it in warm water she must try, without help from the other hand, to enclose it wholly before squeezing the water out, extending her wrist as she does so. She can also be encouraged to wash out anything that must be squeezed. All these activities can be continued at home. She may not yet have tried to write. The correct position encourages wrist extension and this is good treatment. Many women enjoy learning some woodwork and with this there is scope for treating the shoulder, forearm and hand simultaneously.

The Hand

One speaks of someone 'having a good grasp of his subject'. One is urged 'to get to grips with a situation'. So have thought and the movement of the hand been brought together in common parlance. Only by so linking them together in treatment can a successful result be attained. Grasp, or grip, is but one function of the hand. Release is almost as important. So is appreciation of shape and texture; and not only for present advantage. Memory is made more vivid by remembering the feeling of things touched. Hands also express personality, thought and emotion. A patient may be greatly shocked by injury to his hand, the more so if there is disfigurement, and his instinct will then be to hide it. He must learn that the more naturally the hand is used the less it will appear disfigured to himself or to others. He must be given encouragement and opportunity to join in socialising activities, to use public transport, to go to the shops and to the pub. It may be of help when digits have been amputated, to provide a glove padded and wired to simulate the missing fingers in slight flexion.

Immobilisation following trauma should always be minimal, in extent and in duration. If the whole hand is implicated, and unless there are contra-indications, it will be held in the position reached by the initial movement towards closing the fist from full extension and abduction, i.e. the fingertips and the tip of the thumb moving towards each other as if to fit round a large grapefruit, so maintaining the arch across the palm and the web space between the thumb and index finger. The wrist will be extended approximately 10° above the straight position. Subsequent restoration of function is easiest from this position. Gentle active movement of the digits is encouraged at once in most cases. The shoulder must be kept mobile while the hand is out of action, for it has temporarily lost its incentive to move spontaneously. Exercising the shoulder will also help to reduce or to prevent oedema in the hand. With severe lesions the sooner intensive and comprehensive treatment can be started the better the prognosis. If this is not available at the local hospital the patient should be sent to a special unit, for once a hand is allowed to become stiff and the muscles to atrophy it may never regain normal function.

As in all treatment planning, the total demands of the patient's job must be known, for example if he stands and must be active on his legs when at work, his treatment should not force him to sit. The therapist must appreciate the range of movement required of the different digits in using normal grips and the factors which will prevent efficiency in using them. This is based on knowledge of anatomy and kinesiology but above all on practical work and acute observation of skilled craftsmen. The hand itself is used as a power tool and as a precision instrument, and everyone has need of it in both roles. Often too little attention is given to the function of the little finger. When this lacks mobility it is a serious handicap. In the dominant hand it is largely responsible for stability of grip, as on a dinner knife or screwdriver, and unless mobile it can be an inconvenience when writing.

Instead of the aimless movements thought by many patients to be beneficial exercise between treatments, they should try to close and open a fist, having been taught exactly what to aim for. Another good exercise is to crumple a large sheet of newspaper, starting at one corner and continuing until it is reduced to a ball in the hand. Yet another is to dip the hand in water, then place the palm on a plate of dry lentils and rub them off with the thumb and fingers of the same hand.

The finger flexors are normally strong enough to hold the weight of the body against gravity, but strength is not normally required in the extensors. They prepare the hand for picking things up, by extending and abducting the fingers and thumb for large objects or by keeping the digits on the ulnar side of the hand out of the way when precision grip is used. Because of inability to extend the metacarpo-phalangeal joints of the ring and little fingers, the arthritic patient finds himself trying to pick up with the hand fully pronated and the object out of sight. In some jobs the flat of the hand is used; the warehouseman, for example, who pushes bales, or the laundry hand who must be able to smooth out creases. These actions will not strengthen the extensors for it is the flexors that work in pushing or pressing down even when the fingers are extended.

The thumb is said to be 50 per cent of the functional value of the hand. Essentials for its efficient use are as follows:

(1) Full mobility of the ball, so that it can be in the same plane as the palm for a flat hand with wide span, and can also be swung forward and across the palm, to be at right angles with it for opposition to the fingers.

(2) 90° flexion of the tip, so that small things can be picked up from a flat surface.

(3) Strength in the related muscles.

The thumb is used in all the standard grips except one. In the hook grip it is extended as in the flat hand, to be out of the way, e.g. in carrying a sheet of metal. It is rarely used in isolation. (See Plates 7–12.)

Treatment of Hand Injuries

Treatment of specific injuries to the hand is discussed in detail in various other books (see pp. 174-5). Therefore only general principles of treatment are considered here.

Psychological Effects

There is frequently severe personality upset and dissociation with the injured hand, particularly when this is the dominant one. The patient fatigues quickly and this is probably more psychological than physical. A rapid change of work will be needed, plus constant supervision and encouragement to make sure the hand is used, initially, in any way that is possible. This is the most important factor in treatment. A further psychological problem occurs when the patient, often subconsciously, avoids using his hand because a compensation case is pending. If he continues to do this he may never regain maximal functional ability and this should be made clear to him. The therapist may need to help the patient to overcome his fear of moving machinery, electricity or whatever it was that caused his accident. This may prove impossible and resettlement in alternative work will then be necessary.

Activities of Daily Living

Problems of self care are given priority. Some will be temporary but unless there are contra-indications any patient unable to wash, dress and use his knife, fork or spoon should be helped to do so. Grip may be inadequate to control tooth brush, razor, hair brush or pen. Handles may need to be adapted, with care to make them as unobtrusive as possible, but as function improves normal grip will be expected to take over. Buttons, usually done up with the injured hand, may be done by the other one, but an attempt should be made with the injured hand.

Oedema

If possible this should not be allowed to develop. When it is present or likely to occur the hand should work in elevation. Active movement stimulates circulation and is beneficial. Static muscle work impedes it and is contra-indicated. Gentle grip and release action on an overhead lever for drilling (Plates 5 and 6) fulfils both the need for elevation and for movement. (See p. 96.)

Conditions of the Skin

The condition of the skin and any sensory loss should be checked before treatment is begun. Wounds on the dorsum may be opened by movement, and on the palmar surface may be 'traumatised' by contact with tools or materials. Because early mobility is of prime importance a delay in healing is justifiable, but if a small wound is opening into a larger one medical advice must be sought. A crepe bandage mitten will protect the palm, and tubigauze, if necessary covered with a Durex fingerstall, will protect a finger. *Scar tissue* interferes with the elasticity of the skin and may tether it to underlying structures, for example scarring on the dorsum can prevent metacarpo-phalangeal joint flexion. Softening of the scar tissue is the concern of the physiotherapist. *Defective sensation* is discussed on p. 97: final treatment must include *skin toughening*, especially when the patient is a manual worker.

Position of the Wrist Joint

It is impossible to grip with the wrist in flexion and therefore the optimum position is slight extension. If necessary, some form of cock-up splint should be provided. For a normal pattern of picking up and release the wrist is in slight flexion and this should be the secondary aim. Flexion is also needed in many personal activities, particularly washing and dressing.

Developing Span, and Strengthening the Long Extensors

A good span is important because it is difficult to pick up an object if the hand cannot spread over or encircle it first. The initial aim is to increase the thumb web, that is the distance between the metacarpo-phalangeal heads of thumb and index finger and if possible to bring the thumb into opposition, then to increase the web between the little and ring fingers because abduction of the little finger will increase the total span.

Treatment activities will include encouragement of a large encircling grip by picking up big objects, such as boxes or the contents of the store cupboard. Where there is limitation of movement, pressing down with the hand to print lino blocks, holding a rule down while cutting along its edge through card or leather, or stabilising wood on a bicycle fretsaw, will stretch tight structures. If, after tendon repair or recovery from a radial nerve lesion, strengthening is needed, the extensor muscles should be used in their normal capacity, and the normal controlledflexion of the wrist should be encouraged as the fingers are extended. String figures, such as cat's cradles, or the game of Jacks, both require strong extension of the metacarpo-phalangeal joints, so do any games at which there must be forceful release, such as Tenni-quoits or Hoopla. Extensors of the thumb are used strongly in cutting with tailors' scissors and with the non-dominant hand supporting a billiard cue.

Increasing Metacarpo-phalangeal Joint Flexion

This is necessary for all grips except hook grip. Precision pinch grip, tip of thumb to tip of index finger, is impossible unless the index finger is mobile at the metacarpo-phalangeal joint. When this joint is stiff the thumb will pinch in adduction instead of opposition and this will not serve the same purpose. Small tool grip relies on the mobility and strength of the ring and little fingers. The latter is not within the patient's sight and it can get forgotten.

Treatment activities include any pulling action with *palmar grip*, such as cross-cut sawing, work on a bench drill, or any squeezing action as in hand blow football. The palm must remain in contact and the wrist be extended throughout. Metacarpo-phalangeal joint flexion is also essential when exerting pressure between an opposed straight thumb and fingers with minimal interphalangeal joint flexion, as in picking up draughts or $2\frac{1}{2}$ inch wide components for assembly work, holding a paint brush or the mesh stick for netting, pulling up clay to make a pot. By substituting a handle $1\frac{1}{2}$ inches long for the normal one on a plane, or attaching one vertically to a polishing block, the little and ring fingers are responsible for the grip. This is also ensured by fixing a disc guard $1\frac{1}{2}$ inches from the end of the lever of a bench drill. To isolate responsibility to the index and middle fingers, the guard can be similarly fixed to a lever specially made with a crook end.

Increasing Proximal and Terminal Interphalangeal Joint Flexion

This movement occurs in all digits in conjunction with metacarpo-phalangeal joint flexion in cylinder grip, and in all but the index finger in small tool grip. There is partial flexion of the joints of the index finger and thumb during precision work. It occurs in isolation in span and is solely responsible for hook grip. This is concerned with carrying shopping bags, buckets or books rather than 'doing', and the thumb is not involved. To mobilise these joints it may be necessary to block or immobilise the wrist and metacarpo-phalangeal joints during treatment. The flexors will act on the most mobile joints and when the wrist and metacarpo-phalangeal joints are flexed it is impossible to flex fully the interphalangeal joints as the travel of the extensor tendon will have been used up.

Treatment activities include many of those used for metacarpo-phalangeal joint flexion with palmar grip but by positioning the tool in the hand to use hook grip instead. Other activities using this grip are holding a dowel and using it either to work an adding machine or with an attached rubber stamp, cutting by pulling the knife towards the body, using pliers or secateurs with a quick release spring, using spanners, peeling potatoes, whittling wood with a penknife, and picking up playing cards by hooking the finger tips underneath one side while stabilising the opposite side with an opposing thumb.

Re-education of Pinch Grip

This grip may be a light picking up action, thumb tip to index tip; it may be a stronger picking up action, a tripod or three jaw chuck movement with thumb, index and middle finger; or it may be the more powerful key pinch between the thumb and the lateral side of the index finger. The first dorsal interosseus muscle is largely responsible for the stability of the metacarpophalangeal joint of the index finger in the action of pinch grip, especially of the key pinch. If there is ulnar deviation this muscle cannot work strongly, but tripod pinch will partly overcome this.

Treatment will include activities involving putting things into small holes and taking them out, picking up and holding small objects by hand or with tweezers, as in printing, screwing on nuts or bottle tops, using paper clips, folding and tearing paper, paper sculpture, clay modelling, holding the mesh stick when netting, threading beads, writing, holding a cork dipped in bath brick to clean knives, twisting rush for seating, and hand sewing, especially saddle stitch using a leather clamp.

Re-education of Power Grip

Grips vary according to the article to be held and the purpose to which this will be put. In *small tool grip* the index finger stabilises and helps to give direction to the movement, the ring and little fingers provide the main gripping power and the wrist is slightly ulnar deviated, as in using a knife, fork or screwdriver. This is not always a powerful grip, for example, in using a pin hammer, but it may need strength, as in cutting hide. In *light cylinder grip* all the fingers and the thumb wrap round the handle and hold it against the palm. The wrist is in slight radial deviation, as it holds the tool. In action, for example in hammering, there will be lateral wrist movement and elbow movement. This is a more powerful grip but it is possible with some limitation of flexion as in osteoarthritis. In *heavy cylinder grip* the fingers wrap round the handle and the thumb grips on to the index finger, as in wielding a pick axe or pulling up on a bus rail. This is the most powerful grip; the wrist and the hand or hands become 'part' of the tool, the shoulders and elbows being largely responsible for bringing it into action. Grip is relaxed slightly as heavy impact occurs.

Re-education of grip will not be achieved when body weight or shoulder and elbow work are providing the main power, as for example using a rip saw with a sawing horse. But in a pulling action, as in cross cut sawing, the muscles concerned with grip must do the work. Active gripping will be provided by a rachet release mechanism on a lever handle. The resistance can be regulated mechanically, because the effort is not continuous this is suitable for repetition over a period of time. Continuous grip and release is required with metal snips; these must be held in the hand, not in a vice. The resistance is regulated by the density of the material being cut, but greater stamina is required and within a given period the muscles will be doing more work. Metal bending provides good static gripping exercise, but body weight tends to undo the grip. Wedging clay provides both gripping action in gathering up the clay and forceful release action in throwing it down.

Work for Full Finger Extension and a Flat Hand

A stiff flexed finger will be knocked constantly. In some jobs it can be a hazard and may in the last resort need amputation. A flat hand is necessary to take anything out of a pocket and it is also important in certain jobs, for example, the electrician who needs to get his hand in narrow spaces between wiring.

To begin with, assistance will be needed as the comparatively weak finger extensors will be unable to overcome the joint stiffness or contracture, for example, sanding or polishing, with the injured hand on a block with a convex surface and the uninjured hand pressing down on the contracted joints. Night splintage will be needed to maintain any improvement. As range increases this must be used actively during treatment. Care must be taken to avoid hyper-extension of the metacarpo-phalangeal joints when extending the interphalangeal joints.

Sensory Re-education

Compensation for sensory loss is possible if there is some remaining sensation. The patient must learn to use the eyes instead, or to feel with a different part of the hand, for example, using the ring finger instead of the index in a median nerve lesion. It is important to know the prognosis for recovery. With poor sensation in only one digit the patient will automatically use the other fingers, but if several digits are affected sensory re-education is very necessary.

Treatment activities must be given on an individual basis. The therapist will try to re-educate stereognosis by, for example, getting the patient to handle coins, small objects such as pins and paper clips, and different materials without looking at them. When there is sensory loss activities of daily living and work activities may present problems which will need attention. (See p. 97.)

Relating Treatment to the Patient's Work

Treatment is aimed not only at achieving a maximally functional hand in general terms, but one which enables the patient to return to his particular job, for example, a touch typist may be incapacitated because she has residual stiffness in one little finger. A watchmaker who has lost the terminal joint of his thumb, although regaining full movement and strength, may still be too clumsy and slow because he lacks a thumb nail and a terminal joint and will therefore benefit from pollicisation. Careful study of the patient's job will be needed to assess his particular difficulties and to explore ways of overcoming them.

Limited Aims of Treatment when there is Gross Destruction

When there is inability to gain opposition of the thumb because of lack of abduction, try to get pinch grip against the proximal interphalangeal joint of the index finger, by working for thumb extension and adduction.

When the metacarpo-phalangeal joints are fixed, work for interphalangeal joint movement.

When there is fixed flexion of the proximal interphalangeal joints, try to get hyper-extension of metacarpo-phalangeal joints to bring the finger tips into the flat hand position.

Try to use any sensory area to the best advantage.

Assessment for Reconstruction

Assess function in relation to A.D.L.*, work and recreation. Find out what tasks cannot be done and why they cannot be done. Refer this information back to the patient's surgeon and with his help, think in terms of aids and prostheses which could be of value.

Media of Treatment

Because the hand is an undifferentiated instrument which is used in many ways, unlike the foot, which is specialised and consequently easier to re-educate, treatment must be planned to give a rapid change of occupation. This is very necessary to avoid fatigue. It is also important in teaching the patient to use the correct pattern of movement at all times, not just on one piece of apparatus during treatment. The occupational therapist must have a battery of activities from which she can select a suitable programme.

Activities which Guarantee a Particular Action

Ways in which this can be done include the following:

Choosing an activity which can only be done in one way, for example when gripping an object held in the palm, the metacarpo-phalangeal joints must flex.

Positioning the work in relation to the patient, for example placing a box of components on a shelf above shoulder height so that the patient must stretch forward and flex the wrist to take them out.

Teaching the patient to perform a simple repetitive action in the desired way, for example picking up coloured clothes pegs and placing them round a painted wooden cut out to make an Indian head dress, using either key grip or precision pinch as required.

Isolating a movement, for example making a splint to block the metacarpo-phalangeal joint of the thumb and so encourage movement of the inter-phalangeal joint.

Generalised Activities

The department should provide bilateral activities, sedentary and otherwise, suitable for women and for men, during which the limbs will be used in a variety of ways, for example, woodwork, gardening, cooking, modelling. These will be an invaluable form of treatment in the following circumstances: when an indirect approach is needed to draw attention away from the injured part; when there is need to improve the circulation throughout the limb prior to a period of specific local treatment involving only small muscles; when an antidote is needed to the physical and mental fatigue which can result from repetition of difficult localised movements; when opportunity is needed for the patient to take some responsibility for his treatment; and when the therapist is unable to give him individual, specific attention.

Activities with Special Emphasis

Increase of range of movement, by exerting maximum muscle power over a limited joint range to perform a movement that can just be managed with difficulty, for example, using a softly padded handle to facilitate grip (but this padding must be reduced as flexion improves, otherwise it will be impeding improvement rather than assisting it), playing solitaire with large marbles and progressing to pegotty; playing with big, wooden wall draughts and progressing to small lead wall draughts. Such grading must be continuously under review as the hand changes so quickly and what was good treatment can become just an easy, effortless activity.

Increase of muscle strength—this will be mainly concerned with flexion; extensors rarely need strengthening. Stool seating, using either a shuttle or a needle, needs a powerful grip. There is strong muscle work also in the use of spring pliers: the ball of the thumb stabilises one arm while the fingers flexed at the interphalangeal joints stabilise the other. The pliers are operated by further flexion of the fingers, at the metacarpo-phalangeal joints.

Increase of stamina is less of a problem than in the lower limb. The shoulder will tire more quickly than the hand. Blow football is excellent for improving stamina.

Increase of speed is mainly necessary for those returning to repetitive production line work. This may require both hands performing similar movements, as taking rejects off a conveyor belt, or different movements as in car assembly work. Learning to pick up quickly by playing competitive games such as animal grab, or industrial outwork, if possible on a conveyer belt, are indicated.

Increase of dexterity, and the ability to perform fine finger movements concern the thumb tip in opposition to the tips of the index and middle fingers. The ring and little fingers are held up out of the way. Stability and control of the metacarpo-phalangeal joints of all digits are needed and small range movements of the wrist and radio-ulnar joints. Good sensation is important. Model making, e.g. aeroplanes, sailing boats, etc. Meccano construction and small factory type assembly, such as electric plugs or fly-tying—all encourage dexterity. Both hands are involved simultaneously, in much the same way.

Work for the Non-dominant Hand

It is unrealistic to try to exercise an injured non-dominant arm or hand without considering whether the tool concerned is suitable. For example a skill such as sawing is too difficult for most people using the left hand, but a bilateral saw handle, designed for hemiplegics, can be used to provide good exercise for a weak left arm. An overhead drill, which requires no skill, can have a handle adapted for right or left handed use. A paintbrush can also be used with the non-dominant hand provided the painting is simple.

Competitive Activities

Blow football, fairground games, party games, table games and cards are excellent for hand injuries because they can be adapted to provide movements that are difficult to isolate, such as pronation and supination or opening out the hand and throwing. They can also provide an incentive to work quickly and to use skilled movements. They are good psychologically because the patients enjoy them and relax, improvement is quickly apparent and deformity may be less of a handicap than when attempting conventional activities.

Hand Splints

Doctors must agree the need for splints. These are available through the National Health Service* and a patient, anywhere, can be given a splint, but there are certain disadvantages as workshop and splint technicians are only accessible to some treatment centres. Sometimes the technician may never see the patient, the fitter acting as intermediary. This means a time lag in supplying the splint. It is an advantage, therefore, for the occupational and physiotherapy departments to have facilities for making simple types of splints, and for adjusting those supplied from outside the hospital. It may be common for the physiotherapist to make retaining or resting splints and for the occupational therapist to make functional splints. In some hospitals dental technicians give invaluable help. Where the referrals for splinting are numerous it has been found efficient to employ a splint technician or orthotist to work under the supervision of the occupational therapist, using suitable facilities within the occupational therapy department.

It is essential to have a sound knowledge of the functional anatomy of the hand (g), to understand why a splint is needed and to be able to choose the correct splint for the job. The wrong one can do serious harm. The occupational therapist must know and understand the muscle pattern and range of movement of her patient and the physiotherapist will, if necessary, carry out a muscle test. The occupational therapist will also need a working knowledge of leverage and forces of pull. Differing conditions of the hand require differing amounts of force and both the length of the lever arm and the direction of pull will be critical. A working splint should interfere with the palmar surfaces as little as possible, especially the pads of thumb, index and middle finger. Sensation is almost as important to the function of the hand as movement. Constant watch should be kept on pressure areas. Principles of proprioceptive neuro-muscular facilitation should also be considered. Many doctors and therapists have strong views regarding splinting of spasticity. The therapist should be conversant with theories on this subject, e.g. that spasticity is increased by sensory stimulation of the flexor aspects of the hand and forearm, and that finger abduction reduces spasticity.

Hand splints are often needed immediately. They must be simple so that they can be made quickly, yet well made and tailored to fit the individual. The choice of material is important. A standard design of splint may appear not to work, but it is usually because the material is too thick, thin, rigid, flexible or otherwise unsuitable or because the splint does not really fit the individual patient. More sophisticated, permanent splints inevitably have to be made by orthotists or technicians. Ideally their department should always be accessible to the occupational therapist who should cooperate with them at all stages of fitting and training.

The patient must be prepared to wear the splint when he is not under supervision. This will be more likely if:

(1) It provides immediate functional gain.
(2) It has a good cosmetic appearance.
(3) It does not get in the way when he uses his hand.
(4) It is comfortable and especially if it relieves pain.
(5) He understands the need for the splint.
(6) He has a good rapport with the therapist.

Appearance is most important in a day splint. It is easier to tolerate an inelegant and cumbersome night splint or any splint to be worn for only a short period. A splint should, if possible, be easy to put on correctly by the patient himself. Statistics show that patients who are dependent on others for fitting reject splints far more often than those who can fit themselves. Someone, i.e. the patient, the ward sister or a relative should understand, especially with a night splint, not only how it is worn but for how long it should be worn and any difficulties should be reported to the therapist. It is essential to check that a splint fulfils its function, that it is being worn properly and is adjusted as the hand improves or deteriorates. It is not advisable to make splints for patients who can only attend once and cannot return for checking and rechecking.

In some instances, if a splint is to fulfil its function, it may be so cumbersome that the patient will be unable to use his hand profitably. He may then need two splints, for example, if he has tightness of the finger flexors he may work in a wrist cock-up and wear a retaining splint to hold the wrist and fingers in maximal extension between treatment sessions and at night.

Functional Splints

Functional splints are designed:

(1) To place the hand in the optimum position to obtain maximal function from minimal muscle power and range of movement.

(2) To prevent deformity by holding this position when the hand is in repose and so avoid stretching de-nervated muscle and the adaptive shortening of unaffected muscle. (There are however, exceptions; the flexor hinge hand splint actually accelerates shortening and therefore a natural tenodesis is encouraged.)

(3) To enable maximal use of the upper limb in everyday activities thus preventing shoulder stiffness and muscle wasting.

Many such splints are 'lively' in that they allow mobility in the hand, for example, the Oppenheimer radial palsy splint (Fig. 3) which cocks up

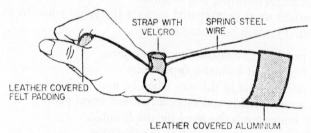

FIG. 3. Oppenheimer radial palsy splint.

the wrist and supports the proximal finger joints [*a*]. This term is however misleading because the amount of movement is not always important. The cock-up splint (Fig. 4) which stabilises the wrist and maintains the palmar arch is made of a rigid plastic, i.e. Darvic/Formasplint. This does not allow wrist flexion but provides a more definite 'fit'. Both these splints are 'functional'.

Splints replacing movement in a fully mobile hand, that is a hand which has full passive range. A splint may be designed to simulate one or a group of muscles as the Chessington thenar paralysis splint [*b*] or the Rancho Los

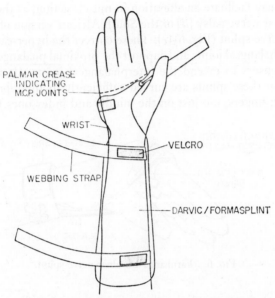

FIG. 4.   Template for wrist cock up splint. There should be only one free end to the strap so that it can be fastened with one hand.

Amigos short opponens splint (Fig. 5 (i and ii)) [c] which substitute for paralysis of the short abductor and flexor of the thumb. Apart from avoiding the deformity of a simian hand these allow the index finger to work in pinch grip. The first dorsal interosseus muscle is a postural one and can waste beyond recovery when not used.

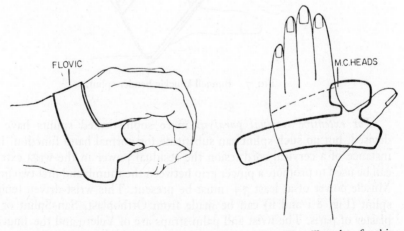

FIG. 5(i).   Rancho Los Amigos short opponens splint.   FIG. 5(ii).   Template for this.

A splint may facilitate an alteration in muscle action, as the Chessington splint for ulnar nerve palsy [*d*] or the South African version of the Farnham Park ulnar nerve splint (Fig. 6) [*e*]. These correct the hyper-extension of the metacarpo-phalangeal joints and support the proximal phalanges, so allowing the long extensors to extend the interphalangeal joints. (It is particularly important that these splints are curved sufficiently to apply pressure on the little and ring fingers, not just on the middle and index ones.)

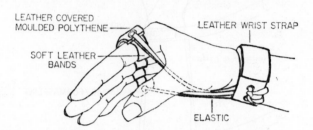

LEATHER COVERED
MOULDED POLYTHENE

LEATHER WRIST STRAP

SOFT LEATHER
BANDS

ELASTIC

FIG. 6.   Farnham Park ulnar nerve splint.

When other factors such as contractures or joint stiffness are involved similar splints will be needed but they must be much more powerful so that the 'stiff' element does not overcome the splint, for example a Bunnell knuckle bender (Fig. 7) [*f*].

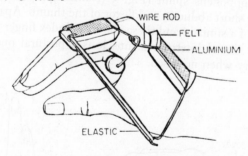

WIRE ROD
FELT
ALUMINIUM

ELASTIC

FIG. 7.   Bunnell knuckle bender splint.

For extensive residual paralysis more sophisticated splints have been devised, but no such splint can substitute for normal hand function. In the instance of a cervical cord lesion the residual power in the wrist extensors can be used to promote a pincer grip between the thumb and first two fingers. Muscle power of at least 3 + must be present. This wrist-driven tenodesis splint (Fig. 8 i and ii) can be made from Orthoplast, San-Splint or thin plaster of paris. The wrist and palm straps are of Velcro and the finger and thumb straps, elastic. A soft cord runs from the front of the wrist, across the palm and up between the index and ring fingers. This cord is slack when the wrist is flexed and tightens on extension, bringing the thumb and fingers into apposition.

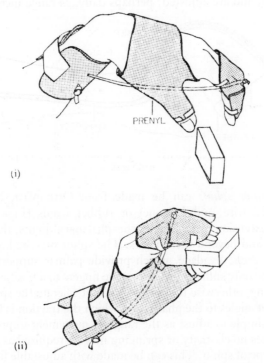

PRENYL

(i)

(ii)

FIG. 8(i) and (ii). Wrist driven tenodesis splint.

When there is no active extension the gas-powered McKibben 'muscle', or electric motor power, can activate the flexor hinge hand splint to give a similar three jaw clinch type of pinch. Such splints are only worn for selected activities when the patient cannot do them in any other way. Thorough and long-term training from the therapist, and positive and determined motivation from the patient will be essential. Only a small proportion of patients will need such splints.

Retaining Splints

These splints assist reduction of contractures and joint stiffness. They do not provide active stretch, but retain stretch that has been acquired by treatment. They are both corrective and preventive.

Serial plaster splints may be fitted to the palmar surface of the hand and forearm to overcome flexion deformities, due to flexor tendon adherence at

the wrist or contractures affecting the metacarpo-phalangeal or interphalangeal joints. These splints are made of Orthoplast, San-Splint or
plaster of paris, and are adjusted, perhaps daily, as range increases.

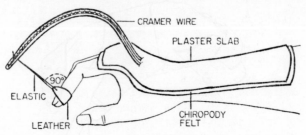

FIG. 9.   Cramer wire finger extensor. Night splint (secured in position by a crepe
bandage).

Dorsal extensor splints can be made from Orthoplast, San-Splint or
plaster of paris, wire, and Lastonet or rubber bands (Fig. 9). To avoid
causing hyperextension of the metacarpo-phalangeal joints, the back slab is
extended over and beyond these joints. The splint may be kept in position
by straps or a crepe bandage, which provide palmar support. The elastic
traction must be only sufficient to return the fingers to a position acquired by
formal stretching, otherwise the patient will not tolerate the splint. The pull
must be at right angles to the phalanx on which the traction is being applied.
This splint is simple to adjust as the range of movement improves. A splint
that incorporates no elasticity or springing may be required as an alternative
to the above type of splint. This can be made with adjustable finger-rods (*h*).

Individual joint splints are also used to retain stretch, for example the
Bunnell safety pin splint which holds the interphalangeal joints in extension
(Fig. 10); a treble finger band which enables the index and ring fingers to
assist flexion of a stiff metacarpo-phalangeal joint of the middle finger (Fig.
11) and the tyre web spreader, a piece of motor tyre attached with Velcro,
which retains stretch in the adducted thumb (Fig. 12).

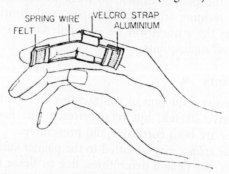

FIG. 10.   Bunnell safety pin finger extensor.

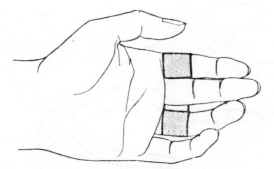

FIG. 11. Treble leather finger bands.

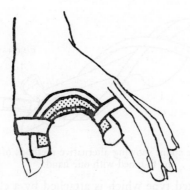

FIG. 12. Tyre web spreader.

Resting Splints

These hold the hand in a functional position. Their main purpose is to prevent pain, for example with carpal tunnel syndrome, and they may need to be worn for some time after the pain has gone, to prevent a recurrence. They also prevent further deformity, as in a rheumatoid hand (j). A good example is a Paddle splint, made from rigid plastic and secured with webbing straps and Velcro (Fig. 13). A piece of Cramer wire, wide enough to take the fingers but not the thumb, padded with chiropody felt and applied with a crepe bandage, provides a quick temporary substitute.

Other Support and Assistance to the Upper Limb

When there is good functional use in the hand, with or without splintage, but weakness or paralysis in the elbow or shoulder, such devices as the Chessington splints for elbow flexion, a gas-powered flail arm splint or mobile arm support, may be prescribed. These latter range from simple gutters which clamp to a table and provide a rocking and swivelling motion

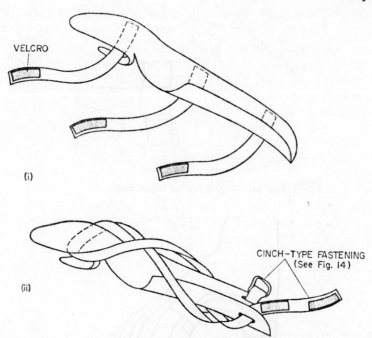

VELCRO

(i)

CINCH—TYPE FASTENING
(See Fig. 14)

(ii)

FIG. 13(i) and (ii).   Paddle splint showing alternative methods of strapping, which can be fastened with one hand.

to the more sophisticated type which is attached by a clamp to an Everest and Jennings wheel-chair. These arm supports not only take the weight of the upper limb but allow free horizontal movement from the shoulder and vertical movement of the hand. Such a support must be fitted for the individual's needs and he must then be thoroughly trained in its use. They are not suitable for anyone with spasticity.

Splint-Making Materials

Handsplints should be made from the lightest weight materials suitable for the purpose. They should be sturdy and able to stand up to hard wear. When choosing a material the following should be considered.

(1) *Rigidity.* Will it support the wrist adequately in the cocked-up position?

(2) *Flexibility.* Will a modified short opponens splint break when the hand is used actively?

(3) *Bulkiness.* Some plastics are too thick to make splints for working in, others become too thick because more than one layer may be necessary to obtain rigidity.

(4) *Cleanliness.* Some materials such as plaster of paris, white elastic or light-coloured leather become dirty quickly.

(5) *Ease of handling.* Plastics are usually easier than metals. Some plastics can be cut and moulded more readily than others, but ease of handling comes with practice and the preceding criteria are of greater importance except where splints are made infrequently.

(6) *Economy.* Although this should not affect the choice, it may in practice do so.

(7) *Heat.* Some plastics can be moulded at very low temperatures. This makes for ease of handling but will be contra-indicated when the patient will be wearing the splint in the heat such as the housewife washing up or an arc welder handling hot metal.

Padding and Lining Splints

Resting and retaining splints, and all splints made from plaster of paris or metal will be better padded, while functional splints made from plastic may be comfortable without. The lining of a functional or a retaining splint which is made to fit the patient's hand should be thin. With a resting splint thicker padding would be suitable. The lining of a working splint should be easily renewable. Plastic foam will stay clean longer than chiropody felt. With night splints there is not the same problem.

Insulation

This is necessary with heat-mouldable splints which are moulded directly to the patient's hand. This method is quite satisfactory, even when there is loss of sensation, provided suitable care is taken, and is much quicker than making negative and then positive plaster moulds. The material chosen, such as expanded polystyrene sheeting, should be as thin as possible while providing insulation. If it is too thick the splint will be cumbersome and the pressures on the hand may no longer be correct. This is especially important when the insulation is not used to line the splint which would then be a loose fit. Insulation material should be cut larger than the splint both to allow for shrinkage and as extra protection. It can be:

(1) Attached to the patient's hand with Elastoplast.

(2) Stuck to the splint with, for example, Copydex. This can be removed after the splint is shaped.

(3) Placed under the splint in the oven and fused by heat (possible with certain plastics only).

Strapping

Strapping should ensure that the splint is held securely in the correct position. Fastenings should be so arranged that, if possible, the patient can do them up himself. Good quality synthetic leathers are more hygienic and durable than real leather, particularly for functional splints, i.e. in dealing with dish-washing, greasy conditions, etc. There are various methods,

(1) Direct Velcro fastening where there is retaining but not tightening of the strap (see Fig. 4).

(2) Cinch-type fastening with Velcro. This is the easiest type to fasten and provides a tight, adjustable fit (Fig. 14).

(3) Figure of eight webbing to hold the hand when there is spasm or contracture, for example, the Paddle splint (see Fig. 13).

(4) Synthetic leather strap with a buckle. This is both hard wearing and cosmetic, especially at the wrist.

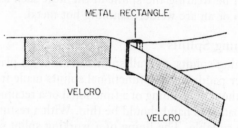

METAL RECTANGLE

VELCRO

VELCRO

Fig. 14. Cinch type velcro fastening.

(5) Synthetic leather strap with snap fasteners.

(6) Crepe bandage for plaster of paris or Cramer wire retaining splints. This gives strong, overall **pressure** which is important when there are severe contractures. It also covers the rough plaster or wire.

(7) Occasionally a retaining splint may be plastered on to the patient to ensure that it is worn.

REFERENCES AND RECOMMENDED FURTHER READING

Anderson, M. A. & Miles, H., *Upper Extremity Orthotics*. Springfield, Illinois, U.S.A., 1970.

Ansell, B. M., Williams, J. G. P., Cheshire, L., Lawton, S. and Haines, R. E. J., Farnham Park modular splint system (See ref. (*h*) in text). *Rheumat. phys. Med.*, 11, no. 7, 1972.

Barr, N. R. *The Hand. Principles and Techniques of Simple Splintmaking*. London, 1975.

Boyes, J. H., *Bunnell's Surgery of the Hand*. See refs [a] and [f] in text. U.S.A., 1970.

Brookes, R. B., *Re-education of the Injured Shoulder*. London, 1959.

Caillet, R., *Shoulder Pain*, Philadelphia, 1968.

Cailliet, R., *Hand Pain and Impairment*, Philadelphia, 1971.

Ebner, J. D., *Orthotic Application, Fabrication and Construction for the Leprosy Patient*, U.S. Publications, Carville Hospital, Louisiana.

Engen, T., *Upper Extremity Orthotics*. A Project Report. Orthotic Dept. Institute of Rehabilitation and Research, Houston, Texas.

Epprecht, E., *Gadgets and Aids for the Treatment of the Upper Extremities*. Basle, 1962.

Flatt, A. E., *The Care of the Rheumatoid Hand*. St. Louis, 1963.

Foster, M., Prenyl hand-splinting with congenital abnormalities, *Occ. Ther.*, 35, no. 10, 1972.

Furlong, F., *Hand Surgery*. London, 1968.

Gilewich, G., Jimenez, J. and Redford, J. B. *Simple Splints, Principles and Techniques*, Univ. of Alberta Hospital, 1969.

Hollis, L. I., *Splint Substitutes*. Chapel Hill, North Carolina, *Proceedings Fourth International Congress*. W.F.O.T.*, 1966.

Houchin, R. and Cheshire, L., Splintage for ulnar deviation, *Occ. Ther.*, **34**, no. 10, 1971.

Jayne, C. F., *A Study of Cats' Cradles in Many Lands*. U.S.A. 1962.

Jimenez, J., *Simple Splints, Principles and Techniques*, Proceedings, Fifth Int. Congress, W.F.O.T.*, 1970.

Jones, M. S., *An Approach to Occupational Therapy*. See ref [c] in text. London, 1964.

Kaplan, E. B., *Functional and Surgical Anatomy of the Hand*, Philadelphia, 1965.

Larson, D. L. *The Prevention and Correction of Burn Scar Contracture*, Shriners Burns Institute, Galveston, Texas 1973.

Lawton, D. S., Hand Splinting in rheumatoid arthritis (See ref. (j) in text). *Brit. J. Occ. Ther.*, **37**, no. 2, 1974.

Licht, S., *Orthotics*, Baltimore, 1966.

Lomax, J. and McLean, P., Splinting the arthritic, *Occ. Ther.*, **35**, no. 2, 1972.

Malik, M. H., *Static Hand Splinting, New Materials and Techniques*, Proceedings Fifth Int. Congress. W.F.O.T.*, 1970.

Malik, M. H., *Manual on Static Hand Splinting*, Monroeville, Pittsburgh, 1972.

Malik, M. H., *Manual on Dynamic Hand Splinting with Thermoplastic Materials*, Monroeville, Pittsburgh, 1974.

Rank, B. K. *et al.*, *Surgery of Repair as Applied to Hand Injuries*. B.M.A.* Aids for the Disabled. London, 1973.

Willis, B. A., *Splinting the Burn Patient*, Shriners Burns Institute, Galveston, Texas, 1971.

Wynn Parry, C. B., *Rehabilitation of the Hand*. See refs. [b], [d], [g], [h]. London, 1973.

Yerxa, E. J. (formerly of Rancho Los Amigos Hospital California, U.S.A.) *The Challenge for the Occupational Therapist in Splinting the Severely Paralysed Hand. Proceedings Fourth International Congress*. W.F.O.T.*, 1966.

Yerxa, E. J., *The Uses and Components of Hand Splints for the Splinting of the Severely Paralysed Hand. Proceedings Third International Congress*. W.F.O.T.*, 1962.

Young, R. R., *Hand Splints and Their Attachments*. See ref [c] in text. Rancho Los Amigos Orthotic Dept., Downey, California.

And see:

Aids to the Investigation of Peripheral Nerve Lesions. H.M.S.O.*, 1966.

Aids for the Disabled. B.M.A. London, 1968.

Practical Surgery of the Hand. The Surgical Clinic of N. America, vol. 44, no. 4, 1964.

The Hand, Journal of the British Society for Surgery of the Hand, published quarterly, Edinburgh and London.

Designing a working frame, *Occ. Ther.*, **36**, no. 1, 1973.

Use of gravity for movement in occupational therapy programme. *Occ. Ther.*, **36**, no. 3, 1973.

Sanding blocks. *Occ. Ther.*, **36**, no. 4, 1973.

Elevated bilateral sander. *Occ. Ther.*, **36**, no. 6, 1973.

Active extension and passive flexion by playing Karam, *Occ. Ther.*, **37**, no. 10, 1974.

Review of upper extremity orthotic systems. *Occ. Ther.*, **37**, no. 11, 1974.

Reading References for chapter 9, this book.

* See *Glossary*, p. 454-6.

CHAPTER 9

Occupational Therapy for the Lower Limb

Normal Use and its Demands on Muscle and Joint Function

Mobility and antigravity muscle strength for sitting, standing and walking are the basic needs for everyday use. Coordination of hip, knee and foot is fundamental for good performance and loss of function in one part prohibits normal use of the others. For example, the patient with painful stiff toes will not bend his knee when walking and the patient with a stiff hip cannot bend his when sitting. The antigravity extensor muscles which are responsible for thrust are also responsible for controlling change of position when gravity is allowed to take effect, as in sitting down. When doing this the weight of the body is taken equally on both legs and is controlled until it is transferred on to the chair. Patients often let go too soon and should practise a soft landing. Coming down stairs is an obvious progression. The weight is on one leg, balance is involved and the height of the step demands more control. Limitation of knee flexion is a common disability and may make normal action impossible. The flexor muscles of the hip with the abdominals as fixators, the knee and the ankle, are jointly responsible for raising the limb so that the foot clears the ground in walking and clears the step when climbing stairs.

A long period of non-weight-bearing is detrimental to muscle tone throughout the limb, especially to the muscle groups which are accustomed to take the full body weight, the glutei, quadriceps and calf muscles. However regularly they may be exercised they cannot be worked hard enough to maintain full function. Therefore, in addition to local treatment for the injured part, the whole limb must be strengthened to regain normal function.

For a comfortable sitting position 90° of flexion is needed in the hip and knee, although a greater range is normally used to initiate the act of standing up. Therefore for all but the young, the exceptionally vigorous or those whose jobs make greater demands, 90° is minimally sufficient. For weight-bearing, extension is the priority. Limitation of foot and ankle movements are rarely a severe disability for men unless there is also pain, although walking on other than level ground may be awkward. Women, according to their choice of shoe can be in difficulty. With limited plantar flexion for example, high heels are impossible, while a low heel may need to be raised when there is residual equinus.

Routine Priorities for the Different Joints.

Hip.

(1) To strengthen the glutei for extension of the joint and for control of the pelvis on the femur when weight-bearing.
(2) To increase pain-free range of flexion for sitting.
(3) To strengthen the hip flexors for walking and stair climbing.
(4) To relate the above to correct walking.

Knee.

(1) To strengthen the quadriceps for stability, for antigravity thrust, and for eccentric control when weight-bearing, e.g. the act of sitting down or coming downstairs.
(2) To increase flexion to a minimum of 90°.
(3) To relate the above to correct walking.

Ankle and foot.

(1) To strengthen the calf muscle for weight-bearing, i.e. raising the heel for push off in walking.
(2) To mobilise dorsi-flexion and plantar flexion.
(3) To mobilise the metatarso-phalangeal joints, especially extension, for the position of weight-bearing on the ball of the foot.
(4) To strengthen the dorsi-flexors.
(5) To maintain and strengthen the arches of the foot.
(6) To relate the above to correct walking.

Mobilisation of inversion and eversion is difficult to achieve by occupational therapy and is therefore not included. Strength of the muscles which produce the movements can be increased if there is good range (see pp. 62-3).

Treatment Priorities for Lower Limbs

The therapist who treats patients after lower limb trauma must understand the mechanics of walking. This is the basis on which faults are identified. One of the best ways of helping the patient to correct a fault is by demonstrating the right action in slow motion, with a walking aid if relevant. The patient must realise that the success of his treatment is not increased proficiency in his sawing or wood turning. It is improvement in the way he sits down, because he now remembers to take weight on *both* legs, and in the way he walks, because he is now able to 'pass' his feet equally. To drive this point home his performance is checked as part of his treatment. After work on the bicycle saw, the O.T.* should call upon the patient to demonstrate his walking, with the reminder to 'try to get the same easy pull up of your hip and knee as you bring your foot forward'. And, after work on the lathe, 'see if you can push forward onto the ball of your foot so that it feels the same as you've just been doing'.

Fractured neck of femur. The patient is usually elderly and the physiotherapist begins general mobilisation within days of surgical fixation of the fracture. The aim is to have the patient walking before the habit is lost and before muscle power deteriorates through disuse. Local treatment for the hip is rarely needed. Instead, after about ten days, assessment of likely A.D.L.* problems and training in safe mobility for home are the priorities, including the minimal essential kitchen activities. The majority of patients are women. The accident and the strange surroundings may lead to confusion and the patient's description of her home may mislead. A home visit, prior to her discharge, is invaluable. Slip mats belong to this generation and if possible should be removed, but other alterations may unwittingly increase hazards by removing a familiar hand hold or resting place.

Arthrodesis of the hip. While immobilised, an overhead work table may be wanted, or, in the case of a patient only interested in reading, prismatic spectacles. These relieve strain on the eyes and neck or on the arms, for the book can be supported on the chest. Later, when mobile, there will be difficulty with some A.D.L., for example dressing below the waist, bathing, and sitting in comfort. There may also be work problems.

Osteotomy or arthroplasty of the hip. Priorities are routine for the joint and the knee, too, must be treated according to routine. The bicycle is ideal. The extensor thrust of the unaffected leg assists hip and knee flexion of the weaker one and the hip flexors can be strengthened by having the foot strapped to the pedal so that emphasis can be put on 'pull up and over'. Prospects for range of flexion depend on how long there has been limitation; full pain-free movement can sometimes be achieved. Until full weight-bearing is allowed adequate strengthening of the glutei is difficult. Sticks are used for walking until pelvic tilt, with its Trendelenburg's sign, can be controlled and this stability may be slow in building up. It can be helped by conscious strong static contraction of both gluteal groups while doing standing work. Initially there is a tendency not to take a half share of the weight on the leg. This must be detected and corrected. The work can be anything that it is possible to do from a standing position, with feet slightly astride for comfort and so that there can be a shift of weight. A high work top is needed. Technical drawing, painting, constructional work, e.g. model making are suitable. When unilateral weight-bearing is possible, short periods of lathe work standing on alternate legs can be given, extended in time as the leg proves its ability to stabilise the pelvis while taking the weight. Heavy manual work is contra-indicated. Sensible 'middle aged activity' is not.

Fractured shaft of the femur. The only joint affected is the knee and its treatment is routine. All body weight-bearing groups of muscles must be built up. The patient is seldom able to walk without a limp and this is caused as much by weak glutei and calf muscles as by dysfunction of the knee. Occupational therapy is not suitable for the patient who is not allowed to take weight, unless he has approximately 60° of flexion. Resistance in the joint will be transmitted up the femur and it is difficult to support the fracture site adequately.

Fracture of lower end of femur. This is treated as fracture of the shaft but in some instances the knee has been partially flexed during immobilisation. This will lead to limitation of extension and the range must be increased.

Fracture of the patella. The knee only is immobilised in the plaster and treatment is routine.

Patellectomy. A fracture no longer exists. Instead, treatment follows routine procedures for any tendon suture, i.e. first, work for the muscle involved, the quadriceps; second, gradual mobilisation to restore full range of the movement during which the sutured tendon is on the stretch, knee flexion. Kneeling may be painful and a patient whose job requires prolonged kneeling, e.g. a carpet layer, may be helped by a protective knee pad.

Injuries to the knee joint other than fractures. The knee is especially prone to injury, being a hinge joint acting between two long bones. It is dependent for lateral stability on its colateral ligaments and to a lesser extent on its menisci. The former can be torn by valgus or varus strain and the latter by rotational strain in flexion. Surgery may be necessary. For antero-posterior stability the joint relies on the cruciate ligaments. Surgical repair is not always practicable. Strong quadriceps are essential for the normal knee joint. When there is injury the muscles deteriorate markedly. Pre-accident strength is always the aim and in the instance of torn cruciate ligaments above normal maximal efficiency is needed as compensation. Hamstrings, too, must be strong. They control hyper-extension of the joint and work in agonist-antagonist relationship with the quadriceps. Effusion is common and may persist. If, exceptionally, occupational therapy should be prescribed at this stage, i.e. when quadriceps work with minimal flexion and elevation is needed, this can be given. 'The patient can sit with his leg in a wide canvas sling supported from above the knee to above the heel. The sling is attached to a hook on the back of the lathe and the patient can easily detach it himself which prevents that feeling of being "tied up" which nearly all people dislike. The patient then works the treadle with the uninjured leg. The muscles of the leg in the sling work as stabilisers of the pelvis, rhythmically in time with the action of the leg treadling.'† If a bicycle saddle is used the muscle contractions will be strong for there is need to stabilise the pelvis on a smaller base. As the rectus femoris comes into action the other muscles in the group contract with it. There is further benefit if the patient can be taught to make a conscious effort to extend the lower leg on the thigh as he contracts his quadriceps, i.e. while pushing down with his knee, raising his heel with the foot dorsi-flexed. Ways of using this movement to operate ratchets or electric push buttons or adapted looms have been devised.

Fracture of the tibial plateau. Only the knee is immobilised and treatment is routine. The articular surface may be involved in the fracture and this predisposes to pain. There is often some permanent loss of flexion and there may be lateral laxity in the joint. There is therefore special need for quadriceps sufficiency.

Fracture of the shaft of tibia. Both the knee joint and foot need routine treatment and often the latter is the greater problem. Practically, too, there may be difficulty in treating the ankle if knee flexion is restricted and the patient is not weight-bearing. Most treadle machines assume that the worker can sit on a chair of normal height and presuppose good range of knee movement. This patient will need a high stool to bring his foot into normal contact with the treadle and his posture must then be checked. If this is strained by an abnormal relationship to the work he will do with his hands, the treatment is unsuitable. The bicycle saw is good, and with careful supervision treatment can be given on the back of a foot power lathe.

Fracture dislocation of the ankle. The ankle and foot are the major problem. The knee may be immobilised initially but its full function can quickly be restored. Treatment is routine. Pain may persist, particularly when moving over rough ground or weight-bearing abnormally, e.g. on ladders. There is a stage when treatment should include working normally in boots or working shoes. Sometimes there is thickening round the joint and the boots will be too tight. New ones should be 'broken in'. Change of work may be unavoidable.

Fracture of the lateral malleolus (Potts fracture). Treatment for the ankle is routine if prescribed. Often occupational therapy is not needed.

Fracture of the os calcis is commonly caused by falling from a height, while at work. It affects both ankle and foot. Treatment is routine. Stiffness may persist and pain, especially when walking over uneven ground. The patient will doubt his ability to climb ladders or to work safely on scaffolding. Periods of treatment, wearing his working boots or shoes, at a bench, using his arms and back strongly are a good preparation for trying outside work. A thick sorbo heel pad in the boot may add to comfort.

Fracture of the metatarsals. This is considered a minor fracture. It is often a disabling one. Both arches of the foot may be disorganised, weight-bearing is then painful and walking poor. Anything putting strain on the foot increases pain, for example, hurrying, pushing, pulling, climbing. Treatment emphasises correct placement and correct weight-bearing through the foot, at whatever activity may be used to strengthen it. Moulded arch supports are sometimes needed when pain persists in spite of treatment.

Injury to the ankle other than fractures. Treatment may be prescribed for a patient with recurrent sprain of the ankle. Women predominate. In addition to general strengthening while avoiding the position of trauma, advice about suitable footwear may be needed. The most important feature is breadth of heel whether it be flat or otherwise. High heeled shoes must fit well, sling backs being avoided.

After injury to the tendo-Achilles or after surgery for tendon lengthening the patient's difficulty is to combine dorsi-flexion with extension of the knee, as in standing. If occupational therapy is prescribed it will usually not be until full free activity can be encouraged. It can include bicycling, the heel up against the pedal to make it easy to emphasise dorsi-flexion when the knee extends, as in the position of preparing to take weight on the heel of the forward leg in walking; pushing a garden roller slowly, or pulling it along behind. When doing bench work there is opportunity for conscious effort to stand correctly and to move with avoidance of limp. Strenuous pushing or pulling, as in pipe bending, works the calf muscle but also encourages good range of dorsi-flexion by transferring weight on to the front of the foot while the heel is down. It may be difficult to re-establish a good walking rhythm with restricted dorsi-flexion. It will help to practise on a slight downward slope, and going up again gives opportunity for increasing the range.

Treatment Potential of a Bicycle for the Lower Limb

Muscle Work

One of the chief assets of the bicycle fretsaw is the familiarity of its action for most people. The reciprocal movement is directly related to walking, it is easily adjusted for different needs and it is suitable both for patients not yet allowed to take body weight and for those who are. Suitable clothing that will not restrict movement is important. Little time is needed, however, to teach how the machine as such works. Careful instruction *is* needed to teach each patient how *he* must use it. For example, the patient with weakness of his left leg might work rhythmically but with over-emphasis on the thrust of his strong right leg. To counteract this it will help him to 'think' *left* and *left* and *left*, the 'and' being the thrust of the right leg. Over-correction is unlikely but the emphasis will become more nearly equal and the muscles of the left leg will contract more strongly. Toe clips are necessary to give the patient confidence that his feet will not slip off the pedals. The prime movers are normally the antigravity extensor muscles but here again there may be need for change. The patient with a stiff knee must learn to contract his hamstrings voluntarily. This is often news to him, for he seldom knows they exist. A good way of doing this is to strap his feet on to the pedals.

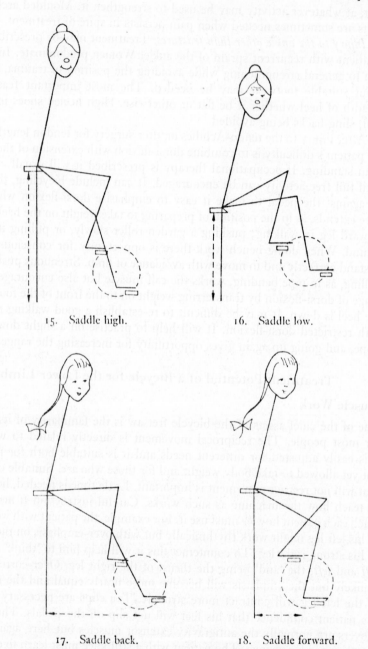

15. Saddle high.   16. Saddle low.

17. Saddle back.   18. Saddle forward.

FIGS. 15–20. Variations in range of movement of the hip, knee and ankle joints obtainable on a bicycle machine. The therapist makes adjustments in one or more respects to fulfil the aims of treatment for individual patients.

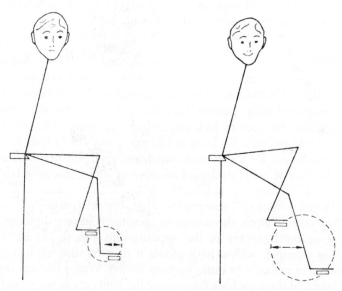

19. Pedal cranks short.   20. Pedal cranks long.

Then, a 'pull back and up' action can be emphasised instead of the usual push action. In this way the flexors of hip, knee and ankle must all work and he can feel the tendons standing out behind his knee.

Every patient must be trained to keep his knee and foot in correct alignment by statically contracting the abductors, adductors and rotators of his hip. Here again teaching is often necessary. The therapist will tell the patient to resist her as she exerts pressure inwards on the outer side of his knee, first while his legs are not moving and then while he pedals. If he can do this and can also resist outward pressure, he can be expected to balance the work of the opposing muscle groups and the knee will be stabilised correctly.

Many adults have stiff feet and toes. When combined with dropped arches there will be a total lack of spring in the walk. Non-weight-bearing exercises are indicated. Unless, for any reason, cycling without a foot plate is contra-indicated the patient will benefit from doing this, without his shoes and with his toes directly on the pedals. With the shanks long there can be good range of foot and toe movements and work for the long and short muscles in the foot, provided that the knees are correctly stabilised and that inversion rather than eversion is stressed.

Some patients, women especially, who must use sticks or crutches to prevent weight being put on an injured leg, are helped to get the feeling of working the depressors of their shoulder girdles by having to hold down the material they are sawing, e.g. wood, metal or plastic.

Mobilisation

With accurate adjustment a good range of flexion and extension can be obtained in the ankle and knee. Because the final degrees of extension of the knee are completed with rotation, this does not occur, for the continuous movement allows no time to lock and unlock the joints. The patient can, however, be told to brace his knee in full extension and to hold it so, with his foot dorsi-flexed, for a few moments before each rest period. The same thing can be done at intervals during a session of sitting watching television. Good range of hip flexion is obtainable; inner range of extension is not.

Two factors govern the movements. First, the relationship of saddle to pedals. Any change alters the degree of movement in one direction at the expense of an equal degree in the opposite one, just as on an ordinary bicycle. For example, with a high saddle it may be difficult to reach the pedals and there will only be outer range of flexion. With a low one the knees are very bent and the muscles ache because the joints are never straightened. The second factor is the length of the pedal shanks. By lengthening them there is equal increase of movement in both directions, i.e. flexion and extension, and by shortening them there is equal decrease (see Figs. 15 to 20).

Compensatory action. The more joints there are moving simultaneously, the greater the likelihood of compensatory action if one of them is stiff. The therapist soon learns to recognise such action, i.e. flexion of the lumbar spine avoiding hip flexion; excessive ankle movement because the knees are held together—a female characteristic; excessive plantar flexion at the point of maximum knee flexion; tilting side to side on the saddle, so avoiding knee extension. These are comparatively simple actions and can often be at least partially controlled by the patient once he realises that they are happening and when given positive instructions. Manual correction may also be needed until the feeling of the right movement becomes familiar. Pelvic movement in compensation for limitation of knee flexion is difficult to control, by any means. It occurs when the knee movement is severely restricted and combines tilting and rotation in such a way that as the knee reaches its limit all the body weight is transferred to the opposite side of the saddle. Short pedal shanks, saddle well back from the pedals, emphasis on the knee being pulled *forward* and up, and on the weight being kept equal on both sides of the saddle are the conditions needed for the best results.

Adaptability

An adjustable work table on a bicycle is important, both so that it can accommodate a tall patient working in maximum flexion with long pedal shanks without hitting his knees, and also to ensure the possibility of good posture for patients of all heights.

To add resistance to a bicycle fretsaw without changing the range of movement or having to give tougher material, many machines are fitted with a braking mechanism graded in pounds weight. Patients like to know how hard they are working. With a milometer they can also know how fast and how far they have cycled as they work and a progressive treatment plan can include a gradual increase of distance daily. If there can be gears, it is possible to treat patients for whom the machine might otherwise not be suitable, for example those with partial spastic paraplegia. The movement is exactly what they need as re-education for walking but with difficulty in relaxing they cannot work at normal speed and need a higher gear. At the other end of the scale a young athlete should be expected to work at speed in low gear.

Treatment Potential of an Ankle Treadle

Muscle Work

The action of an ankle treadle is usually that of a first order lever, movement is kept going by pushing down alternately in front of and behind the fulcrum. The standard foot plate, for example the treadle sewing machine, is in one piece. This allows for simultaneous action of the feet, placed side by side, toes in front of the fulcrum and heels behind it. The knees should always be kept together too: this is often difficult. Once the action is learnt, and when strength and range are adequate, some patients can be progressed to keeping the movement going with one foot only. This will have to be well stabilised in a position of mechanical advantage for the rocker movement. Even so the muscle work is demanding and frequent changes of foot may be needed. The prime movers are alternately the posterior tibial group which plantar flex, and the anterior tibial group with, perhaps surprisingly, the hamstrings, which exert downward pressure on the heel. Emphasis is put on the dorsi-flexors if the forepart of the foot is strapped down.

It is less easy to ensure that the intrinsic muscles work. A specially shaped wooden foot piece on the treadle used with bare feet is helpful. This conforms at the front to the line of the metatarso-phalangeal joints. Shaping at the heel in not necessary. The wood must be thick enough to allow for flexion of the toes. With a retaining strap over the dorsum the patient can try to shorten his foot by pulling up the longitudinal arch as the treadle is brought up into dorsi-flexion. The strap must have 'give', and be fastened at just the right tension; a piece of $2\frac{1}{2}$-inch elastic bandage serves well. The foot piece itself can drop on to the footplate with strong dowel pegs reciprocating with a choice of holes.

When the patient cannot maintain the longitudinal arch actively, a wedge foot piece raised on the inside and with the same dowel fittings will prevent a valgus position. Its use will not strengthen the weak muscles but as a preliminary step towards doing this it may improve position sense provided the knee is correctly positioned too. But with concentration on the foot, the knee can be forgotten and will tend to roll outwards.

Mobilisation

A treadle action is good for mobilising and full range movement can be achieved. It is essential to be able to adjust the range of the treadle. Making this possible is a simple engineering job. It is also useful to be able to adjust the length of the 'pitman' which joins the treadle to the wheel. The ankle treadle is suitable for patients not yet weight-bearing, with one proviso. There must be enough movement and power to work rhythmically without strain.

Compensatory action. Unlike the bicycle there are no other joints working simultaneously so there is no alternative possibility of adequate compensatory movement should the range be inadequate. With lack of plantar flexion the foot loses contact with the foot plate and so loses power but there is no forcing of the joint. If there is lack of dorsi-flexion there is no escape from the rising foot plate, and this will exert pressure on the ball of the foot even if the heel loses contact, as it will. The pressure is then transmitted up the lower leg and in some cases this would be contra-indicated. To prevent this the patient's range of movement must be assessed accurately, the treadle action adjusted to it and the patient's foot correctly placed and maintained on the treadle. These points can be checked by the therapist moving the treadle slowly by hand while the patient allows his foot to ride on it. It is easy to see if the ball of the foot and the heel can both be kept in contact throughout. If neither can, the treadle needs adjusting; if either one loses contact the foot can be shifted slightly in the opposite direction. This may be the answer. If not, there will be loss of contact again, this time by the other part of the foot, and adjustment to the treadle is indicated. Some local compensatory movement is possible and it must be recognised. Extra flexion of the toes with arching of the forepart of the foot will provide contact with the foot plate as a substitute for plantar flexion. This can be acceptable only if the maximum movement has been made. If it has not, the patient can be told to push down with the whole *ball* of his foot. At the extreme of dorsi-flexion a mobile foot can be pushed into valgus. Active prevention, by keeping the weight on the outer side of the foot, or adjustment of the machine is needed.

A patient's foot should never be strapped to the treadle unless his ankle is mobile enough to maintain, or marginally maintain, contact without. Correctly used, the strap both stabilises the foot on the treadle and directs the muscular effort.

An alternative way of treadling is to have one foot fully in contact in front of the fulcrum, the other foot behind it, with the heel raised. There is value in both actions and the patient will be instructed to change his feet. Pressing down through the ball increases range of toe extension and this is often needed after a period of non-weight-bearing.

Some treadles have separate foot pieces. They are worked by reciprocal action of plantar flexion and dorsi-flexion, the calf muscles being the prime movers unless a dorsum strap is used.

Adaptability

It is essential to be able to alter the range of movement. It is an advantage if the height of the work top can be changed too, not only to ensure good posture but for the patient who must sit on an exceptionally high seat because of very limited knee movement.

Treatment Potential of a Footpower Lathe

Muscle Work and Mobilisation

Normal working of a lathe is directly re-educative for standing and walking and as a rule the patient should change legs at intervals. Both sexes enjoy turning and like the things they can make, while also subjectively appreciating the treatment as such. Suitable clothing, which allows unrestricted movement, should be worn. The patient stands with most of his weight on one leg; pelvis level, hip extended and knee straight, weight on the forepart of the foot, arches of the foot braced. Because part of the body weight is taken by the leg on the foot plate, the demands made on the hip abductors of the standing leg are less than those made when walking. Therefore a patient who must still walk with a stick, because of Trendelenburg weakness, can be treated successfully on the lathe, provided that he can control the tilt of his pelvis and that he does so when turning. The action of the moving leg is alternately an extensor thrust, and control of the upward return swing of the foot plate by the same muscles. The foot should either be fully supported, or with the heel held slightly raised so that the thrust from the hip and knee passes down through the ball of the foot. Weight should never be taken transversely through the longitudinal arch on to the front edge of the footplate. This happens when the patient allows his foot to slip back from the fully supported position with the result that the heel drops down, or when the calf muscle fails to keep the heel raised as intended.

There is good hip movement round the mid point of its full range. Knee flexion will be little more than a right angle, the range partly depending on the patient's proportions. In full knee flexion the heel is in contact with the ischial tuberosity, and to reach it the foot moves backwards and upwards. Because the working foot on the lathe is in front of the standing one, and the swing of the foot plate is forward and up, the range of knee flexion can never be full. Nor is there full knee extension, and this should not be expected for the action is a continuous one. There is no time to lock the knee in extension and such jarring action would be strongly contra-indicated.

Most lathes have three gears. (The largest wheel on the headstock is the lowest gear.) These gears regulate the speed at which the lathe turns and the strength of action needed to work it. Although the low gear calls for less power and in that sense is easier, the faster treadling required by the low gear may be just as difficult, or more so, for certain types of patients. Those with marked muscle weakness or instability of the knee, and those with poor coordination due to spasticity are examples. They are better treated in a higher gear and given physical assistance. When there are different lathes in a department some may be easier to work than others. This is worth discovering.

Although not standard practice, work from the back of the lathe has great treatment value, providing for well balanced, rhythmical and therefore comfortable ankle movement and so also for calf strengthening. Partly because of the mechanical disadvantage of poor leverage there is strong rhythmic contraction of the quadriceps, as stabilisers, statically or in small range, according to the relationship of the ankle joint to the fulcrum. This is invaluable for strengthening when movement as such is perhaps painful, e.g. with fracture into the knee joint or osteo-arthritis. It is also useful in treating the patient who is apprehensive about his knee. He can be told of the importance of having a strong calf muscle and his attention directed to the ankle movement. Working from the back, sanding and polishing can be done. Turning adds resistance but as the patient is then likely to need some assistance, this is no great problem.

Compensatory Action. Patients whose aim of treatment is mobilisation will need help in avoiding compensatory action. Working from a standing position there is great scope for this and the following examples are common when there is limitation of knee flexion. First using the normal foot plate:

(1) The working foot may slide forward; a horizontal footstop can prevent this.
(2) The patient will tend to compensate by bending the hip of the standing leg and transferring his weight from the *front* of the foot to the *heel.* He should be told: 'brace your knee, tighten your seat muscle, and let me see that you're able to raise your heel.'
(3) There can be pelvic tilt and rotation as on the bicycle. Tell him to 'bend your knee *forward* and up'.

The therapist must always be on the look-out for faulty alignment of hip and knee and ankle. This can cause lateral strain on the joints, usually valgus. A patient at serious risk to such a strain to his right leg should probably not turn a bowl or a lamp base on a standard lathe. In twisting to adjust to his work, being at 90° to the ordinary position, his foot and therefore his knee will be tipped over into the valgus position by the slope of the footplate. A short chain will lessen the risk.

The patient aiming at increase of ankle movement and working at the back of the lathe, will inevitably swing his body forward and back, and in so doing barely move his ankle at all if the muscular effort required is beyond him. It is easy to forget to check the gears. Given the right amount of assistance he can be expected to keep his knee still. As always, it is best to teach the patient the thing that may be difficult with his sound leg first, pointing out special treatment points.

Adaptability

Lathes designed as treatment equipment are adaptable for range of movement and any standard lathe should be so adapted. A standing block is sometimes useful in addition. This has the same effect as raising the bicycle saddle. It increases extension of hip and knee with corresponding decrease in flexion. As with the saddle, if raised too high, the patient would be encouraged to stretch for full extension of the knee and as the foot plate moves beyond reach he would drop his pelvis on that side, and adjust to this by flexing his lumbar spine to the opposite side. All of this is contra-indicated. To prevent it, the height of the block is never quite as high as the lowest position of the foot plate. For a standard lathe it is helpful to have at least two different lengths of chain. These have the same effect as the blocks and there is a safeguard. The lathe cannot be worked unless the foot plate clears the ground at its lowest point.

A simple alteration to the foot plate makes it possible to achieve full knee flexion. This is shown in Plate 14. At the bottom of his stroke the patient's knee is already flexed to approximately 90°. Because his heel is in line with his ischial tuberosity the movement will be increased still further as the foot plate rises.

Instructions for the alterations which must be made to a standard lathe in order to achieve full knee flexion are as follows:

(1) Shorten the foot plate by approximately 1 foot.

(2) Fix two 1 foot lengths of 1 inch bore barrel to the upper surface of the remaining foot plate, one at each side. Fit into each, near the front end, a counter sunk metal thread grub screw, preferably with a wing nut or tommy bar.

(3) For the new extension foot plate:
1 foot by $4\frac{1}{2}$ inches of $\frac{7}{8}$ inch deal and 2 feet of $\frac{7}{8}$ inch barrel; 2 steel plates 4 inches by 1 inch by $\frac{3}{16}$ inch. Drill a $\frac{3}{16}$ inch hole at each end of each plate. Weld the plates across the barrel 8 inches apart. Screw the plates on to the deal so that the barrel projects 1 foot at one end. Cover the top of the foot plate with ribbed rubber.

For treatment purposes the extended foot plate can be fixed into the barrel at the right or left of the original section, as required. To restore the full length normal foot plate, two pieces of $\frac{7}{8}$ inch barrel are fixed, one each, to the sides of the section originally cut off. These will slide into the lengths of barrel on the shortened section.

The single extension foot plate depends on a correct working position for its success. There are two ways of getting this wrong:

(1) It is treated like the normal foot plate, i.e. standing foot back, working foot forward.

(2) Having been right at the start, i.e. feet level, the working one is moved forward. The patient must learn to stand to the *inside* of the extension foot plate, and to have the working foot out of sight underneath his hip. It feels quite different from the normal stance and it is less stable due to the side to side alignment. The hip joint moves less; the knee joint more, and it can give full range. (See Plate 14.)

There are occasions when an additional foot piece on the foot plate will help to achieve the aim of treatment. Although of different size and shape, according to their purpose, these should have a common method of attachment to the foot plate. For example, holes can be drilled on the foot plate at 3-inch intervals, equidistant vertically and horizontally. Into these, two equally spaced dowel pegs on the underside of a foot piece will fit.

Examples. A foot stop 12 inches long by $1\frac{1}{2}$ inches high and $1\frac{1}{2}$ inches wide will stabilise the toe or the heel if horizontal, and will prevent rotation of the foot if vertical; a heel wedge, 1 inch or $1\frac{1}{2}$ inches high at the back, will teach position sense prior to working with the heel unsupported; an inner border wedge, the length and breadth of a boot and with a $\frac{3}{4}$ inch or 1 inch raise, will prevent valgus and train position sense. It is intended that such measures will only be temporary and that responsibility for maintaining the corrected position will be taken over by the patient's muscles.

Treatment Potential of Other Media

Ankle Rotator Machine

This is a misnomer, for the action is a sequence of ankle, subtaloid and midtarsal movement. The prime movers can be built up very adequately but the action is a strenuous one and it is necessary to have the foot strapped to the foot plate. It is contra-indicated after local trauma or if there is restriction or pain in any of the joints involved, or in adjacent joints.

Brazing

The bellows can be worked by hand or foot. The leg action is fundamentally like the lathe. Quick pumping is needed to keep up the pressure and the range of movement is small and around mid range. Stamina and control are the essentials. In a department making A.D.L.* equipment for patients at home there is good scope for the work.

Foot Power Looms

Some models have their pedals on a back spindle, i.e. the second order of levers. Others are on one in front, the third order. This affects both the amount of power needed and the mobility of the pedals themselves under the feet of the weaver. With the second order the pedal must be 'found' and stabilised before it can be pressed down. No such problem arises with the more stable third order. Range of movement is not great in any joint, taking sitting as the starting position, but the muscle work is significant. Hip flexors lift the limb against gravity unassisted; they hold it up while the hip is abducted to allow the foot to select the right pedal and to become stable on it; hip and knee extensors depress the pedal; hip and knee flexors return the limb to base. Traditional weavers work barefoot and this, too, has value in mobilising the forepart of the foot, especially on narrow pedals.

According to the tie-up the legs can work alternately or for every heddle change. Other factors which influence the work effort for the lower limbs are the type of shuttle and the design of the weaving. One patient might need periodic rests and her design would include small sections woven in purely by hand. Another might weave in tabby or twill with a time target to be beaten for a given length of cloth.

Patients with osteo-arthritis of the hips or after hip surgery need this type of treatment, giving muscle strengthening but without weight-bearing. If increased range of flexion is wanted this can be encouraged by leaning forward towards the beater. The weaving stool may need a firmly padded top. Unfortunately lack of space precludes the possibility of having such equipment in many departments.

Hand Machines Adapted for Lower Limb Operation

Machines intended for hand operation can be converted successfully for lower limb action. A given range of movement can be assured for a particular joint by mechanical adjustment, and effort can be accurately graded. Skilfully carried out and with the right patient, one who is or can be made exercise minded, it is highly efficient. Because of the repetition and isolation of joint and muscle action there can be certainty that the patient has had his quota of local treatment in a given time. It is also successful with the patient who responds best to something obviously not available at home. In this respect the technique shares a common aura with some forms of electrical treatment given by a physiotherapist. The method has its critics. Isolation of joint movement is unnatural and emphasis on the subnormal limb is undesirable.

The therapist must be available to tie the patient up and to make adjustments. Some people, however, dislike the restriction of being tied up.

Examples of apparatus suitable for conversion include printing press, bench drill, bench mortice, spring vice, hand press, table loom.

Bench Work and General Workshop Activity

This is valuable from two points of view, firstly, as indirect treatment for improvement of local function. According to the activity given, the working positions and the direction of the effort needed will determine the way the joints and muscles are used. Although unlikely to be repetitive the value of this for a patient who is over anxious about his disability is clear and if the work can be with others, in a group project so much the better. Secondly, this is a positive means by which a patient can get used to being about on his leg and can forget that it has been injured. When first fit for such activity, fully weight-bearing, there will be obvious dysfunction, showing mainly in faulty walking. Improvement in spontaneous movement, as the patient goes about a job in the workshop, is one of the best yard sticks of the efficacy of his other treatment.

Walking Aids

These are used:

To take full or partial weight from a limb. Axillary or elbow crutches will be indicated and these will be held in an approximately vertical position.

When there is an habitual limp or poor pattern of walking although the patient is now fully weight-bearing. Two sticks will be indicated until this has been overcome.

To assist balance when there is incoordination, as in disseminated sclerosis. Crutches or some form of stick will be indicated. These will be used in a wide apart and slightly forward position to give 'an extra leg'.

For moral support and protection in the case of a painful or unstable joint, or with an elderly nervous patient. A stick will be indicated here. This will be especially valuable out of doors as other people will recognise a handicap and show consideration.

The occupational therapist must understand the selection and correct usage of walking aids in order to reinforce the physiotherapist's teaching. This will perhaps involve her in giving physical help and she must know from what position to do so. Patients are afraid of falling forwards but this is, in fact, rare; they more often make the mistake of leaning too far back. The therapist in such a case walks behind the patient with hands lightly on the iliac crests. Many patients are unfit to practise their walking without supervision when they first start with their aids and although perhaps coming to the department primarily for something quite different, opportunity to walk should be given. But the therapist must be realistic. An old lady of ninety with a fractured neck of femur will not achieve the same walking pattern as a boy of eighteen who has had a meniscectomy. Safety is more important than anything else. When a patient is discharged with a walking aid he should be taught the importance of non-slip ferrules and how to get them replaced before they become too worn.

Axillary Crutches

The standing position must be with crutches in front, i.e. a stable base. The patient should stand upright with the head up, shoulders pulled down, gripping the top of the crutches with the pectoral muscles, the elbows slightly flexed, taking the weight on his hands. Weight-bearing on the axilla may result in a crutch palsy.

The crutches should be adjusted to fit when the patient is wearing shoes, not slippers or plimsolls. The non-slip ferrules rest on the ground about 6 inches laterally to the shoes; the hand piece should be level with the ulnar styloid; the tops should reach two inches below the axilla when the shoulder girdle is depressed.

For non-weight-bearing walking, take the weight on the sound leg, bring the crutches and the injured leg forward together and then take a step with the sound leg. Aim at paces of equal length, not too long and therefore unsafe, not too short and so lacking in rhythm. 'Crutches and injured leg, then sound leg.'

To climb stairs, take the weight on the crutches and the injured leg, step up with the sound leg, lean slightly forward and then bring the injured leg up to the same step, followed by the crutches. Going downstairs, take the weight on the sound leg, step down with the crutches and the injured leg followed to the same step by the good leg. 'Good leg up to heaven, bad leg down to hell.'

For partial weight-bearing, use the same pattern of movement but take some weight on the injured leg and only use the crutches for additional support.

Elbow Crutches

These are less cumbersome but less stable than axillary crutches. They also take the weight on the hands but rely heavily on the strength in the muscles of the elbow joint. They are used for partial weight-bearing as a progression from the axillary type and for non-weight-bearing for young and active patients. Being less of an inconvenience on stairs, public transport or in cars they are also indicated for patients with long-term need, e.g. after poliomyelitis or, now also relatively rare, with osteomyelitis. Some patients prefer to negotiate stairs holding both crutches in one hand and the hand rail with the other. In other respects they are used like axillary crutches.

Gutter Crutches

When the hands cannot take weight, for example in rheumatoid arthritis or after trauma involving the wrist or hand, a gutter crutch taking weight along the forearm may be indicated. This has a handle beyond the gutter. Often this is vertical. It is more comfortable bent forward to conform with the normal alignment of the wrist and with the palmar crease (i.e. with slight ulnar deviation). Straps are the usual fastening. Velcro may be easier and can be asked for. The arthritic patient with painful hands may also have painful elbows and painful 'bumps' along the ulnar border of the forearm. Extra padding will then be needed in the gutter.

Sticks

For taking weight the stick is used close to the body, and the grip must be forward on the handle, not at the back of the crook. The handle should be level with the ulnar styloid. (Measure the stick by turning the stick upside down and marking the end.) For helping balance a stick will be used in front or to the side, sometimes both. It may be used with a straight or bent arm and the length will vary accordingly. A better pattern of walking is achieved by using two sticks. When one is used, it should be on the opposite side to the affected leg.

When walking with sticks to relieve weight from one leg, stand on the sound leg and swing both sticks (or the one stick) forward and take a medium sized step with the affected leg. Then take an equal sized pace with the good leg. When two legs are 'bad', move the right leg with the left stick, and the left leg with the right stick. To climb stairs, either use the technique for axillary crutches or hold a banister and one stick, or the banister alone. The unwanted stick may be hooked onto the patient's clothing. For winter use the hook must fit over the sleeve of a great coat.

Tripods and tetrapods are more stable than sticks, and are preferred by old people rather than crutches. They are ideal for hemiplegics as they stand on their own when left, instead of falling over. According to the different makes these come in different weights, with different sized bases (important when there are stairs) and in varying stability.

Walking Frames

These are available in a wide variety of designs. Some are rigid and must be lifted forward in the order of; 'frame, first leg, second leg'. Some have castors or gliders, or a combination of both and can be pushed on a smooth surface or continuous carpet. Others are hinged to allow for normal walking sequence 'left hand and right leg, right hand and left leg'. Elderly patients often feel more confident with walking frames than with other forms of aid.

They find them helpful when standing from sitting, as well as for walking. It is always hoped that the patient can become independent of a frame before being discharged for it is too wide for many people's homes and useless for stair climbing, but when the patient is going to a Home or a geriatric unit a frame may provide the only means of independent mobility.

Walking Trolleys

A trolley of suitable height can substitute for a walking aid in some environments, thus serving a dual purpose. Other forms of aid will make it difficult to carry anything and until keeping conscious tally, the amount of carrying done during the day is not realised. The trolley is designed to allow freedom of leg action, and the patient's sticks hook over the sides. It can, if necessary, have gutter crutch supports added for those unable to take weight on their hands (see Plate 16).

Gaits

A therapist who is experienced will find herself unconsciously assessing abnormal gaits both at work and elsewhere. Until she is skilled she should perhaps make a conscious effort to recognise them, for this will be part of her responsibility. It is not enough to notice an abnormality in a patient. Unless the cause for it is appreciated, correction in positive terms will not be possible and this is the only form of benefit to the patient.

Some abnormalities are unavoidable and will be permanent; others must be accepted temporarily but will resolve as function improves with treatment. This is not automatic however. A patient rarely knows why he walks badly and a fault can easily become a habit. It may persist even when the original cause no longer exists. At this stage it is particularly important that treatment be related to functional use. People walk in spite of difficulties. Sometimes unaware of what they do, and certainly not knowing why they do it, they find ways of overcoming their difficulties. Most of them find the standard way, i.e. that which others with the same problems have found, and many of these are easily recognised. The solutions all have one thing in common. They are logical and their rationale can be worked out. There is often more than one possible reason for any single walking abnormality and examples follow:

Difficulty in clearing the ground with the foot. Weak dorsi-flexors; spasticity of calf; inability to flex the hip because of limitation in the joint or because of lack of power in the hip flexors.

Lack of 'push off' with the back foot. Weak calf muscle; painful stiff toes; externally rotated hip.

Dropping on to one foot more heavily than on to the other. Weak calf muscle on the other leg; painful forepart of foot.

Inability to 'pass' the feet equally. Painful limitation of dorsi-flexion of the foot which is not passed as much as the other; weak quadriceps of the same leg.

Heel does not reach the floor. Short leg; shortening of calf muscle; flexion deformity of hip or knee.

Feet turned out. Painful feet; fixed external rotation of the hips.

One foot turned out. As above: external rotation deformity at fracture site in lower leg—the patella still looks forward.

Foot swings out and round instead of passing close to the other one. Bad habit after temporary immobilisation of the knee; arthrodesed hip; inability to compensate for a stiff knee by an extra lift onto the ball of the other foot.

Patient rolls from side to side. A pain avoiding action, when knees are painful as a result of degenerative disease.

Knee is bent. Flexion deformity; adjustment to flexion deformity of the hip; adjustment to adduction deformity of the hip; spasticity of hamstrings.

Knee is hyper-extended. Weakness of hamstrings; weakness of quadriceps, with hyper-extension as a safeguard against instability.

Hip flexed, when weight-bearing as the other foot passes. Weakness of quadriceps; adjustment to flexion deformity of the knee.

Pelvis dropped on one side with marked body swing to the other—Trendelenburg's syndrome. Weakness of hip abductors on the side to which the body weight swings.

Dropping of shoulder and bending to the side of the weight-bearing leg. Weakness of hip abductors, less marked than the above.

Lordosis. Flexion deformity of the hips or adjustment to instability of the hip joints, for example, bilateral congenital dislocation.

Uneven rhythm. Pain in the leg from which weight is relieved quickly; lack of confidence in the same leg.

Adaptation of Footwear

The occupational therapist may be asked to make a temporary adaptation so that the patient can be taught a correct walking pattern without delay while a shoe is sent to the fitter for permanent adaptation. Occasionally the therapist may want to try this out as a treatment aid.

Full Shoe Raise

A raise is usually built half an inch less than the actual shortening; when this is only half an inch a raise may not be required. A markedly short leg will cause the pelvis to tilt when walking. This leads to abnormal mobility of the lumbar spine and to back pain later. A method of making such a raise is fully described in *An Approach to Occupational Therapy*, p. 170 *et seq.* With modern adhesives raises can now be made from balsa wood soled with leather, stuck on to shoes with composition or rubber soles, using a contact glue.

Heel Raise

This may substitute for a full shoe raise when there is not a great deal of shortening. According to the height required there may be, for example, $\frac{3}{4}$ inch on the heel and $\frac{1}{4}$ inch on the sole, or $\frac{1}{2}$ inch on the heel and none on the sole. (A small raise will be of leather only, not balsa wood and leather.) A heel raise may also be needed when, for any reason, the heel does not reach the ground. This may be through calf muscle shortening, either adaptive or from spasticity; joint stiffness, as after severe trauma of the ankle joint; or as a result of fixed flexion deformity in the knee, as in arthritis. The patient will lack stability because with the heel off the ground, the base is smaller. It will be difficult to take a normal sized step forward with the sound leg because this would require further dorsi-flexion of the affected ankle. The raise is thicker at the back then at the front so that the centre of gravity falls within the base and there is maximum contact with the ground.

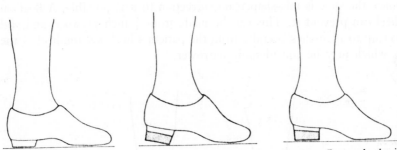

FIG. 21. Normal low heel.   FIG. 22. Incorrect heel raise.   FIG. 23. Correct heel raise.

Temporary Toe-Raising Splint

This may be needed as a temporary measure in the early stages of hemiplegia or peripheral nerve lesion or may be experimental, for example an attempt to improve the gait in disseminated sclerosis. A simple version of this is shown in Fig. 24. The screw eyes are inserted just proximal to the metatarsal heads and at an angle following the line of the metatarso-phalangeal joints. The degree of valgus or varus is adjusted by tightening the relevant strap.

Float

This may be needed when there is instability at the ankle and the patient 'goes over' at each step. Ill fitting shoes with narrow heels encourage this

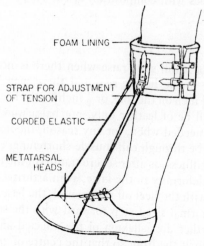

FOAM LINING

STRAP FOR ADJUSTMENT
OF TENSION

CORDED ELASTIC

METATARSAL
HEADS

FIG. 24. Temporary toe-raising splint, heel-toe action in walking.

and once the shoe is mis-shaped no correction to it is possible. A float on
the heel can prevent it. This can be made from $\frac{1}{4}$ inch plywood and will
project up to $1\frac{1}{2}$ inches laterally from the patient's heel, *not* the heel of the
shoe, which may be considerably narrower.

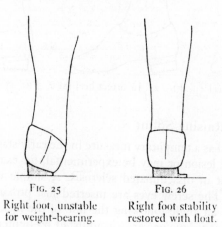

FIG. 25   FIG. 26

Right foot, unstable   Right foot stability
for weight-bearing.   restored with float.

Wedge

This is needed to correct a mobile valgus (or occasionally varus) deformity.
It can be made from $\frac{1}{2}$-inch wood chamfered to a minimum half way across
the sole. This is generally made the length of the shoe because if it is only
on the heel or the forefoot it will force rotation at the mid-tarsal joints.

Metatarsal Bar

This is needed when there is pain on transferring weight from the heel to the ball of the foot because of hallux rigidus or metatarsalgia. It is sometimes needed when there is a heel raise. It is made from a strip of $\frac{1}{8}$ to $\frac{1}{4}$-inch soling leather, $\frac{1}{2}$ inch wide, glued beneath the sole of the shoe proximal to the metatarsal heads and at an angle dictated by the line of the metatarsophalangeal joints.

Foot Pads Worn Inside the Shoes

These are described in *An Approach to Occupational Therapy* p. 167 *et seq.* When the shoe is roomy enough, they can be glued to a thin insole which will keep them in the correct position.

Note. It is important to remember that all these adaptations are only temporary and as normal function returns with treatment the raise or float or wedge can be pared down. If needed permanently they must be replaced by a skilled fitter. In the case of the wedge or float a new shoe with a wider based heel may be sufficient.

REFERENCES AND RECOMMENDED FURTHER READING

Apsley, G., *A System of Orthopaedics and Fractures.* London, 1967.
Aston, J. N., *A Short Textbook of Orthopaedics and Traumatology.* 1972.
Crabbe, W. A., *Orthopaedics for the Undergraduate.* London, 1968.
Crawford Adams, J., *Outline of Fractures.* London, 1972.
Davies, W. T. & Stone, E. M., *Orthopaedics for Nurses.* London, 1971.
Jones, M. S., *An Approach to Occupational Therapy.* London, 1964.
Powell, M., *Orthopaedic Nursing.* Edinburgh and London, 1967.
Saywell, S., *Physiotherapy in Major Knee Surgery.* London, 1965.
Stewart, M., *Rehabilitation following Fracture of the Femoral Neck.* London, 1965.
Wiles, P., *Fractures, Dislocations and Sprains.* London, 1969.
† Quotation from Jones, M. S. Occupational therapy equipment for treatment of the lower limb. *Br. J. Phys. Med.* 8, 54.
* See *Glossary*, p. 454.

CHAPTER 10

Occupational Therapy for Neurological Conditions

Head Injuries [1]

The significance of a head injury lies in the site and extent of the resultant brain damage. There is therefore a wide range of possible neurological damage depending on the mechanics of the blow and the anatomy of the head. The problems which arise from brain damage are:

(1) Mental disturbance.

(2) Post-concussion syndrome.

(3) Personality disorder.

(4) Physical disability.

(5) Communication difficulties.

There are also special problems in treating patients who have survived as a result of treatment in Intensive Care Units, now common throughout the country.

Mental Disturbance

The patient may experience difficulty in concentrating and complain of poor memory. There may be intellectual blunting or more marked thought disorder such as disorientation, confusion and dementia. Exaggeration of normal personality traits may amount to mental disturbance in which anxiety, obsession, suspicion, etc., become disabling. Sometimes psychotic symptoms are evident and the patient is paranoid or deluded to the extent that mental hospital care is necessary. Apraxia—a disturbance of visuo-spatial relationships—presents particular problems as the patient may not recognise familiar objects, e.g. he may be physically capable of dressing but cannot recognise a garment nor remember how to put it on.

The level of concentration can be improved if attention can be held. Suitably quiet surroundings, free from distractions, will be needed. An activity simple enough to ensure success but complex enough to be interesting should be given. Note the length of the attention span and do not make excessive demands on concentration but aim at a gradual improvement. A variety of activities may have to be used to prevent loss of interest. Assessment should be made of a patient's present level of attainment in basic arithmetic, spelling and vocabulary compared with his standard of education and employment. Coaching in these subjects may improve performance and should be attempted before making a final work assessment.

Apraxia may prove difficult to overcome, but repetition of a simple task, e.g. putting on a sock until it is achieved, is helpful.

Post Concussional Syndrome

The patient complains of 'headache' associated with exertion of sudden activity or emotional stress; of lassitude and fatigue; and of vertigo, particularly on stooping. Concentration is poor and memory for day to day things is unreliable.

A personality change may be noticed by the patient's family and associates, in particular increased irritability and intolerance of environmental noise and activity. If there are no accompanying physical signs to account for this, he may be labelled a malingerer or as suffering from 'compensationitis.' Evidence shows however, that this may have an organic cause. It appears that this group of patients will improve if given the benefit of rehabilitation where encouragement and gradual build-up of activity in stimulating work will help them to function more normally in spite of persistence of some of their symptoms.

Personality Disorder

Personality change as the result of brain damage is usually associated with permanent intellectual deterioration. It may be mild, showing only an exaggeration of the pre-accident personality traits, e.g. inertia, depression, euphoria, tension, anxiety, obsessions, etc. A previously anxiety-prone man may present a 'catastrophic response' under stress—crying, banging, shouting, and becoming generally uncontrolled. General irritability and intolerance to noise are often evident and anti-social behaviour causes embarrassment to family and friends. Emotional lability and childlike dependence may also be evident.

Personality re-education is difficult and prognosis is uncertain. Considerable tolerance and free rein may be necessary initially (unless it is too disrupting for other patients). To become exasperated and attempt to discipline or remonstrate continuously with a patient who has no insight and with whom it is impossible to reason only aggravates the situation. Within a week or two some rapport will probably be established and once the occupational therapist has his confidence he is more likely to cooperate. Most of all at this time he needs to be shown understanding by someone who will talk to him and encourage the more stable facets of his behaviour. He is not insensitive to other people's attitudes towards himself. Gradual introduction of routine, discipline and responsibility should be planned.

Physical Disabilities

These are caused by severe head injuries and are most frequently seen as hemiparesis of varying degrees, showing ataxia, incoordination and poor balance. There may also be sensory disturbance affecting light touch, pain and sense of position; and visual disturbance—diplopia or hemianopia. In addition there may be loss of sphincter control. All cases of head injury are put on prophylactic doses of anti-convulsants for a time but between 2 and 3 per cent of cases develop epilepsy.

Treatment of these physical symptoms are discussed elsewhere, but certain points are worth emphasising. The use of a standing harness for bench work is valuable in the early re-education of postural sense and standing balance. Weight can help reduce ataxia; for instance, writing may be made easier by fixing a weighted strap to the patient's wrist. Double vision is helped by covering the affected eye and as with hemianopia the patient must learn to turn his head to compensate for lack of vision on the affected side.

Patients may compensate to some extent for other sensory loss by using their sight instead. It is not unusual for the affected side to be ignored or even disclaimed. This makes re-education of dressing difficult. Attempts should be made to toilet train incontinents by keeping to a strict habit routine. This can only be done by a team effort involving everybody in touch with the patient during the 24 hours.

Communication Difficulties

Damage to the dominant hemisphere will often cause disturbance of speech and comprehension, i.e. executive and receptive dysphasia, and difficulty may be experienced in reading and writing, i.e. dyslexia and dysgraphia. Extreme isolation and frustration is experienced by patients with speech and comprehension disturbance and it is usually this above all other disabilities that the patient is most anxious to overcome. At certain levels of recovery scrabble and other word games are valuable. If a patient is dysarthric and so incoordinated as to be unable to write, but not dysphasic or dyslexic, an alphabet board on which he can spell out his needs should be provided.

General Principles of Rehabilitation, as Applied to Patients with Head Injury

(1) Initial assessment of physical and mental abilities.
(2) Activities designed to improve physical and mental abilities.

(3) Re-education in activities of daily living in both physical and social aspects.

(4) Final assessment and resettlement.

Head injuries are most common in young men, as a result of road accidents, and there may also be other injuries. If the patient is referred for occupational therapy soon after consciousness has been regained little more can be done than to give reassurance and to show understanding. Stimulation of interest is needed where apathy persists or reassurance where there is agitation and anxiety. The patient will tire easily and lucid thought may be short lived. Anticipate fatigue and do not overstress the patient at this stage. Note his attention span, mood and degree of insight. Assess his physical disability, his sense of posture, his ability to use his hands. This is best done by giving him familiar objects to handle.

As soon as is permitted, get the patient out of the ward, but until this can be done, build up tolerance to physical and mental fatigue by use of games: dominoes and scrabble are suitable activities for increasing co-ordination, joint movement and muscle power. Encourage independent feeding, washing, shaving and writing.

It is extremely important to cooperate with all others treating the patient so as to draw up a balanced programme of rehabilitation. It is also important to be in touch with the family. They can advise on the patient's previous interests and abilities and they can see for themselves his present abilities, and can learn what to do when he needs help. The families of patients with personality problems are often subjected to tremendous emotional stress. In units treating head injuries it has been found that if relatives can get together to discuss their problems they derive much support from one another and benefit from compared experiences.

Rehabilitation of the severely brain damaged patient presents a special problem because of the combination of physical, intellectual and behavioural difficulties. Ideally the patient should have a full day's programme of rehabilitation, attending daily from home or as a weekly in-patient.

The period of attendance for medical rehabilitation must be guided by progress. An initial period of at least a year may be needed. This in itself creates problems for it is difficult in any one centre for optimism and enthusiasm to be stimulated for so long, and once either is lost progress stops. Special centres usually restrict attendance to a few months. Since maximum improvement may not be attained for 5 years, it is often best for the patient to be discharged after the initial treatment period and to be re-assessed after 3 or 4 months. In some cases arrangements should be made for the patient to attend a Day Centre to provide continued stimulation and social contact, and also to relieve the strain on the family. On reassessment further treatment may be prescribed if there are signs of worthwhile improvement. Once maximum function is achieved resettlement plans are discussed as for any type of patient. Many will be able to do work of some kind but others present both work and social problems, and when there is severe residual disability—either physical or mental—the patient's family may need continuing support if he is to be looked after at home. The responsibility for providing this will usually be allocated to the Local Authority Social Services Department. In addition the hospital authorities may recommend periods of in-patient care at regular intervals. Even if these are relatively short they may be an invaluable contribution to the social resettlement plan.

Hemiplegia [2]

The Patient's Symptoms

In addition to the motor defect of spastic paralysis or paresis there may be sensory loss, with superficial anaesthesia or loss of position sense, or both. There may also be perceptual defect shown by loss of body image and inability to relate to things outside the body. With organic involvement of the frontal lobes there may be deviations in behaviour or changes in personality. Damage to other areas can affect vision, memory and facilitation. Emotional disturbance is common, the patient being labile and depressed. This is not always organic, rather it may be a reactive depression which will lift with successful rehabilitation. Speech defect is also common.

The onset of illness is sudden and the severity of the disability is a shock to the patient and to his family, especially when there has been no previous illness or when the patient is young. They think of it as an acute illness from which there will be recovery.

The Patient's Problems

On referral for treatment the patient may present any of the following problems:

(1) Inability to move the affected arm or leg, to change position in bed or in a chair, or to balance unsupported in sitting. Often there is preoccupation with the paralysed arm.

(2) Inability to feel the affected limbs, to appreciate movement of joints or to appreciate their relationship to the body. Inability, too, to recognise the limbs as part of himself.

(3) Inability to understand terms of direction, e.g. right, left, forward, back. Instructions are misunderstood and re-education of movement patterns, e.g. walking, and those of activities such as dressing, are difficult and frustrating.

(4) Loss of initiative, poor memory, confusion, depression and emotional instability. This last causes distress and anxiety. With time it

decreases but while it lasts choice of placement for treatment will be affected. Usually it is best not to comment on it.

(5) Inability to understand the spoken word or to recognise the written one. Inability to express thought in words. Inability to articulate.

(6) Self-consciousness relating to physical ineptitude (including loss of use of the dominant hand), to speech difficulty and to emotional lability. Incontinence may be an added source of embarrassment. The patient is often acutely aware of loss of personal dignity.

The disability of one-handedness is easily assumed and every therapist should prepare herself for treating hemiplegic patients by experiencing it herself for at least a day. She will soon discover the frustration and may also find some of the solutions. What she cannot experience is the general clumsiness, the slowness and the sensory deficit but in treating her patients she must remember these handicaps and their implications.

General Policy of Physical Treatment

Treatment is begun in the ward by the physiotherapist, usually after two or three days. Prophylactic passive movements to the affected limbs are important at this stage and, if later there is no recovery, they will continue to be so. In particular the shoulder joint must be kept mobile, for a stiff shoulder becomes a painful one. Later on it may be the occupational therapist's responsibility to see that the patient does not allow the joint to become stiff. She must therefore know the technique of moving it passively through its full range. An early start is made on re-education of sitting balance and as soon as practicable the patient is helped up on to his feet. It is generally at this stage, approximately 2 or 3 weeks after the stroke, that occupational therapy can be added.

In the ward, bed and chair heights may be inappropriate for training in general mobility and for undressing and dressing. Treatment is best given in the department where there will also be greater stimulation than in an acute ward. Within the limits of fatigue treatment should be intensive, but planned rest periods are as important as periods of activity. Therapists must be ready to adjust a patient's programme if he becomes fatigued or if his efforts are unproductive. Dressing training, for example, may have to be postponed if a patient has insufficient balance or loss of body image.

Most patients on intensive treatment will walk again. Comparatively few will recover a useful hand and the degree of recovery present three weeks after the stroke is a fair indication of what can be expected. It is right to persevere with treatment while the patient shows improvement which will increase independence or decrease dependence. Increased ability to co-operate, return of pride in personal appearance and growth of a realistic adjustment to the disability are also important signs of improvement and while they continue so should treatment. At this stage emphasis will increasingly be placed on achievement in spite of residual disability. Aims must be broadly based to cover as many aspects of daily life as possible. It is hoped that both the patient and his family will be able to accept this policy and to take pride in the patient's increase of independence. The doctor should be involved in this stage, for explanations and encouragement are much needed, especially when the patient has interpreted, 'It will take a long time', as an assurance of ultimate recovery.

Treatment programmes must be realistic. For example, in treating elderly patients it is helpful to know their previous physical capacity and habits of daily living. Without this, targets could be set too high or too low. Long-term prognosis is also a guide and plans for the patient whose hemiplegia is the result of trauma can be more ambitious than those for the patient who is hypertensive.

Pattern of Recovery and its Implications

Gross movements return first; only later, if at all, can fine coordinated movements be hoped for. Gross movement in the lower limb can be of functional value but in the upper limb this is rarely the case. Without ability to place the hand for use and to release grasp, the ability to grasp is of little practical use. Knowing this, nurses and therapists should encourage the use of the unaffected hand as a substitute for the affected one as soon as possible, for example cutting up food with a Nelson knife. If such practice can be initiated early it may be accepted as a temporary measure, while in fact laying the foundation for essential adjustment to one-handedness.

Re-education of the trunk muscles is possible before that of the limbs. It follows that some degree of sitting balance should be possible before occupational therapy is prescribed. During treatment this should be furthered by expecting the patient to sit with his back unsupported for short periods. The same principle applies later when the physiotherapist is training the patient in standing balance. It would be wrong for the occupational therapist to treat him sitting throughout in his wheel-chair. It is beneficial for him to stand up and sit down again if only once and with physical assistance. Each reminder of the correct method and each experience of it helps to re-establish the movement patterns involved.

For a patient with whom communication is difficult because of receptive aphasia or of confusion, methods of individual therapists within a department and in different departments should be integrated as fully as possible. This is of special importance in aspects of treatment such as walking where there is overlap of treatment. Even so it is clearly best for the patient if, instead of two therapists sharing responsibility for one part of treatment (for example, the initial assessment and training of personal care aspects of daily living, which includes mobility), it is covered either by the occupational therapist or the physiotherapist. In some centres this is accepted practice.

Even when intensive speech therapy is available the speech therapist is usually glad if the occupational therapist can help the patient to practice his current vocabulary and his writing.

Content of an Occupational Treatment Plan

If the patient has problems, so has the therapist:

(1) Until return of function is adequate for use, the techniques of occu-pational therapy cannot help the patient towards the three things he most wants, i.e. to use his hand, to speak, and to walk. Yet referrals for treatment may be made at this stage and rightly so, for the sooner he can be stimulated to activity the better.

(2) Important aspects of treatment which can be tackled often seem to the patient to be pointless, i.e. learning to do everyday things for himself one handed, e.g. dressing, shaving, etc. Similarly he may think it childish to be given activities to assess and retrain perceptual function.

(3) The patient may be mentally unable to cooperate and until his interest is roused there can be no progress. This may be a matter of personal relationships and a change of therapist might make all the difference. If so, it should not be considered as failure by the original therapist.

Activities of daily living. These involve general mobility, handling ability and concentration. They are complex and demanding both physically and mentally. Although it is right for the patient to be dressed for his treatment, it may have to be accepted that as part of treatment he will achieve little at an early stage. Even so the daily repetition of simple dressing procedures is therapeutic if done always in the same routine.

The therapist must be able to break down each activity into its com-ponents. The plan for any one treatment session can then avoid unprofitable attempts at difficult sequences. For example, practice in crossing the affected leg over the other, by lifting it with the opposite hand, purely as an exercise, will make it easier to put on the sock and shoe in a few day's time. After this practice the patient might be taught the method he will use to tie his laces, the shoe being stabilised at knee height.

What has been said so far applies to cases referred for treatment early after the incidence of the stroke. Many patients are sent much later, after initial care at home. The first need then is a thorough assessment of func-tional ability, of the disability, of the personality and the capacity to co-operate. If the patient has had no previous physical treatment an intensive short course of physiotherapy and occupational therapy may be prescribed

to improve local function in the arm and leg with a view to better performance in walking and possibly in two-handed activities. It is important that
the patient understands that this is a short term measure. The doctor should
also make it clear that the major part of treatment will be training to achieve
maximal competence in spite of the residual handicap.

Treatment to improve hand function. For a hand to be of functional value
there must be control of the shoulder, elbow and forearm, and also good
position sense and body control. Treatment for the hand cannot be isolated
from any of these and all are difficult for most patients with hemiplegia.

In a minority of cases where individual finger movements recover early,
prognosis is good and treatment, if needed at all, includes general strenthen-
ing of total grip for stabilising and carrying; re-education of release and the
preparatory movements for pick-up; coordination in two-handed activities
needing accurate hand placement and finger precision, especially those of
everyday importance, e.g. doing up small buttons, tying shoe laces, handling
a newspaper, etc. There will also be retraining of special skills as relevant,
e.g. writing, using scissors, sewing, use of tools, etc. Treatment for improvement of general mobility may be needed if full use is to be made of the
restored hand skill, e.g. crouching and bending as needed by the housewife,
the amateur motor mechanic or the gardener.

Something considerably less than normal efficiency is of functional value
in the non-dominant hand. Provided there are signs of ability to grasp and to
release, or of ability to place and maintain a position in which the weight
of the forearm could substitute for stabilisation by the hand, treatment is
justified. Shoulder and elbow mobility and active control will be encouraged.
Ironing, hand duplicating, planing, self-assisted sanding or polishing, double-
handed sawing, bench drilling or morticing are all useful. Unreliable grip
can be augmented by using a special mitten. (See Ref. 2. Epprecht.)

To overcome spasticity, which might lead to flexion contracture of the
fingers, thumb and wrist, the hand can be held in position for sanding or
polishing on a block, hollowed out but convex for the palm with the fingers
in extension and abduction. Initially the patient will sit while working but as
stamina and balance improve he will benefit additionally by standing. With
one foot forward and one back in opposition to the affected arm, transfer of
weight will be encouraged and with it contraction of the knee, hip and
spinal extensors. If the working height was right when he sat, there will be
need to make adjustments when he stands. Increased extension of his wrist
might force clawing of the fingers. Either raising the work or having it on a
downward slope solves this problem.

Training in mobility. Safety depends as much on awareness of position as
on muscle strength and control. When there is sensory deficit, the patient
must learn to compensate by checking the position of his limbs visually.
Suitable glasses are important. Bi-focals are contra-indicated. A further

safeguard for the patient walking is to wear a small, metal toe cap which can be heard as it strikes the floor.

Standing from sitting and sitting from standing is the first mobility training the occupational therapist must give. The need for it will be evident early in assessment of activities of daily living.

Once walking is reasonably safe with just one helper, the patient should have opportunity to practise during occupational therapy sessions, at first perhaps only from wheel-chair into the department, standing up and adjusting balance, and then walking. Initially most of the weight will be on the walking aid and the unaffected leg, gradually more on the affected one. Flexion of the hip and knee are weak, and with the toe catching on the ground help may be needed in bringing the leg through. The therapist, standing sideways, facing the patient on his paralysed side can push the leg forward with her own. Support to straighten an unstable knee can be given by exerting pressure on the front of the joint, or on the upper part of the lower leg, with the inner side of her knee, slightly bent.

A temporary toe-raising splint may be needed, made by the occupational therapist or physiotherapist as agreed between them (see Fig. 24). Muscle power and coordination may be improved by working a bicycle, the foot strapped to the pedal, and with emphasis on control of the position of the knee, and on even rhythm.

When the patient can walk unaided he must learn how to open and shut doors, how to move sideways in a confined space and how to walk safely in spite of hazards in a workshop. As he becomes competent he should be encouraged to discard his walking aid indoors so that he can carry things. When progressed to a stick, a wrist thong will help, especially when climbing stairs and shutting doors. He must also learn how to pull his chair up to the table, transferring his weight forward over his feet then pulling the chair forward by gripping the seat between his legs. Standing and moving away from a table also needs practice. The relationship of the chair or table leg with his own may be misjudged or not considered at all by a patient with poor position sense or loss of body image. Turning quickly before standing balance is assured, is another common fault. The patient will not learn except by repeated practice and nor will the therapist. Hers should be with fellow students, developing skill in positioning and handling and in making the emergency moves needed to counteract a patient's loss of balance. Falls destroy confidence. She must also be able to explain to the patient *why* he lost balance, and to give him positive correction. When possible, progression will be made to stair climbing and walking on slopes. Later on some patients will be trained to use public transport and to get in and out of a car. A small minority will qualify for an invalid tricycle as a means of getting to work.

Treatment to help social adjustment. First contacts will be with other patients. Placement in the department near the 'right' patient can be as valuable as the 'right' occupation. Solitary activities must be avoided, and those which encourage sociability encouraged, for example cooking, community singing, games, shopping expeditions, a bus journey, or a joint project in the workshop with a patient briefed to encourage conversation. It is obvious that the treatment programme must be reviewed frequently in view of the diversity of aims to be covered.

Assessment and Preparation for Resettlement

The first phase of resettlement is discharge from the ward. The patient's immediate family is naturally apprehensive about his return home, fearing for his safety if he tries to move on his own and being impatient with his slowness. Everything possible must be done to alleviate this. Necessary adaptations such as rails for the stairs, must be installed before his discharge. His limitations and his abilities must be explained and demonstrated and methods of giving necessary help must be taught. The patient himself might have neither the energy nor the words with which to resist 'help' mistakenly forced upon him.

Out-patient treatment increases the overall demands on the patient. He will be expected to take more responsibility both in planning and in carrying out his programme. With improved fatigue tolerance he will be expected to extend his activity to his home. Both women and men should be encouraged to take some part in the work there: shoe cleaning, caring for pot plants or for the budgerigar, and certainly washing up or, better still, cooking. If deterioration is to be prevented when treatment stops, active participation in something is essential. Attendance at a day centre or club is recommended.

Apart from the housewife who, if well adjusted, can be helped to overcome most of her problems patients with professional or clerical backgrounds have the best chance of returning to their former jobs. Gainful employment for the majority of others is an unrealistic target. Training is seldom possible. When hopes are realistic there must be a comprehensive assessment. Slowness and fatigue may be inevitable. Each will increase the other and both must be corrected as far as possible, the former by work study methods applied to the full day's activities and the latter by building up and consolidating stamina by progressive effort.

Paraplegia [3]

The most common cause of paraplegia is spinal injury and of the patients who suffer this young adult males predominate. Their disability is a stable one and the prognosis for leading an active life is good. When the cause is a progressive disease not only is the prognosis different but the occupational therapist will need a less dynamic approach. The aim of treatment in both cases is for physical and psychological adjustment to a wheel-chair life, so that

·the patient can be independent in self care and mobility and can hope for satisfactory resettlement at home and in work.

It is usual for treatment to be given in a special residential centre. During the period in bed, nursing care and intensive physiotherapy occupy most of the day. This will include dressing and transferring exercises. The occupational therapist may or may not be involved in the basic personal care aspects of A.D.L.*, for example dressing, but if she is she must have special training which can only be obtained in such centres. Sometimes, usually because of resettlement problems, a patient will be referred to a hospital with rehabilitation facilities in his home area. When fit enough the patient will attend the department in his wheelchair.

The occupational therapist's first aim will be to strengthen or maintain the muscles which must compensate for loss of power in the legs when transferring to and from the wheel-chair and when crutch walking. Treatment must be physically demanding, for example, using metal snips for strong hand grip with other muscle groups acting as stabilisers; bilarteral overhead drilling or morticing against spring resistance for strengthening arms, shoulder girdle and trunk muscles; bench work at a suitable height providing for a variety of trunk and upper limb movements, practice in correct positioning of the wheel-chair and good sitting balance. The patient should try to fetch tools and materials for himself and put them away afterwards. This is not only physically therapeutic but builds up self reliance and self esteem.

Women patients often enjoy, and will certainly benefit from, the same workshop activities. It may be by finding out that they can still work satisfactorily in a kitchen and can carry out other domestic duties that their morale is best built up, and occupational therapy should provide for this. Every encouragement should be given to the patient who wants to explore any reasonable avenue of potential achievement or interest and he should be given time in which to do it. New recreational, social and hobby activities may be needed. Archery and table tennis commonly feature as treatment in many centres.

Sometimes standing practice is requested. It will be important for the occupational therapist to know the technique by which the patient has been taught to stand wearing his calipers and helpful to have seen him doing it. His competence in balancing will determine what he can attempt while standing and details of optimum positioning and of necessary safeguards must be understood.

Patients are trained to take responsibility for preventing damage to their skin. During prolonged sitting they should frequently push up on the arms of their chairs to relieve pressure on weight-bearing areas. They must also avoid burning themselves, by carrying a hot plate across the thighs, for example, or bruising by coming into contact with the pipes under a basin.

The layout of the home often restricts the chairbound patient limiting his mobility, putting him at risk and forcing him to accept help he would not need in suitably designed surroundings. This is especially true in relation to bathroom and lavatory. Home problems may have to be tackled before re-settlement in work is possible. This is markedly true of the housewife whose home is her work place. Lack of access to her sink, to her work preparation area and to her storage in addition to difficulties of access from room to room may prevent her from running her home. Without major alterations or resettlement in a purpose-built flat or bungalow the problems are often insoluble and detrimental to health and morale. A well-adjusted woman will have little difficulty in managing after a period of training in new and safe methods, provided she has reasonable stability in sitting, good use of her arms and a home in which she can be mobile.

Assessment for resettlement in work outside the home follows the usual pattern. For many jobs, being chairbound creates no special problems and training is available through the Department of Employment for such jobs as precision instrument making, watch and clock repairing, draughtsmanship, typing, bookkeeping, dressmaking and teaching. Higher education is more possible now than formerly and some institutions are planning to provide facilities for disabled students.

Paraplegics with their excellent upper limb function are good candidates for hand controlled vehicles and many of them, having learnt the technique, will need no help in getting either themselves or their wheel-chairs in and out of their cars or tricycles.

Progressive Paralyses [4]

General Principles

Progressive locomotor dysfunction is a symptom common to many diseases. Most are neural in origin, the lesion being in the brain, e.g. Parkinson's disease, or in the spinal cord, e.g. Friedreich's ataxia, or in both, e.g. dis-seminated sclerosis. Muscular dystrophy is an exception. It is caused by intrinsic dysfunction of muscle. In other respects too, the individual con-ditions are different, the age of incidence, the distribution of paralysis and the prognosis. The incidence of sensory and mental involvement also varies. While planning treatment for the present and for the immediate future, the long-term implications must be remembered.

There must be a balance between a too hopeful outlook and one not bold enough to plan for the future. Sometimes there are appreciable periods of remission from all symptoms and a patient is able to return to his former work. At others, substantial improvement in the early stages may lead to disappointment when this does not continue. Considerable variation in performance may occur from day to day, e.g. the patient with an ataxic gait being unable to walk unaided the very day after a marked improvement. His programme must be pliable enough to adjust to these variations: when it includes a period of work to improve standing tolerance, the work itself should be equally suitable for positions of sitting or of perching on a stool. In this way the patient is less aware of the down grading. At the same time he should be helped to be realistic, to conserve his energy and to think out safe methods. A housewife, even if she can walk about in her kitchen, should sit on a stool when preparing food, washing up, or working for any length of time at the stove.

Early treatment will aim to improve function followed by assessment for return to work. The total of the day's activities must be easily within the patient's capacity, for fatigue is contra-indicated and performance is variable. With a deteriorating condition return to work should be initiated as soon as possible, and with the same employer if this is practicable.

In some cases deterioration is gradual, over many years. Occupational therapy may play no part until increasing disability creates a problem in the patient's normal routine. This may be related to work, use of public transport or handling of tools and materials. Alternatively it may relate to self care activities and indicate the need to have help with bathing or with cutting up food. Sometimes physical deterioration is rapid, with the patient fully aware of his increasing dependence on his family for maintaining standards in personal appearance and for safe mobility. The resulting depression is not unreasonable. With other patients mental deterioration is marked; personal standards fall and there is little realisation of the physical and mental strain imposed on those who must provide care. In the advanced stages of illness the occupational therapist can only hope to help the patient and his family to manage in spite of his increasing disabilities: lack of mobility, loss of coordination and perhaps mental deterioration. These produce practical problems which are only a part of the total social problem.

The longer the patient can keep some independence, the better for his self respect. If, however, he takes so long to dress that he is exhausted, chilled and dishevelled, his energy is better spent in cooperating with someone who will help him. It would certainly be unwise to suggest alteration of an efficient domestic routine where one exists. Special equipment may be needed. This includes the right type of wheel-chair and other aids, for example, a bath seat or a hoist which will relieve the helper of some of the physical strain of moving the patient. The size of the total problem depends as much on the layout of the home and of the availability of care as on the patient's condition.

When his attendance at the hospital stops, the patient will benefit from some form of stimulation and outside contact. If this can be regular attendance at a day centre or club his family will benefit too. The hospital occupational therapy department should not be expected to supply a maintenance service, but it can and will expect the patient to be referred back for re-assessment if a change in his condition makes this necessary.

MULTIPLE (DISSEMINATED) SCLEROSIS

This disease is usually first diagnosed in the young adult. It is characterised
by remissions and relapses. In some cases a plateau may be reached; in
others deterioration is rapid; in most, disability increases over several
decades. Although mental changes develop, the first symptoms are physical
and it is often a feeling of heaviness in one or both legs and perhaps unsteadi-
ness in walking which first brings the patient to hospital. Visual disturbance
and abnormal sensations in the trunk or limbs are also common early symptoms. Although there may be clinical evidence of intention tremor, this
textbook symptom rarely seems to be a problem until later. Physical treatment is not always indicated at first. If it is, and occupational therapy is included, advice on safety measures for travel may be the main need. The
overall aim will be to get the patient back to work as soon as possible. Often
the symptoms clear up altogether and there may be no recurrence for several
years.

As the pattern of the disease becomes established there is increased
spasticity in the legs and frequently ataxia of cerebellar origin in the limbs
and the trunk, sometimes presenting as a hemiplegia. Walking requires a
conscious effort and balance is unreliable. Arm movements may be difficult
to control and ability to hold good posture is dubious. Although the course
of the disease cannot be influenced, the overall deterioration will be lessened
if rest during a period of exacerbation can be followed by a short course of
progressive treatment during the early stages of remission. The timing of
this is vital; the patient with realistic hopes of going back to work should do
so while functioning capably and with reasonable prospects of continuing
to do so. This will partly depend on the overall routine of his day's activity
being within his fatigue tolerance limits. To keep his job, other activities
may have to be curtailed and the wear and tear of travel reduced by any
means possible, e.g. his wife might drive him to work or, in the case of the
housewife, local shops might deliver goods to save her struggling with
shopping. These principles are also observed in planning treatment. With an
in-patient this is easy. With an out-patient home commitments must be
taken into account, particularly those of the housewife who could easily be
overtired by household chores when she gets home.

Occupational Therapy

Build up stamina by decreasing rest periods and by gradually increasing
the effort content.

Improve coordination. Special attention is given to posture training. Any
patient who is unsteady on his feet is liable to slump in his chair, but this is
especially true of one with generalised ataxia. Training is first a matter of
motivating the patient to make conscious effort to sit well so that this be-

comes a habit even while thinking about something different. This form of treatment can immediately be continued at home. When trunk muscles are strong enough to maintain an upright sitting posture, progression can be made to standing work in a special harness. This can be used at a bench or a sink, and is adjustable. It can give either physical support and stability to the pelvis or psychological support to build up confidence.

Assess the current problems of personal independence, giving help in finding alternative methods or in using aids and special equipment to overcome them.

Assessment for resettlement. Maximum abilities can only be estimated if fatigue can be avoided and use of work study methods are indicated. At home for example, a list of the items required for setting the table can be attached to the trolley to avoid frequent journeys. Contact with an understanding employer may also lead to appropriate measures being thought out at the patient's place of work.

With further deterioration other symptoms increase the disability:

(1) Frequency and urgency of micturition becomes a major problem when mobility is restricted and slow.

(2) Double vision adds to the difficulty of using the hands accurately. An eye patch sometimes helps.

(3) Dysarthria hampers communication which is already restricted by difficulty in writing.

(4) Depression, although seldom cited, is not uncommon at the stage when prospects for continuing at work deteriorate and when the job is lost. Later there may be a feeling of well being inconsistent with the patient's physical state—euphoria.

Inability to travel, lack of alternative means of getting to work, inability to stand at work or to work quickly or neatly enough ultimately make employment impossible. General fatigue is frequently a contributing factor. The housewife without need to travel or to keep to a rigid timetable can often carry on satisfactorily for longer, taking at least part of her former responsibility if given appropriate help in adapting her methods to safeguard herself against accidents.

From the physical and psychological point of view activity should be continued for as long as possible. The male patient who can no longer work should be given every encouragement to be active in his home with some household tasks which make regular demands upon him. It may be increasing incoordination or mental deterioration which curtails and finally stops such activity, or both. The patient may still be relatively young and it will be necessary to find a means of freeing his family from their responsibilities and ties at regular intervals and meeting the patient's need for change of environment and for social stimulation.

Ultimately spasticity in the legs increases until rigidity and spasm prevent voluntary movement and contractures develop. The patient may be in-continent and will become fully dependent. Admission to a home able to provide full care or to a long-stay hospital may be the only solution.

This term describes a group of symptoms associated with disease or damage to the basal ganglia. It is characterised by inhibition of movement:

(1) Lack of facial expression, control of saliva, and movement of the head.
(2) Poor articulation of speech; monotonous, festinant and lacking in volume.
(3) Loss of the automatic swing of the arms in walking, a position of flexion and adduction with the hands held close to the front of the the body, replacing this.
(4) Shuffling festinant gait with the knees flexed; sometimes retropulsion.

The paralysis produces rigidity affecting the whole body which is held in flexion; there is also a tremor, e.g. typical 'pill rolling'. This is present when the patient is at rest but not when he is asleep. Mental retardation is common but it is easy to assume this wrongly because of the physical slow-ness and the Parkinson mask. There are also psychological symptoms, all of them reasonable in view of the form and severity of the incapacity, i.e. anxiety which increases the symptoms, despondency and frustration because so much effort is needed to achieve so little, and depression. The patient is embarrassed by his appearance and difficulty in communicating and tends to become withdrawn. The relations have emotional problems too. They are distressed by the patient's difficulties, frustrated by his slowness and anxious for his safety when walking. This adds to his lack of confidence.

Occupational Therapy

(1) To stimulate endeavour.
(2) To improve physical ability to the maximum, i.e. general mobility and purposeful activity with the hands.
(3) To encourage clear speech.
(4) According to the extent of disability, to assess ability to return to work or to assess ability to manage at home with the help available there.
(5) To contribute to plans for continuing support both for the patient and his family. The need for stimulation to maintain the patient at his best level of physical and intellectual performance must be met.

In addition to the above aims there will need to be performance testing of patients before and after treatment with L-dopa and associated drugs, or, where surgery is carried out, pre- and post-operative assessment. The therapist will record performance, using standard dexterity tests and also practical achievement in everyday activities. The tests should be timed.

Following operation a programme of re-education in normal patterns of movement and use of the limbs now free of rigidity and tremor is rewarding. Considerable improvement can be expected in mobility and general independence and equal improvement in the patient's morale.

Mobility. In most cases general physical ability can be improved. Patients are stimulated by taking part in group activities and these should be carefully upgraded. Sustained effort is particularly tiring to them, however, and they cannot tolerate fatigue. Allowance must be made for this and there must be close supervision. Good posture and large movements are to be encouraged, and activities should be suitable for the patient's intellectual level.

Getting up from a chair, particularly from a low one, is a frequent problem, due to inability to initiate the necessary preparatory body movement. If, with a chair of suitable height, with arms, and using the correct pattern of movement, there is still no success, a grab rail or a sturdy piece of furniture in lieu may answer. An ejector seat is helpful to some. Others are too nervous to use it.

Taking big steps improves walking as does stepping over or on to pre-marked positions on the floor by kicking at a walking stick or by having something to push or carry. Some patients who are unable to 'pick their feet up' on the level surprisingly have no difficulty in climbing stairs and can continue successfully on the level for a number of yards while remembering the 'feeling' of climbing them. Obstacles such as doorways may cause hesitation and an increase in symptoms, and meeting someone in a doorway might precipitate retropulsion.

Activities of daily living. One of the difficulties in treating parkinsonism is the variation in performance from day to day. For a realistic assessment of ability the patient must be judged on his days of poor performance as well as his best days. The effect of stimulation and encouragement provided by the therapist must also be taken into account when judging ability to overcome akinesia. It is the slowness of performance and rapid onset of fatigue which defeats achievement rather than inability to perform the required movements. In dressing, the patient may be capable but takes so long over it that it is not reasonable to expect him to manage unaided if help is available.

Communication. Emphasis on the consonants is needed when there is dysarthria and slow speech is necessary for practising this. Singing can help to overcome monotone and correct breathing is essential both for this and for speaking loudly. The patient should be encouraged to work at his speech but opportunities for spontaneous speaking should also be created, e.g. playing 'snap' with someone else turning up the cards. Writing can improve by practising large letters, stopping when tremor or micrography interferes with the rhythm and formation of the shapes.

Advanced Parkinsonism. The problems of advanced Parkinsonism are manifold. Unable to communicate verbally or in writing, with field of vision severely restricted by his kyphosis deformity—chin on chest—and virtually immobilised by akinesia, the patient is cut off from his environment and fellow beings except for those who tend to his needs. Mental stimulation in these circumstances is urgently needed to combat mental retardation and depression. Being able to partake even passively in a group situation, whether at home or in a larger community, will afford some mental stimulation and may give at least some feeling of participation and social contact.

Sometimes it helps to have a high backed chair which can be tilted safely backwards to such an angle that gravity no longer acts on the forward droop of the patient's head. If in addition a soft and pliable scarf can be tolerated with comfort round the forehead and fixed to the back of the chair, the position of the head is much improved. It is possible to see and easier to be fed and to drink. It also improves respiratory function. The feet of course must be supported.

Lower Motor Neurone Lesions [5]

The lower motor neurone may be damaged at any point from the anterior horn cell as in poliomyelitis, to the periphery as in lesions of the common peroneal or ulnar nerves. Peripheral lesions in the upper limb, partial or complete, occur more often than any other form of lower motor neurone lesion. The paralysis is flaccid and with time there is obvious muscle wasting and change in contour of the part. Trophic changes may occur in the skin. Damage to the anterior horn cells results in loss of motor function only, but most lesions are complicated by some degree of sensory loss.

Basic Principles of Treatment

During the stage of paralysis no form of physical treatment can effect recovery or prevent atrophy, nor can it affect the rate of recovery if and when this takes place. Joints must be kept mobile and unaffected muscles must be exercised maximally to prevent disuse atrophy. After a period of treatment, its length depending on individual factors, some patients can take responsibility for maintaining residual function for themselves. In the instance of an upper limb lesion they must be taught how to move the joints through their full range using the other hand, and how to stretch the muscles in which contractures might develop. They must then come back at regular intervals for a therapist to check that this is being done satisfactorily. If return to work is practicable, so much the better. With a functional splint this may prove possible in instances of isolated lesion either in the upper or in the lower limb, e.g. of the radial or common peroneal nerves.

When there is gross weakness of grip and consequent inability to use the hand, the incentive to move the arm is lost. Regular treatment is then needed for without it, stiffness, particularly of the shoulder and the hand, would develop, together with disuse atrophy of the unaffected muscles.

Both physiotherapy and occupational therapy are indicated to counteract these. In addition, the occupational therapist should check on the patient's need for help with A.D.L.* Any increase of independence is good, because use of the hand normally involves use of the arm also.

As and when recovery takes place, progressive re-education of function is the aim of treatment. If ultimately there is insufficient recovery to be of functional value the patient must be helped to achieve maximal competence in every aspect of living, despite the residual disability. The handicap imposed is not necessarily proportionate to the extent of the paralysis. It depends rather on the way of life of the individual. A watch repairer would be seriously handicapped by loss of precision grip in his dominant hand, the result of paralysis of one small muscle, yet be able to do his work without difficulty from a wheel-chair. A good opposition splint could compensate for lack of the opponens muscle. When there is extensive paralysis, self care activities and general mobility are major problems for the patient and his family. These are best dealt with at a treatment centre with experience and special knowledge of the equipment available to meet such needs, e.g. hoists and chairs of different designs and, if necessary, adapted for the individual; electronic aids to communication and for control of doors and window curtains etc. See Possum* and P.I.L.O.T.*

POLIOMYELITIS

Although rare now in Great Britain, patients who contract this disease abroad may come to this country for medical treatment. Facilities for comprehensive physical treatment which are available in some centres may be less good in others. The occupational therapist may have to take the initiative in providing the special equipment needed by severely paralysed patients, especially those who must be supine and have little use in their upper limbs, i.e. an overhead mirror to bring more of the ward into sight and so reduce the feeling of isolation, a book rest and page turner (the latter in some cases operated by a microswitch and in others being simply a length of dowel with a rubber thimble tip strapped to the forehead), taped books which are available from special libraries, etc.

There is no typical poliomyelitic patient. Treatment is planned individually according to the distribution and degree of the paralysis. It is based on principles common to the treatment of all lower motor neurone dysfunction. The occupational therapist must be adaptable as her role will differ from patient to patient. Those with functional use in their upper limbs or in one limb will benefit physically and psychologically from making use of that function, but if there is extensive paralysis elsewhere, nursing attention and physiotherapy must take precedence. Any occupation suggested must be one from which there will be pleasure with only short periods of attention and for which equipment is minimal. An easily removable work table will certainly be needed if only for writing purposes. The choice will be influenced by the patient's position in bed, his respiratory function and by his interests. Even if the occupational therapist were not treating him it is helpful to get to know the patient at an early stage.

Patients with upper limb dysfunction must be helped to make use of returning function. Any method of achieving independence in eating, in moving a stray hair from the eyes or in wiping the nose is invaluable. The therapist must understand the fundamentals of correct positioning of limbs and trunk, and skill and confidence in handling such a patient.

As functional use returns, occupational therapy to encourage this and to build up further strength will be needed. This must be coordinated with physiotherapy both in content and in its timing during the day. The patient must not be overtired in himself although maximal effort up to and including the point of fatigue will be expected of the affected muscles. Functional hand splinting may be an important part of treatment both as an aid to normal functioning, e.g. an opponens splint to enable the patient to pick up with precision grip, and as a trial prior to possible surgery.

These patients are usually willing and well able to take a responsible share in planning and carrying out a comprehensive programme to cover their needs. Many return to a normal or near normal way of life. For those likely to be severely handicapped by residual disability the programme might include any of the following in addition to long term specific physical treatment: training and practice to achieve maximal independence in self care and mobility; a wide variety of general activities giving opportunity to discover and adjust to new methods, e.g. one-handedness or those made necessary by being chairbound; assessment of the problems relating to return home and to the possibilities of work; consideration of social, recreational and hobby interests and needs. Adjustment to disability is both physical and psychological. The occupational therapist can contribute towards both aspects, neither of which can be wholly achieved without the other.

POLYNEURITIS

Treatment is the same as for poliomyelitis. The paralysis is usually symmetrical; often it is proximal only. There may be sensory loss; more often this is related to position sense than to tactile sense. When the latter occurs it usually corresponds with the site of paralysis. The patient may therefore have problems of hand placement.

PERIPHERAL NERVE INJURIES

Some peripheral nerves are motor, others sensory and some are mixed, having both motor and sensory fibres. Loss of sensation can be almost as great a handicap as loss of power, especially when it affects the palmar surface of the hand. Picking up, grasping and manipulative actions are clumsy and unreliable. The patient will also be at risk from damaging himself. Sometimes there is hyper-aesthesia and this complicates treatment for it deters the patient from attempting to move and the joints become stiff.

Basic principles of treatment are the same as for all lower motor neurone lesions. Training to avoid damage to insensitive areas may be needed, and sometimes protective covering. For example a carpenter with an ulnar nerve lesion needed a specially designed handpiece to protect the ulnar border of the hand and little finger against injury at work.

REFERENCES AND RECOMMENDED FURTHER READING

1. **Head Injuries**
   Potter, J. M., *Practical Management of Head Injuries*. London, 1974.
   Case report on the rehabilitation of a farm worker following head injury. *Occ. Ther.*, 36, no. 6, 1973.
   Treatment of head injury in its later stages. *Occ. Ther.*, 36, no. 7, 1973.
2. **Hemiplegia**
   Bobath, B., *Adult Hemiplegia: Evaluation and Treatment*. London, 1970.
   Epprecht, E. D. L., *Gadgets and Aids for Treatment of the Upper Extremity*, p. 12. Basle, 1962.
   Gardner, W. H., *Text Manual for Remedial Handwriting*. U.S.A., 1966.
   Jay, P. E., Ellison, A. & Walker, E., *Help Yourselves. A Handbook for Hemiplegics and their Families*. London, 1966.
   Richardson, N., *Type with One Hand*.
   Ritchie, D., *Stroke: A Diary of Recovery*. London, 1966.
   Smith, G. W., *Care of the Patient with a Stroke*. London, 1963.
   Wareham, T., *Return to Independence*. London, 1970.
3. **Paraplegia**
   Thompson, M. & Murray, W. A., *Paraplegia at Home*. London and Edinburgh, 1967.
   Walsh, J. J., *Understanding Paraplegia*. London, 1965.
4. **Progressive Paralyses**
   McAlpine, D., *Multiple Sclerosis*. London and Edinburgh, 1955.
   Onuaguluchi, G., *Parkinsonism*. London, 1964.
   Friedrich's ataxia. *Occ. Ther.*, 35, no. 10, 1972.
   Parkinsonism; Diagnosis of parkinsonism; Some individual cases of parkinsonism; Surgical treatment of Parkinson's disease; General medical aspects of parkinsonism; Functional assessment; Living with parkinsonism. *Occ. Ther.*, 35, no. 11, 1972.
5. **Lower Motor Neurone Lesions**
   Wynn, Parry, *Rehabilitation of the Hand*. London, 1973.
   And see:
   Aids to the Investigation of Peripheral Nerve Lesions. H.M.S.O.*, 1966.
   Refs. chapter 7, Collins, D. W. re P.I.L.O.T.* and Maling, R. G. re Possum.*
   General
   Brain, R., *Clinical Neurology*. London, 1973.
   Sandifer, P. H., *Neurology in Orthopaedics*. London, 1967.
   Spillane, J. D., *An Atlas of Neurology*. Oxford, 1968.
   Walshe, F., *Diseases if the Nervous System*. London and Edinburgh, 1969.
   Walton, J. N., *Essentials of Neurology*. London, 1971.
   And see:
   Approach to Treatment of Patients with Neuromuscular Dysfunction. Study Course VI. Third International Congress. W.F.O.T.*, 1962.
   * See *Glossary*, p. 454.

CHAPTER 11

Occupational Therapy for Other Physical Conditions

Rheumatoid Disease [1]

Rheumatoid arthritis is a systemic illness of a progressive and chronic nature which produces inflammation and pain in many joints, with involvement of associated tissues, particularly tendons and their sheaths, with subsequent muscle weakness.

The course of the disease is variable: in some cases it progresses steadily and remorselessly to increasing incapacity; in others progress is slow occurring only in acute phases followed by periods of remission. The patient's prognosis is ascertained by whether he has rheumatoid factor in his blood. If this is positive then active disease is likely for a long period, with joint erosions and nodules occurring early in the course of the disease, and a persistently raised ESR.* Spontaneous complete remission of activity sometimes occurs but is not common in the type of case seen in occupational therapy departments, in most of whom the disease is severe, painful and crippling.

In the acute phase, pain in joints is the main symptom; this will persist at rest and will disturb sleep unless treated by drugs. Stiffness, particularly on rising, and especially after a good night with little change of position, is another troublesome symptom and may make for more disability at the beginning of the day. Rheumatoid disease in children—Still's disease—is usually more acute with more severe systemic signs and shows greater tendency to natural remission.

Patients attending an occupational therapy department will have had various forms of treatment: bedrest, splintage, physiotherapy and drugs. In some, orthopaedic procedures, such as arthrodesis, synovectomy or correction of contractures, will have been carried out. Most patients will still be taking drugs of various kinds and having physiotherapy. It is important to be aware of these other measures and to ensure that occupational therapy is coordinated with them.

Comprehensive Treatment

Rest. In the acute phase of rheumatoid disease physical activity should be restricted, as excessive attempts to keep moving may cause exacerbation of joint symptoms. Simple, gentle mobilising exercises and passive movements within the limits of pain are enough to maintain joint movement. Bedrest may be necessary for some patients for a short time and is usually followed by a striking, if temporary, remission of symptoms, but care must be taken during this period to ensure that good posture and joint alignment is maintained.

Splints. Splinting has two functions, to rest inflammatory joints and to maintain them in a good position, thereby avoiding deformity. Splints should be light and carefully moulded and should be reviewed frequently. The fastenings should be so designed that the patient can put them on himself.

Splinting consists of four main types:

(1) *Rest splints* for night wear, which hold the involved joints in correct alignment and a functional position.

(2) *Day splints* provide support and protection to joints which are vulnerable to strain during daily tasks of lifting and walking, particularly where there is muscle weakness or joint destruction.

(3) *Serial splints*, to correct residual flexion deformities particularly of the wrists and knees.

(4) *Special splinting* following hand surgery, to restore function quickly and maintain correct alignment.

Static splints only should be used for these patients unless the surgeon specifically requests another type. Dynamic splints are seldom tolerated and can cause strain to affected joints. Splints should be light and carefully moulded to give a very accurate fit and should be reviewed frequently. Fastenings should be so designed that the patient can put them on himself.

Physiotherapy may include heat in some form (infra-red, diathermy, wax, etc.) for this effects local relief of pain and helps muscle spasm. It is usually followed by exercises which, in the patient with active disease, must be graded carefully. Where joint movement is painful, exercises should be mainly static ones as the object is to maintain good muscular tone.

Occupational Therapy

General principles. Occupational therapy should be planned on a long-term basis. It should provide a service for the patient over a period of years, whilst he remains under the care of the hospital or domiciliary occupational therapist. The patient should feel that this help and support will be available to him when difficulties arise due to changes in circumstances or increase in disability.

Because of morning stiffness and the effort of attending hospital for treatment, appointments are best arranged for late morning or afternoon sessions. The patient, in receiving understanding supportive as well as physical treatment, is helped to face the loneliness and frustration which accompany the disease and the tensions which arise in the family situation. For example, by helping the patient to overcome his problem of getting in and out of bed, relatives may be spared disturbed nights, and if difficulties of dressing can be solved, a relative may avoid delays in getting off to work. The patient himself may also benefit by not having to get up so early.

Assessment of the patient. The best assessment can be made if it is combined with a home visit, particularly when there is a gross disability. Consideration of details of the patient's daily routine may suggest that some changes are advisable. Initially, an A.D.L.* assessment chart may be used. This should be completed with the patient, not presented as a questionnaire to be filled in by him. He may hesitate to mention some problems, thinking them too trivial or too intimate to discuss. A formal form, carefully presented, may help to uncover these. Patients do not always realise in what areas help can be given, nor the best ways of helping themselves.

Surgery is being used increasingly, as new techniques are developed· Pain can be relieved and function improved. In some centres occupational therapists are developing functional hand tests for use pre- and post-operatively. These are based on the grips normally used in handling everyday objects (see plates 7 to 12). The findings of the first ones may be of help to the surgeon in deciding whether or not to operate. Following surgery to the hands or lower limbs, specific treatment will be required in the occupational therapy department to restore full range of movement and to re-educate the patient to use his hands correctly to diminish the possibility of deformity recurring. The principles of joint protection should be thoroughly understood by the therapist, and every patient should be instructed in the correct methods of doing everyday activities.

The importance of posture. The importance of good posture should be stressed continually. To prevent stiffness and deformity the patient should be discouraged from:

(1) Standing with bent knees and hips.
(2) Sitting without moving for long periods, however good the sitting position may be.
(3) Sitting on the edge of the chair.
(4) Sitting still for a long period with head bent over work.
(5) Sitting with hips and knees at right angles for long periods.
(6) Sitting in a wheel-chair with a sagging back support and badly set foot rests.

(7) Sleeping on a sagging mattress.
(8) Sleeping with hips and knees bent.
(9) Sleeping with heavy bed clothes weighing on the feet.

Relief of pain in a weight-bearing joint will improve mobility and may open up possibilities of activities formerly impossible. A review of these may be helpful.

Treatment aims. These are to encourage normal activities within the limits of the handicap and to help the patient to find the most efficient methods of tackling his problems, so that he may achieve maximum independence. Treatment is planned following a comprehensive individual assessment. These patients may have to accept aids to overcome lack of grip, lack of manipulative ability or lack of reach and they must be trained in using them. The relatives must also understand the purpose, and method of use, of anything introduced into the home. In addition they will need practical instruction in how to give such physical help as is needed by the patient in, for instance, bathing. Attendance for one or two sessions may be adequate, followed by the offer of more or of a home visit later. Other patients may need a longer course of treatment. Assessment for work either in the home or outside it is another possible need.

Social rehabilitation is also important. Tiredness, a common symptom and one to be expected with the conscious effort needed to accomplish simple ends, is a deterrent to social activity, especially if this involves going out. Yet the need for it is great, both for the patient and for his relatives. Introduction to an interesting hobby, i.e. embroidery, painting, model making, sweet making, etc., are valuable. Gardening can give great pleasure if these considerations are extended to the problems of indoor, or specially adapted outdoor, gardening.

Space and equipment. Adequate room for the patients to move about easily with their walking aids, and chairs and working surfaces of suitable heights are all essential. Cantilever tables on mini-castors can be adjusted and pushed away easily. Recently increased independence has been achieved with the use of a 'glideabout' chair, particularly in the kitchen. The importance of the correct height, stability, firmness, weight and positioning of chairs, stools, beds and other equipment cannot be over-emphasised (*see* Plates 1 to 4). These considerations may help to overcome problems of mobility in the home and, if relevant, at work.

Osteo-arthrosis [1]

Osteo-arthrosis is essentially a degenerative process affecting articular cartilage; to some extent a natural 'ageing' process, it may be hastened by abnormal stresses, by injury, or by other disease in or around the joints. Changes occur in the cartilage and secondarily in the capsule and are of importance, mainly in weight-bearing areas, the hips, knees and spinal apophyseal joints. Gross limitation of movement, with pain on weight-bearing, may lead to severe disability. Patients with limitation of movement of the hips will benefit from advice on activities of daily living, and so also will the occasional patient, usually with unilateral disease, who has had an arthrodesis of the hip.

Affected hips are treated surgically with increasing success, as techniques improve, and post-operative rehabilitation after arthroplasty remains of great importance. Physiotherapy is prescribed in the immediate post-operative period, but the occupational therapist has an important role to play in the later stages of return to function and when necessary in resettlement.

Occupational Therapy

It is advisable for the occupational therapist to work out with the physiotherapist a daily programme, so that the combined exercises for abduction, flexion and extension of the hip are balanced.

The bicycle fret saw can be used to good effect, and later, when full weight-bearing, the foot power lathe and standing activities to build up tolerance. During rest periods, time can be utilised to assess manual skills, through some sitting activity. This may be important for resettlement. The patient should be encouraged to get up and move about at intervals. When the residual ability can be determined, an assessment for work can be made by the occupational therapist.

Ankylosing Spondylitis [1]

Ankylosing spondylitis occurs most commonly in males, with onset usually in the second or third decade. Stiffness is severe and ankylosis, particularly of the spinal and costo-vertebral joints, occurs readily and often early on. In a severe case the end result is often complete immobility of the spine and ankylosis or gross limitation of movement of the hips. Hand function is not affected. The main problems are those of daily living, dressing and bathing in particular, and sometimes of work. In severe cases it is difficult for such patients to sit with comfort in any standard chair.

Low Back Pain [2]

This is commonly given as a diagnosis without stating the cause. The aim of treatment will however be defined: strengthening of the back muscles, mobilisation and toning up for return to previous work, or assessment for alternative work. There are typical patients, i.e. the older man on heavy work whose back is put to sudden extra strain; the sedentary worker called upon to shovel snow; a woman with no knowledge of how to lift who must give physical help to an invalid; a man or woman who turns and bends down suddenly to pick up a fallen brief case or umbrella. Sometimes there is no precipitating incident. In an acute phase a period of bedrest is prescribed, with fracture boards under the mattress. Sometimes there is no acute pain, but instead chronic, low backache in the lumbar region and across the sacrum. Some patients can tolerate this, others are so disabled as to be unable to work. When there is no clinical justification for it the term 'functional overlay' is given in explanation. These patients are often depressed, and hopeless about their future. They are difficult to treat and diversion in its true sense is needed to stimulate some interest in something, before any routine assessment can be made.

Methods of Strengthening Extensor Muscles

The main responsibility of these muscles is to stabilise the spine, so it is best to work them statically. A stable spine is needed for all strong upper limb action and especially for movements of wide range or overhead. At first the patient may need to sit at least part time. He should sit high, perhaps on a stool with a comfortable saddle top, for it will then be easy to maintain a normal lumbar curve. When sitting low the hips are more flexed and this predisposes to flexion of the lumbar spine which is contra-indicated. Patients should be fit for moderate activity before being referred. Wood or metal work are suitable, as is stool seating. The choice between wood and metal may depend partly on the patient's height, e.g. a tall man can stand erect at a metalwork bench on which the vice stands proud whereas the relatively lower woodwork bench would encourage stooping. Also from a high seat, a woman can do washing using an old fashioned dolly board, for this works the back muscles in the same way if good posture is emphasised. It will be a progression on washing by squeezing, for when doing this, weight can be supported on the forearms and there is then a smaller range of arm movement. This type of treatment may not be direct enough for some patients and both men and women can be treated by *overhead work* on a bench drill or mortice adapted to take double levers:

Starting position. On a high stool with feet firm on the floor, apart and slightly in front of the knees; normal lumbar curve maintained jointly by the extensors and abdominal muscles controlling the pelvis; dorsal spine and head erect; arms relaxed.

Preparatory action. Both hands raised to grasp the overhead levers, at least shoulder width apart, with the hands and elbows both slightly in front of the shoulder joint and above shoulder level.

Action. The levers are pulled down by bending the elbows and working the depressors and adductors of the scapulae. Simultaneously the spinal extensors and abdominals contract strongly to maintain the correct position of the spine. The strength of the muscle work is graded by the use of springs attached between the levers and a firm point of fixation overhead. The drill must be adjusted so that the levers cannot be pulled below shoulder level, as a safeguard against flexion of the spine.

Release. The return of the levers to their original position is controlled by eccentric work from the same muscles.

Someone else must feed in the work for the patient and with morticing this is easy. Fixed in a jig, dense metal such as steel can be drilled. This will need repeated action of the lever before the drilling is completed so the patient can change it for himself.

A printing press can be similarly adapted and departments where there are upright rug looms can use these successfully. The loom may have to be raised to provide a correct starting position. Painting at shoulder or head height is also good, on plain flat surfaces for choice, to encourage big movements. If there are outdoor facilities, raking and hoeing are suitable for patients who have learnt to work with a flat back and can be relied upon to do any bending that may be needed, from the hips.

Methods of Mobilising

Mobilisation is first given by physiotherapy, with gravity eliminated, and closely supervised. Later, when referrals come for occupational therapy, they are best interpreted as an all clear for full free activity which will include changes of position, picking up, putting down, reaching, bending, crouching, twisting, as could happen when executing a large collage, playing table tennis, doing housework or when working out of doors.

Methods of Toning up before Returning to Previous Work

Toning up after a period of incapacity can be done by some people for themselves. Many others, and in particular town dwellers, have no facilities for doing it. The aim is to restore capacity as needed by the individual, but if possible with a margin of safety. Recurrence of strain is less likely if activity is making less than maximal demands. The rate of progression depends on results and especially with back patients it is better to err on the side of not pushing hard enough than to push too hard. Assessment of work tolerance is best made by working to a plan agreed to by patient and therapist. The plan for an office worker might begin with 45 minutes of copy typing with special attention to correct seating and posture; then 15 minutes rest before standing at a filing cabinet for an agreed time. The rest period is an essential part of the scheme and should be taken. If, in reviewing the day's results it is clear that activity can be stepped up, adjustments are made but not necessarily by removing the rest period. It might be more relevant to extend the daily treatment period. When standing tolerance is below par, treatment to strengthen leg muscles may be needed, with care to avoid strain on the lower back. If bicycling is given for example, the pedals must be reached easily without having to tilt the pelvis from side to side on the saddle.

Back Care

Restoration of strength or mobility may be the primary aim but training in back care is equally important if the chance of recurrence is to be minimised. Responsibility for this should be shared by the physiotherapist and the occupational therapist. The former will concentrate on teaching correct lifting techniques, i.e. feet diagonally apart, knees bent, back flat; the elbows, and the load supported by the palms, held close to the body; then the knees straightening to take the weight and the back foot pushing off to initiate walking. A quadriceps build-up may be necessary. For many patients, class instruction is enough but it is one thing to repeat these actions as an exercise and quite another for them to become habitual. Occupational therapy contributes by providing a situation in which lifting can be incidental, for example the housewife cleaning out her kitchen, having to move table, chairs, etc. For a man a short period helping in the steward's stores may answer.

Many people are unable to lift according to the rules. Stiff or painful hips, knees or feet will prevent it, and obesity. Those who must return to their heavy work can perhaps work out a compromise; when the acute symptoms clear up, they do return to it—until the next time. Housewives should be referred for help in finding ways of avoiding unnecessary strain. For example: beds and heavy armchairs can be put on castors; the bath can be cleaned from half kneeling; anything weighty in regular use should be stored between waist and shoulder height; the bucket of water used for washing the floor can be pushed along on a small wooden platform with castors; the milk should not be put on the back doorstep unless into a carrier which can be hooked up with a walking stick; ideally the oven and refrigerator should be on work top level. The therapist will demonstrate and teach the appropriate methods.

For the patient who must be able to move an invalid or push a wheelchair, instruction and realistic practice with a similar size of invalid will be arranged. While the occupational therapist may be more likely to see the need for this, the physiotherapist may give better tuition.

Anyone whose job involves long hours of driving should sit well back, with the lumbar curve supported.

Cardiac Conditions

Congenital defects which cause circulatory disorder are now treated surgically in childhood. If previously the child has been much restricted in physical activity it is not easy for him or his family to adjust at once. It is even more difficult for an adult with longer memory of disability, and some adults who were not treated as children are now having surgery and are being referred for occupational therapy. They should be helped to consider themselves no longer disabled and to work up gradually to live reasonably active lives. Aims are the same for patients who have surgery for such conditions as mitral stenosis. They, too, may be apprehensive and anxious. These symptoms are often shown prior to operation during in-patient treatment while tests are being carried out. Even if this is short, the patient will greatly benefit from appropriate occupational therapy, anything sufficiently interesting to him individually to distract him from thinking of his heart sensations and of the operation. Later, when attending as an out-patient post-operatively, the treatment programme is planned to increase tolerance to activity in general, to develop self confidence and to stimulate an expansion of interests. Potential capacity may be greatly increased after surgery and consideration of work possibilities will be part of treatment, both for the patient who will be going out to work, and for the housewife who wants to increase her activities at home. The patients themselves have no reason to know what their new capacity will be: the occupational therapist must be watchful without being seen to be watching. With signs of fatigue the tempo of work must be slowed down and with an anxious patient this must be done without his realising it.

If patients who have had serious cardiac disorder, e.g. coronary thrombosis, are sent for treatment for any reason their limitations must be appreciated. Return to work is recommended medically but with restrictions of varying degree. Such patients may have been frightened by their illness and they may retain an interest in their past symptoms. Discussion of these amongst patients should always be discouraged and with cardiac patients this is especially important.

Bronchitis [3]

The patient with bronchitis may need help from the occupational therapy department in these ways:

(1) Consideration for his breathlessness during treatment for some other condition.
(2) Opportunity to build up to his former work capacity after a period of illness or unemployment.
(3) Help in resettlement.

An "afternoon's only" programme is helpful initially to enable him to get under way in the morning in his own good time. For the same reason, eventual resettlement in night work can be considered. Much night work is also less strenuous than daytime work which is an added advantage. Outdoor work is contra-indicated; good indoor conditions being preferable to the uncertainties of temperature, wind and wet. Those who need to change their jobs are usually in heavy manual work and of middle age. They are therefore unsuitable for retraining, but will need some form of resettlement.

Pulmonary Tuberculosis [3]

The advent of effective chemotherapy in the treatment of tuberculosis has led to a reappraisal of old methods of treatment. The previous régime of sanatorium treatment, with its segregation from the community for periods of years, emphasis on complete bedrest in the early stages and subsequent slow up-grading of activity, has been greatly modified. Operative procedures are also less frequently required.

Effective treatment by chemotherapy is, however, of at least one year's duration for the mildest case, and part of this time is usually spent in hospital. The patient's level of morale affects the rate of progress, and constant encouragement is necessary to ensure that he cooperates in all his treatment including taking his drugs.

The occupational therapist can contribute to the treatment by providing an activity programme of increasing intensity both physically and mentally. It may range from a light interesting bed activity such as stamp collecting to a full day's work. It should always be related to the patient's cultural, home and work background, so that he can see the relevance of it to his future life.

Throughout treatment, training should be linked with the establishment of good postural and working habits, the avoidance of fatigue and worry, and the benefits of fresh air and a balanced diet.

For the long-term patient, who may have contracted the disease prior to the advent of antibiotics, a programme which includes high-class craft-work or work of pocket-money earning potential is of value. This will help the patient to keep his self respect, as will care of his appearance and interest in local and national events. Music and play reading groups help some patients both socially and mentally. Assessment and retraining for suitable employment is sometimes required and a few patients may benefit from correspondence courses and other forms of organised study.

Diabetes

Patients with diabetes will not usually be sent to the department unless there is need for treatment for some other condition, a fracture for example. It is to be hoped that there will be reference to the medical diagnosis in the treatment referral. The occupational therapist must watch for any signs of hyper- or hypo-glycaemia and deal with them promptly.

In the later stages of the disease complications may arise which require treatment, such as adjustment to failing eyesight in early cataract or retinopathy, re-education of function and training in compensatory action when there is peripheral neuropathy with sensory functional loss. Peripheral vascular disease may necessitate lower limb amputation.

Occupational Therapy for the Amputee [4]

Patients who have had an amputation fall into two main groups, lower limb amputees and upper limb amputees. The lower limb group is the larger in the ratio of 9 to 1. This imbalance is caused by increased incidence of peripheral vascular disease in the elderly, leading to lower limb amputation in many cases. Trauma and congenital limb deficiency still account for an approximately equal number of cases in each group.

LOWER LIMB AMPUTEE

Trauma

In the *pre-prosthetic stage*, and when the stitches are removed, about ten days after the operation, pressure bandaging [4a] together with a régime of exercise is begun by the physiotherapist. At this stage activities should be commenced by the occupational therapist.

Aims of treatment. Single amputee:

(1) To improve and maintain joint mobility above the level of amputation, particularly extension of the hip and knee, e.g. with sling and pulley circuit attached to printing or weaving.

(2) To increase muscle tone and power, particularly in the range of extension of the hip, knee and trunk, e.g. with temporary pylon, on the bicycle fretsaw or lathe (4b) or with sling and pulley circuit for printing or weaving with added resistance.

(3) To reduce oedema in the stump. This is achieved by active movement in 1 and 2, which improves the circulation.

Aims of treatment. Double amputee:

(1) To encourage independent mobility, teach transfers from:

(a) bed to wheel-chair and the reverse. A sliding board may be required to achieve this, but should not necessarily be needed permanently;

(b) wheel-chair to toilet and the reverse. Rails are normally essential;

(c) wheel-chair to bath and the reverse. Bath overboard and inner seat are normally adequate. Some patients ultimately achieve this transfer without bath aids.

(2) To assess for a wheel-chair. Most double amputees require a wheel-chair if only for emergency use.

(3) Consider (a) home conditions and (b) future employment.

In the *prosthetic stage* all amputees are first fitted with a temporary walking pylon before progressing to a fully articulated prosthesis.

Occupational therapists who treat patients at this stage should familiarise themselves with the application of the prosthesis so that they appreciate the correct weight-bearing areas, and they should learn the correct methods of walking in a prosthesis [4c].

Aims of treatment:

(1) Cooperate with physiotherapists and remedial gymnasts in enabling the patient to put on the prosthesis independently by modifying fastenings and clothing if necessary.

(2) Improve standing balance and tolerance by (*a*) working at optimum height and within the inner range of shoulder movement (using a pelvic sling if necessary in the early stages) and (*b*) working in the same standing position and increasing shoulder and elbow range of movement to encourage weight transference and lateral trunk rotation.

(3) Encourage independent walking by suitably selected activity. This should only be attempted when the doctor has given his approval that the patient is safe to balance on his own.

(4) Relate this mobility to employment and hobby interests and co-operate with the disablement resettlement officer in planning the patient's future.

(5) Make a home visit if necessary and cooperate with the local social services when alterations are required in the home.

Geriatric

When treating this group of patients in the pre-prosthetic stage consideration must always be given to the causal disease necessitating amputation with its possible sequelae.

The whole tempo of the treatment programme must be dictated by the patient's general physical and mental condition. Many of these patients are single leg amputees, but unfortunately a number become double leg amputees.

Aims of treatment: single amputee. The same principles can be followed as for the traumatic amputee but usually cannot be begun so soon. They may not be appropriate at all if the general physical condition is poor. The treatment should also include:

(1) Independent mobility. Transfers from:

(*a*) bed to wheel-chair and the reverse. A sliding board is not normally needed;

(*b*) wheel-chair to toilet and the reverse;

(*c*) wheel-chair to bath and the reverse. A bath overboard is normally adequate.

(2) Assessment for a wheel-chair when it is felt that the patient's

general condition or the condition of the other leg will limit the amount of walking undertaken after a prosthesis has been fitted.

Aims of treatment: double amputee. Particular emphasis must be placed on independent mobility as some of these patients never progress to the stage of prosthesis and must be made independent in a wheel-chair. The aims of treatment are:

(1) To assess for a wheel-chair. This should be self propelling with removable sides. A body retaining strap is advisable if the amputations are above knee.

(2) To teach transfers from:

    (*a*) bed to wheel-chair and the reverse. A sliding board is normally required;

    (*b*) wheel-chair to toilet and the reverse. Rails are essential and patients should be taught to transfer forwards and remain seated that way. A commode chair with arms may be used as an alternative where accessibility to the toilet is difficult;

    (*c*) wheel-chair to bath and the reverse. Bath overboard and inner seat are essential. Safety must be considered and a helper should be available, either a relative or the district nurse.

(3) To carry out dressing practice, with appropriate adaptation to clothing when necessary.

(4) To consider home conditions and make appropriate recommendations in liaison with local social services.

(5) To instruct relatives in the methods of independence used by the patient.

(6) To encourage hobby interests and work participation within the home environment.

For the *single amputee* in the *prosthetic stage* the same principles can be applied as for the traumatic group, depending on the patient's general physical condition and associated complications. Particular emphasis should be placed on sections 1, 2, 3 and 5 (p. 233).

When the condition necessitates *double amputation*, patients are fitted with bilateral rocker pylons [4d]. The same principles of treatment apply as for the traumatic group, but the therapist must remember that the patient will be severely reduced in height and therefore optimum work heights must be considered. It is unrealistic to expect this group of patients to walk and stand all day on pylons and many will still carry out a number of activities from a wheel-chair.

Only if the patient succeeds reasonably well in mobility on rocker pylons will he be fitted with longer fully articulated prostheses. It is then essential to start a complete prosthetic treatment programme again, carrying out the principles as for the traumatic group. The number who reach this stage are relatively small.

UPPER LIMB AMPUTEE [4e]

It is impossible to replace the normal intricate functions of a human arm and hand by a prosthesis. The patient must, however, be encouraged to realise that a prosthesis will not be just a sleeve-filler, but for the single arm amputee a practical aid to the remaining hand and for the double amputee the principal means of leading an independent normal life.

In the *pre-prosthetic stage*, and as soon as immediate post-operative tenderness subsides (approximately five days), activities to exercise the stump should be started. These should continue throughout the period of stump bandaging and exercise carried out with the physiotherapist. Bandaging is done to control oedema and to condition the stump to prosthetic wearing.

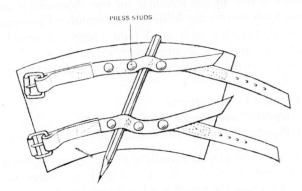

PRESS STUDS

FIG. 27. Pre-prosthetic gauntlet.

Aims of treatment:

(1) To maintain normal neuro-physiological movement patterns.
(2) To maintain joint movement and improve muscle tone above the level of amputation.
(3) To improve circulation and help reduce oedema.
(4) To encourage the patient to appreciate the usefulness of the stump related directly to prosthetic wearing.

In order to achieve these aims a light leather gauntlet should be made to fit snugly round the stump and over the bandage. Into this a variety of aids can be slotted as follows:

(a) A pencil or paint brush for writing and drawing, painting and word games. Careful positioning of the paper, etc., can help grade the range of movement.

(*b*) Cutlery

    (i) *Single below-elbow amputee.* Knife and fork. The knife is best used in the gauntlet because pronation/supination is not required and this will probably be absent. Spoon and fork. The fork is best used in the gauntlet as a pusher for the same reason.

    (ii) *Single above-elbow amputee.* Bilateral feeding is very difficult at this stage and is not usually attempted because of the difference between the length of arm and stump.

    (iii) *Double amputee.* These patients must start as soon as possible with a spoon or fork, using the longer or the dominant stump, progressing to bilateral feeding later. They will need a plate buffer and non-skid mat.

(*c*) Typing peg. This appliance can be used for all levels of amputation.

(*d*) Table tennis bat. This appliance is good in the later stages as it isolates flexion of the shoulder for the above-elbow amputee plus elbow extension for the below-elbow amputee. These movements are essential, together with good joint range and muscle power for efficient control of a prosthesis (see Fig. 28).

(*e*) General activities which encourage the use of the stump to assist the sound arm, e.g.:

    (i) Holding down objects.

    (ii) Knitting with needle through gauntlet.

    (iii) Planing, if a below-elbow stump is sufficiently long.

Activities must be graded according to the degree of sensitivity in the stump and the tone in the muscles around the joints above the level of the amputation. These are the muscles normally used in gross movements as in manual work. They frequently have to be re-educated to control and co-ordinate finer precision movements and this can cause mental as well as physical fatigue.

In the *prosthetic stage* it is essential for the patient to have a course of training in the use of his limbs. At present this is carried out by the occupational therapists in special departments either within the limb fitting centres, or in selected hospitals within easy reach of limb fitting centres.

Aims of treatment and training. These cover:

(1) Checking that the prosthesis is fitted correctly for maximum use with minimum effort in all forms of activity.

(2) Encouraging the patient to use the prosthesis in the most natural way possible and showing its potential value.

(3) Gearing the training to the patient's individual needs related to:

    (*a*) Activities of daily living.

    (*b*) Employment.

(c) Hobby interests.
For the double arm amputee activities of daily living always take priority.
(4) Advising on the most suitable appliances to be used in the prosthesis for specific activities.
(5) Cooperating with the disablement resettlement officer when necessary.

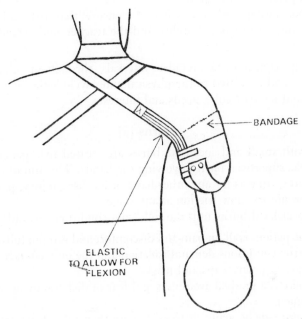

FIG. 28. Adaptation of a pre-prosthetic gauntlet for table tennis.

CONGENITAL LIMB DEFORMITY

The most common form of congenital limb deficiency is the absence of part of *one* limb. Although this may appear to be a minor functional disability to the child, it is a major tragedy to the parents who inevitably feel guilty for their child's deformity. If the child is to grow into a normal psychologically balanced person the parents must learn to accept the child's disability during the early months of its life. There are a proportionately small number of children who present gross deformities, involving two or more limbs and in these cases the parents acceptance of the disability is even more difficult.

Early referral to a limb fitting centre or better still to a specialised unit is important. At such a unit the coordinated services of specialists working as a team are available.

The role of the occupational therapist as a member of this team is:

(1) Initial assessment of function without prosthesis.
(2) Training in the use of a prosthesis when prescribed.
(3) Training in functional activity without a prosthesis when appropriate.
(4) Training in activities of daily living with and without a prosthesis. Modification of clothing where necessary.
(5) Involving the mother in the treatment programme throughout, as her cooperation is essential.
(6) Cooperating with the school to ensure that the child maintains maximum functional ability and the teacher understands the problems.

Training continues at regular intervals throughout childhood and adolescence and is related to the physical and psychological development of the child and his particular needs and interests.

Burns [5]

Patients with small and localised burns are treated in a general hospital for example, superficial burns involving the hands. The aim of occupational therapy is the same as for any other hand or localised injury, particular care being taken not to allow friction at any stage.

In a specialised burns unit the following conditions prevail:

(1) The patient is ill, in pain and discomfort and is often fully dependent.
(2) Sterile conditions demand isolation and the only contact is with staff wearing gowns, caps and masks.
(3) There is a gradual awareness and fear of disfigurement, especially in women.
(4) There will be acute distress if more than one of a family has been involved in the incident.
(5) The attitude of the patient's relatives and friends, and his financial situation are of paramount importance.
(6) The patient may be undergoing a series of surgical operations.

Early Treatment

The occupational therapist has an important role to play at the stage when the patient can first be expected to use upper limbs which have been burned. Special equipment may be needed:

(1) To encourage him to perform tasks for himself, e.g. by using a wrist strap holder into which a spoon will fit if he cannot grip.
(2) To make possible any activity which will provide interest outside himself and so encourage purposeful free movement, e.g. provision of a book rest, page turner or provision of an overhead work table for writing, painting or playing patience.

Frequently, on medical grounds, the movements which are permitted vary from day to day and the therapist will need ingenuity to make continuation of previous activities possible. Although the appearance of the patient may cause aversion the therapist must not show emotional reaction. Sometimes the patient is reluctant to become independent and resents any pressure to achieve this. Some patients have personality problems: the mentally ill and the aged amongst them: the epileptics are at special risk. Psychological trauma following burns will increase the difficulty of carrying out treatment and resettlement.

After body burns, clothing should be loose and allow good ventilation; cotton is most suitable. Following burns of the feet soft shoes are recommended. Plastazote may be used to make shoes and pad handles of cutlery, tools, pens, etc. for those with burnt hands.

When the patient is well enough in general terms to tolerate a routine of treatment this should include physio- and occupational therapy, both specific and general. Ideally both forms of treatment should be given twice or more daily and for a minimum of 20 minutes. Contractures developed during the resting period must be corrected by progressive manual stretching and exercise by physiotherapy, followed by specific occupational therapy, for example gripping with maximum span, playing draughts with big convex topped pieces and model-making which requires pick-up and manipulation. When the joint tissues have been burnt, movement cannot be restored but where restriction is due to contractures a degree of improvement can be achieved by treatment.

Continuous splinting between treatments is usually necessary, and it is advantageous to use 'Orthoplast', which can be altered easily to maintain improvement, and which provides a climate most likely to reduce contractures. Hypertrophic scars can be treated by splinting and pressure dressings.

Local mobility is not the only aim. The whole limb should be kept as functionally competent as possible. The incentive to move may be lacking and for example a stiff shoulder may result when the hand is affected. Special measures must be devised such as playing table tennis with a bat with a lengthened handle fitted into a leather cuff on the forearm. (See p. 237.)

Treatment when there is Skin Grafting

Pre-operatively good personal contact should be made with the patient and he should be encouraged to be as active as possible so that the effects of post-operative immobilisation will be minimised. Contact with heat or wet should be avoided and loss of tissue fluid or oedema prevented by encouraging him to work in elevation if practicable. Within these limits any clean activity is permissible and interest will be the best incentive to activity.

Post-operatively treatment may be reordered after only a short period of inactivity, and general function is then quickly restored. It will also be possible to improve local function, e.g. metacarpo-phalangeal joints can be mobilised when skin loss on the back of the hand has been replaced by new skin. Friction and pressure must be avoided and the patient must learn to safeguard insensitive areas. The donor area may be tender and cause additional temporary limitation of function. Former problems in A.D.L.* in its widest sense should be reviewed, for the patient can now be expected to use his hand more effectively.

When pedicle grafting is necessary the patient may be much in need of diversional occupational therapy. He may be forced to tolerate positioning which is abnormal and restricts natural activity. Imagination and ingenuity may be needed on the part of the occupational therapist.

Final Stages of Treatment

What follows applies to all patients whether or not they have had surgery. When healing is consolidated physical treatment is stepped up. In some cases normal function may be achieved but deep burns can lead to permanent deformity in spite of expert treatment. The typical claw hand is a major handi-cap. The disability is not one of lack of mobility and power only. Sensory discrimination may be lacking, for example difficulty in identifying coins in a pocket. This can sometimes be re-educated by treatment. It is also important that the skin is toughened enough to tolerate reasonable wear and tear before discharge. Tendon grafting may be necessary at the later stages of re-constructive surgery.

Resocialisation is an equally important part of treatment. This begins in the treatment departments, then in the immediate vicinity of the hospital —visits to a local shop or public house—and finally in the home and the community. Some patients remain self conscious and apprehensive of their acceptance by the public and perhaps because of this are reluctant to prove increasing physical and social independence.

Patients should be encouraged to regain confidence in an environment similar to that in which the accident occurred—the housewife in the kitchen, the electrician working with power. A home visit may be necessary to ensure that any aids which may have been supplied are useful and used. This will especially apply to the housewife.

The final concern is with work prospects, whether in the home for the housewife or outside it. The therapist must help assess whether the patient can manage his own job, whether he can do alternative work for the same employer or whether he must change to some other field. Many factors will complicate resettlement.

(1) The possible need for further and perhaps repeated surgery.
(2) The patient's physical competence for his job.
(3) The suitability of the environment. A shop assistant with obvious disfigurement might present a problem either because of self consciousness or because her employer feared the reaction of his customers.
(4) The personal attitude of the employer, whether sympathetic or hostile, and whether there is a case pending.

Children with Burns

Burns in the case of children are as likely to be on the body and the front of the legs as on the upper limbs. Special considerations for the application of occupational therapy will be found in chapter 18.

Leprosy [6]

Leprosy is a widespread and slightly contagious disease affecting about fifteen million people, mainly in the developing countries. It is caused by a micro-organism called *Mycobacterium leprae* which attacks the skin, the peripheral nerves and the mucosa of the upper respiratory tract.

The commonest kinds of leprosy are: (*a*) *tuberculoid*, in which a few light-coloured patches occur in the skin and one or more peripheral nerves are often damaged; (*b*) *lepromatous*, which is a generalised infection of the skin, respiratory mucosa and peripheral nerves; (*c*) *borderline*, an intermediate form which shows itself in a variety of skin and nerve lesions. The main nerve trunks most commonly damaged in leprosy are, in order of frequency, the ulnar, the posterior tibial, the median, the external popliteal, the facial and the radial.

If the patient with leprosy is treated early, nerve damage should not occur, and if such damage is already present, appropriate treatment will often prevent further damage. The standard drug used is dapsone, a simple (and cheap) sulphone. Various measures are employed to control acute neuritis, drugs, splinting, local injections of anti-inflammatory compounds, etc. Tests of motor activity and sensation are regularly performed to assess the patient's progress. The physiotherapist is the person who usually undertakes these tests, but sometimes the occupational therapist is called upon to do this in the absence of a qualified physiotherapist, perhaps using less sophisticated techniques. A large part of the work is concerned with educating patients in the use of their anaesthetic extremities, and in the recognition and immediate reporting of early signs of neuritis.

Despite the increasing emphasis on early treatment, it is still true that in most countries leprosy patients present themselves for treatment when they

9

already show evidence of nerve damage. In some cases, treatment has been given inexpertly, or early signs of nerve damage have been overlooked, or the patient is suffering from a very severe form of leprosy that progresses despite everything that is done.

Surgical measures, such as correction of foot-drop, are often successfully undertaken, also tendon transplants for the hand. These require post-operative physiotherapy to educate the patient in the use of the transplanted muscle.

The role of the occupational therapist is to extend this activity to the patient's daily living and work. She helps the patient to recognise sensory loss in hands and feet, and to prevent unfelt injuries that would damage anaesthetic parts. She instructs him to check hands and feet regularly for early and slight signs of damage, and to develop a sense of anticipating and avoiding actions that might injure his tissues. 'Is it hot?', 'Is it sharp?', 'Would it hurt me if I could feel it?' These are questions that the patient must constantly be asking himself.

With the help of the occupational therapist, the patient must devise ways and means of continuing to do his job without incurring injury. Thus, tool handles are adapted to spread pressure or facilitate grip; methods of work are changed; protective gloves and footwear are introduced and commended, despite the risk that they may single out the worker as suffering from a stigmatising deformity. Some ingenuity is needed for the resettlement of patients living in poor rural areas, or in situations where there is little chance of alternative employment, or where specialised training or sheltered work-shops are non-existent.

Special measures must be taken to deal with the special needs of the patients. Thus, to prevent cracking and infection, dry skin will need soaking in water baths and oiling, or wax baths (provided by the physiotherapist). The patient must learn the methods he has seen applied successfully to his case, and should continue to practise what he has been taught when he goes home. When the facial nerve is partly or completely destroyed, special precautions must be taken to prevent damage to the eye that is constantly exposed.

In the world as a whole, centres for the total treatment of leprosy patients are pathetically few and chronically understaffed, and the available staff must try between them to cover all the needs of the individual patient, physical and social. Education of the public, at all levels, is urgently needed if the fear, superstition and ignorance that still surround leprosy are to be dispelled.

REFERENCES AND RECOMMENDED FURTHER READING

1. Rheumatic/Arthritic Conditions
Copeman, W. S. C., *Arthritis and Rheumatism*. London, 1967.
Flatt, A. E., *The Care of the Rheumatoid Hand*. St. Louis, 1968.

And see:
Handbooks for Patients; Ankylosing Spondylitis, 1966; *Lumbar Disc Disorders*, 1966; *Osteoarthritis*, 1967; *Rheumatoid Arthritis*, 1967. Published by Arthritis and Rheumatism Council.
And see the Rheumatology Issue of *Occ. Ther.*, **35**, no. 2, 1972, covering: Rheumatoid Arthritis. Current drug treatment of rheumatoid arthritis; Still's disease; Research in rheumatology; Pathogenesis of osteoarthrosis; Joint replacement; Splinting the arthritic; Crystal synovitis.
Footwear in arthritis. *Occ. Ther.*, **38**, no. 6, 1972.
Understanding the arthritic hand. *Occ. Ther.*, **35**, no. 7, 1972.
Surgical treatment of arthritis of the knee. *Occ. Ther.*, **35**, no. 7, 1972.
Pre- and post-operative assessment of hip function. *Occ. Ther.*, **36**, no. 2, 1973.
Joint replacement prosthesis, particularly knees. *Occ. Ther.*, **36**, no. 8, 1973.
Rheumatoid arthritis: hand assessment. *Occ. Ther.*, **36**, no. 11, 1973.

2. Low Back Pain
Eklundh, M., *Spare Your Back*. London, 1965.
And see:
Lumbar disc disorders and reading refs. on posture. *Handbook for Patients*. Arthritis and Rheumatism Council, 1966.

3. Respiratory Conditions
Heaf, F. & Rusby, N. L., *Recent Advances in Respiratory Tuberculosis*. London, 1968.
Kemp, R., *Understanding Bronchitis and Asthma*. Tavistock Publications. London, 1963.
And see:
Tuberculosis today. *Brit. Hosp. J. Soc. Service Rev.* (Apr. 1966).

4. The Amputee
Humm, W., *Rehabilitation of the Amputee*. Chapter 3, ref. [a]; chapter 7, ref. [c]; chapters 11 and 12, ref. [d]. London, 1969.
Jones, M. S., *An Approach to Occupational Therapy*. Pp. 124 to 135 ref. [b]. London, 1964.
Wellerson, T., *A Manual for Occupational Therapists In the Rehabilitation of the Upper Extremity*. See ref. [e]. U.S.A.

5. Burns
Larson, D. L., *The Prevention and Correction of Burn Scar Contracture*, Shriners Burns Institute, Galveston, Texas, 1973.
Muir, I. F. K. and Barclay, T. L., *Burns and their Treatment*, London, 1962.
Willis, B. A., *Splinting the Burn Patient*, Shriners Burns Institute, Galveston, Texas, 1971.
Willis, B. A., Orthoplast isoprene for burns. *Occ. Ther.*, **32**, no. 11, 1969.
Yeakel, M. H., *The Role of the Occupational Therapist within a Burn Centre. Proceedings Third International Congress.* W.F.O.T.*, 1962.

6. Leprosy
Brand, M., *Watch Those Eyes*. Leprosy Misson, London.
Brand, P. W., *Insensitive Feet*. Leprosy Mission, London.
Brand, P. W., *Deformity can be Prevented*. Hind Kosht Nivaran Sangh, Delhi.
Cochrane, R. E. & Davey, T. F., *Leprosy in Theory and Practice*. Bristol.
Mendis, M., *Physiotherapy in Leprosy*. Bristol, 1965.
And see:
Physiotherapy. **54**, 9. London, 1968.

* See *Glossary*, p. 454.

Part Three

CHAPTER 12

Introduction to Occupational Therapy for Psychiatric Conditions

---

In psychiatric occupational therapy, the patient is encouraged to develop those aptitudes and attitudes which will enable him to live as full, useful and satisfying a life as possible. If he is to become a competent member of his community, in or out of hospital, his previous history and present illness must be considered in relation to his personality, intelligence, and social and economic background. Scientific means of assessment are valuable, but should never obscure the fact that patients are people, with the common basic needs for *security, adventure, recognition* and *response* [1]. By creating as normal an environment as possible in occupational therapy, patients will not be tempted to take refuge in over-sheltered conditions and will be better prepared to return to the demands of life outside hospital.

With the implementation of the Mental Health Act, 1959, many new types of unit have been set up [2], and occupational therapists are working in more and widely differing situations. Even so, the fundamental approach to treatment involves knowledge of:

(1) *The framework for treatment* through Regional, Area and District Health Authorities* with particular reference to Mental Health Care Planning Teams* and Paramedical Committees, as well as the more immediate resources available in the therapist's own sphere of employment.

(2) *The social aspects of mental illness*, which include the social and economic aspects of rehabilitation, particularly the relationship between the patient and his family and work group, and methods of group treatment.

(3) *The clinical details of mental illness.*

These aspects are described in consecutive chapters, but effective treatment involves all three in varying degrees, according to the need of the patient. This section of the book should, therefore, be read as a whole.

Access to text books on psychiatry and allied subjects is assumed, and because research into the cause and treatment of mental illness progresses steadily, it is necessary to keep informed of current developments and experiments published in books and journals.

Implications of the Mental Health Act, 1959

Implementation of the Mental Health Act, 1959, has contributed to a more comprehensive psychiatric service, covering both hospital and community needs. It classifies the four main categories of mentally disordered patients as follows [3]:

In this Act:
(1) 'Mental disorder' means mental illness, arrested or incomplete development of mind, psychopathic disorder, and any other disorder or disability of mind; and 'mentally disordered' shall be construed accordingly.
(2) 'Severe subnormality' means a state of arrested or incomplete development of mind which includes subnormality of intelligence and is of such a nature or degree that the patient is incapable of leading an independent life or of guarding himself against serious exploitation, or will be so incapable when of an age to do so.
(3) 'Subnormality' means a state of arrested or incomplete development of mind (not amounting to severe subnormality) which includes subnormality of intelligence and is of a nature or degree which requires or is susceptible to medical treatment or other special care or training of the patient.
(4) 'Psychopathic disorder' means a persistent disorder or disability of mind (whether or not including subnormality of intelligence) which results in abnormally aggressive or seriously irresponsible conduct on the part of the patient, and requires or is susceptible to medical treatment.

Flexibility is the keynote to this Act. It makes it possible for patients to be admitted to the type of hospital best fitted to treat them [4]. The Act also encourages the setting up of psychiatric units in general hospitals, providing more easily accessible facilities, and dispelling the differences in attitude felt by patients or relatives, between physical and psychiatric illness [5]. The informal admission of psychiatric patients to hospital means that they may be admitted under the same conditions as the physically ill, that is, 'without any application, order or direction' [6]. The legal details of the admission of patients who refuse treatment but are in urgent need of it are complicated and not the direct concern of the occupational therapist, although she should be familiar with their implications regarding precautions to be taken described on p. 261.

Emphasis on maintaining or re-establishing more patients in the community, envisaged in the act, has resulted in:

(1) In-patient treatment becoming shorter, a number of repeated short admissions often being preferred to a long stay. [7]

(2) An increase in the number of day patients.

(3) Prominence being given to graded rehabilitation schemes for long-stay patients in hospital.

The long-stay population of psychiatric hospitals is an ageing one. By 1980 there will be a substantial increase in the number of people in the general population over 65 years of age so that the demand for occupational therapy for psycho-geriatric patients will increase [8].

The Mental Health Service

In the re-organised National Health Service* [9] it is envisaged that the mental health care professions will be involved in planning and management at all levels. The maintenance of professional standards and judgments in psychiatric occupational therapy will remain the responsibility of the occupational therapist and it will be increasingly important for the therapist to be able to define her particular role and aims of treatment, because of more involvement in paramedical and multi-disciplinary discussions concerning psychiatric care. Already occupational therapists are contributing at Regional level as well as in Area and District Mental Health Care Planning Teams. Although major policies will be established at Regional level, it will be as a result of consultations from many sources [10] and will be flexible to allow adaptation to particular situations.

At local levels, in the hospital and community services, the occupational therapist will become involved in certain structured team discussions. As a result, a more comprehensive service will evolve with much closer links between hospital and community work [11]. Psychiatric occupational therapy should be seen as a continuing treatment, increasingly community centred except in cases of special need. Although considerable advances have been made in the community care of the physically disabled much still needs to be done for psychiatric cases. The number of day centres, day hospital units, sheltered workshops and group homes will increase. The large psychiatric hospital will still provide treatment for acutely ill patients, the rehabilitation of long-stay patients, and for psycho-geriatric patients.

The Rehabilitation Team

It is as important (if not more so) that the liaison should be as good between staff in a psychiatric hospital as it is in a physical hospital because the patient is less able to develop interpersonal relationships for himself. In planning and carrying out treatment, the occupational therapist works in cooperation with the patient himself, the team of medical specialists and other skilled persons, as well as with lay people who are concerned in his rehabilitation. These may include the following persons and organisations:

Doctors   General Practitioners
Psychologists   Social Workers and Health
Nurses   Visitors
Occupational Therapy Aides   Industrial Managers
Hospital Chaplains   Employers
Disablement Resettlement   Education Authorities
   Officers   Voluntary Organisations
Employment Officers   Relatives of Patients

In a therapeutic community, the concept of team work is widened to include all staff, i.e. a ward orderly, a gardener, or the catering staff.

Psychiatric Treatment

In considering the application of occupational therapy for psychiatric conditions the occupational therapist must be familiar with the psychotherapeutic, physical, surgical and other treatments [12] given to patients individually, and be aware of the contribution her speciality has to make in maintaining and mobilising improvements gained through them. Methods of group treatment are discussed in the following chapter.

Psychoanalysis and Psychotherapy

Psychoanalysis and psychotherapy depend on a special relationship between the trained psychiatrist and the patient. When occupational therapy is prescribed for patients who are also undergoing either of these treatments it is essential that the occupational therapist should confer with the doctor regarding the role he wishes her to adopt in relation to the patient (i.e. permissive, submissive, dominating, etc.). She should also be aware of any particular observations the doctor may require her to make. Apart from these, she must be quick to appreciate subtle changes in the patient's attitude and behaviour, and if her general observations and reporting are perceptive and accurate, she may do much to increase the value of psychoanalysis and psychotherapy.

Chemotherapy

It is essential that the occupational therapist should be aware of the aim of, and any possible side effects arising from, the use of drugs in the treatment of her patients. Each patient may react differently to any one of these drugs, whether sedative, stimulating or tranquillising, and although some general precautions and contra-indications affecting occupational therapy may be mentioned, it is necessary for the therapist to make herself cognisant of the details in each case.

Sedatives, such as barbiturates, have an action upon the cerebral cortex and will cause drowsiness, slowness in comprehension and, in sufficient doses, sleep. Tranquillisers are believed to have an action on the midbrain and, while reducing psychomotor activity, do not produce sleep in the doses usually employed. Some lethargy may result from larger doses but the effect varies not only with the individual personality but with his environment. Parkinsonism is a fairly common side effect and occasionally some fall in the blood pressure may occur. The former may well become apparent in the occupational therapy department and should be reported at once. Some disturbance in the heat regulating centre may occur and exercise in the hot sun may produce pyrexial reaction. Certain stimulants increase motor and cerebral activity, counteract fatigue and reduce appetite. Although confidence may be improved, there is also an increase in distractibility and a tendency to develop overdependence on the drugs. Others relieve depression but have to be prescribed with care and dietary warnings to prevent physical aberrations.

The occupational therapist must be alert for any changes in her patient's condition. Her approach, and treatment methods may have to vary considerably, and success will lie in her careful observation of the changing abilities and needs of each patient and in her cooperation with other members of the treatment team.

Electroconvulsive Therapy

Patients receiving electroconvulsive therapy, which is given for manic or depressive conditions, may attend the occupational therapy department within a short time of regaining consciousness. Almost invariably, however, they suffer from varying periods of confusion or amnesia after each treatment, which, when clearing, may cause them some alarm and anxiety regarding subsequent treatments.

The occupational therapist must be prepared to modify activities while confusion persists. Afterwards reassurance may be necessary, and this is often better given by another patient who has benefitted from electroconvulsive therapy. Grouping of patients for this purpose should be considered. Other after-effects may include headache and stiff or aching muscles. The latter are less common now that relaxant drugs are used in conjunction with the treatment. If, however, the patient complains of pain, due care must be taken during his occupational therapy.

Prefrontal Leucotomy [13]

This has, in the past, been performed only when other treatments have proved ineffective. In consequence the condition of the patient at the time of operation was poor and the subsequent rehabilitation was prolonged and often unsuccessful.

More recently, modified forms of this operation have been applied to carefully selected patients at an earlier stage of illness before deterioration of intellect or personality has taken place. In such cases the results are claimed to be much more successful, but in order to obtain the maximum benefit the rehabilitative measures must be most carefully planned for each individual. Much of this planning will rest with the occupational therapist, as the clinical recovery of the patient is useless without occupational and social readjustment.

The aim is to relieve tension and anxiety, but even where the modified operation is performed there may be a personality change, which some believe to be permanent, with a loss of the more subtle perceptive and reasoning abilities. Reintegration may occur up to eighteen months after the operation. The immediate post-operative state is not always a good indication of the eventual degree of improvement.

Patients who are selected for leucotomy often attend the occupational therapy department prior to the operation. This serves two purposes: firstly, the occupational therapist is able to observe and report upon the patient's performance and behaviour *before* the operation takes place—final selection of the patient for this treatment may depend on such observations; secondly, it may be possible for the occupational therapist to gain the patient's confidence at this stage, thus making subsequent treatment easier. Some occupational therapists like to help the patient to select and learn an activity before operation, so that it can be resumed afterwards. They claim that it is easier for the post-operative patient to carry out previously learned activities. Others prefer to interest the patient in new work graded to his post-operative abilities.

Occupational treatment aims ultimately at helping the patient to acquire a sense of responsibility and an awareness of social obligations, but in order to achieve this, his concentration, persistence and initiative must be re-trained, and to combat lethargy and self-indulgence, a daily work and re-creational programme should be drawn up after consultation with the doctor and nursing staff: adherence to it should be considered an important part of the patient's re-education. Treatment may be given while the patient is still in bed (two or three days after operation) and at this stage only light activities should be undertaken as he may suffer from headaches and giddi-ness. As soon as he is well enough he should be expected to undertake activities in the ward or occupational therapy department, and punctuality, regularity, good habits and appearance should be expected. In many cases it will be found that the patient is quite capable of understanding the purpose of such a plan and will gain confidence in his treatment if it is explained to him.

While individual work is necessary to stimulate the patient and help him to concentrate, group activities will provide a means of increasing his awareness of the needs of others and his own responsibility in the group effort. It is important, however, to see that he does not rely on, or expect to be carried by, other members of the group. Work for others will help to direct his attention towards general social responsibility. While frequent changes of activity are unwise it is necessary for the programme to be flexible enough to allow for regrading, if the patient shows sudden improvement, as this may be delayed if he is kept for prolonged periods on work which makes insufficient demands upon him.

If resettlement outside hospital is anticipated it may be necessary to encourage work of a pre-vocational nature, such as typewriting, dressmaking, cooking, gardening, etc. At all times a high standard of workmanship must be insisted upon, however simple the job may be.

Follow-up of leucotomised patients shows that slovenliness and lack of initiative and responsibility in carrying out everyday tasks are at the root of social and domestic breakdowns which sometimes occur after the patient returns home. It is toward the remedying of these characteristics that the main effort in rehabilitation should be directed.

Stereotactic Tractotomy [14]

An yttrium implant involves the insertion of radioactive seeds, which have a limited range of radioactivity, at the point of conversion of fibres concerned with normal emotional reaction. The operation preserves the benefits of leucotomy without personality change or post-operative epilepsy. The intellect remains unaltered and normal emotions previously suppressed can be expressed. The operation has been used successfully with intractable cases of agitated depression and psychoneuroses and with chronic alcoholics and barbiturate drug addicts. Occupational therapy should begin as soon as possible with a suitable rehabilitation course which takes immediate advantage of improvement.

Insulin Treatment

This treatment, where still used, is now given in modified form to selected patients, mainly those suffering from schizophrenia. Those who are given insulin will require occupational therapy daily, after treatment, when a programme of activities offering mental and physical stimulation should be provided to keep them in contact with reality and to promote exercise to combat increase in weight occurring during treatment.

When several patients are receiving insulin, it is often convenient and therapeutically valuable to deal with them as a group with one member of staff in charge. Glucose should always be available to counteract hypo-glycaemia if this should occur.

Behaviour Therapy [15]

This is a term given to a form of treatment by conditioning for neurotic disorders. It is based on the postulation that these disorders are demonstrated in overt symptoms resulting from habits and obsessions developed by anxieties and manifesting themselves in compulsive reactions. The treatment seeks to replace the unacceptable symptom or behaviour by the substitution, through conditioning, of more appropriate reactions which lessen the anxiety of the patient and if this is effected improve his adjustment to his environment. The tenets of this treatment differ markedly from those of the Freudian and other analytic schools and its value and significance have yet to be established. An occupational therapist may be asked to collaborate with the doctor and others in developing and implementing a conditioning programme with and for the patient.

General Aims of Occupational Therapy

The aims of treatment should be discussed by the rehabilitation team, and it is helpful to define a broad aim for each patient. This may vary from rehabilitation for return to home and former work, or to home and a lighter job, or attendance at a day centre, to living within the hospital and working outside it, to living and working within the hospital either in a utility department or sheltered industrial unit, or to total care in a psychogeriatric unit (see chapters 15, 20). More immediate aims may then be defined which may change from week to week as, for example, in helping a patient to overcome a particular anxiety at work or to deal with a difficult working relationship with another patient. Aims of treatment may also be related to a specific activity designed to evoke a particular response at a certain stage of treatment as, for instance, in a painting group, held to promote discussion. With increased specialisation and grouping of patients with similar problems, such as drug addicts, neurotic patients, psychopaths and epileptics, etc., and graded schemes for long-stay patients, the aims of treatment will be closely related to the type of group formed. Reference is made to these in the following chapters.

Allocation of Staff

With the current shortage of trained personnel, the occupational therapist should use her training to the maximum either by working with special groups of patients in a close therapeutic relationship or by organising a wide range of activities, some of which may be supervised or taught by other grades of staff. Here, she will act as a consultant [16], providing the medical link and therapeutic advice. Personnel with different interests and training can fulfil a valuable function, as long as they work under the direction of, or in full cooperation with, the occupational therapist. Help may be obtained from:

(1) *Technicians and industrialists*, who are essential when a professional standard of training and production is required.

(2) *Occupational therapy helpers or aides*, who may have a specialised skill, or general interests and skills and an aptitude for learning and can be trained to supervise industrial work or similar activities.

(3) *Teachers* supplied through a local education authority. Such classes can cover a wide range of activities, and are particularly useful if held in the evenings to stimulate interest in hobbies. As most teachers hold only one or two sessions a week, however, their relationship with the hospital may be remote, and they will need support and encouragement from hospital staff.

(4) *Voluntary helpers* [17], who can perform a most useful and unique function by befriending patients who have few outside contacts, thus forming an important link between hospital and community. There are numerous ways in which volunteers can help in occupational therapy, e.g. by offering special skills, taking patients out, helping with long-stay patients, and providing holidays or accommodation. In some hospitals there is now a coordinator of voluntary help with whom the occupational therapist should work closely. If there is no coordinator, she must be prepared to give her voluntary helpers direction, support and encouragement.

Patient-Therapist Relationship

In occupational therapy the relationship formed between patient and therapist is of the utmost importance, the activity being only the medium of contact used to establish a therapeutic relationship. The occupational therapist having studied the phases of development from childhood to maturity, will note that many patients may still be immature. She must have a mature outlook herself, being aware of her own problems and having her own emotions, motives and beliefs in perspective. A sound relationship can only be built by the occupational therapist's ability to understand the patient's reactions from *his* situation, based on observation of his general behaviour, rather than on isolated incidents. True understanding only comes by disregarding superficial reasons for inappropriate behaviour, and by making a full and careful assessment of the causes for it. When a patient is uncooperative, it is not enough to regard his behaviour as 'part of his illness' or as 'his usual reaction'. The occupational therapist should consider:

Why the patient is reacting this way.

Why it is important to him to be like this.

What he gains by adopting this attitude.

How the patient sees himself as an individual. [18]

Very often the therapist will find that the patient needs *security* in which to develop as a mature person, as well as *reassurance* and *consistency*. As most psychiatric illness is based on emotional disorder, it is useless to attempt to rationalise with patients unless they show positive signs of insight into the subconscious motivations affecting their thoughts, feelings and behaviour. Nor should they be exposed to situations likely to give rise to extreme over-anxiety. The therapist must be prepared to understand and accept the deviant ways in which patients react, through aggression, withdrawal, the use of obsessional rituals or physical disability. Once an understanding relationship has been formed, further observation is necessary to carry out a course of rehabilitation, and the following are suggested points to observe, record and report upon when treating patients with psychiatric disorders:

(1) *Presentation*	Appearance
	Habits
	Speech
(2) *Physical condition*	General physique
	Posture
	Sight
	Hearing
	Any specific disability (including fits)
(3) *Intellectual response*	Alertness
	Comprehension
	Concentration
	Initiative
	Imagination
	Judgment
	Persistence
(4) *Learning ability*	Perception
	Retention
	Recall
	Application
(5) *Degree of maturity and control*	Response to incentives (praise, reward, success)
	Response to stress (criticism, interruptions, frustration, noise, discomfort)

(6) *Relationships*

Individual:
    With therapeutic team members
    With fellow patients
    With those in authority
    With the outside community
Group:
    Within the hospital
    In the community outside the hospital

(7) *Overt symptoms affecting behaviour*

Hysterical features
Depression
Thought disorder
Obsessional traits, etc.

(8) *Effects of other treatments*

Confusion after E.C.T.*
Side effects of drugs, etc.

Activities

Activity is basic to life, and occupation offers release from tension, anxiety and grief. For psychiatric patients, occupational therapy not only involves this normal aspect of life but can strengthen resistance to breakdown through purposeful attainment and satisfying personal relationships, by encouraging new skills, perfecting poorly used ones or relearning forgotten ones, resulting in restored self confidence and a more mature sense of responsibility. The use made of activities in occupational therapy is sometimes misunderstood. An occupation cannot cure a patient by itself; it is the use the patient is able to make of it through the relationship formed with the therapist and other participants that progress is made. Numerous subtle factors surround involvement in an occupation as well as its inherent value, and it is because of the complex forces at work that the therapist needs to be highly trained. Communication, with its social implications and consequences, verbal and non-verbal, emotive and detached, must be recognised and understood, and distinctions made, not only between signs and symptoms of psychiatric illness, but between the differing personalities and reactions of the different communicators. Some will try to manipulate the therapeutic situation and the therapist: others will be subtly hostile or parasitically dependent, or will convert their pressures into aggression, domination or other defensive protest forms. The occupation, then, is an instrument of treatment only, used by the patient and therapist to contribute to the resolution of these and other psychological problems.

For some patients, for example long-stay patients whose illness has reached a plateau, an occupation may be therapeutic in itself, as in a domestic rehabilitation scheme, where the standard and skill in organisation and budgeting are important because the patient is to return to independence in the community outside hospital. For other patients, psychoneurotics in particular, the inability to work consistently is due to emotional conflict rather than lack of practice, and a wide variety of activities not necessarily concerned with a patient's normal occupation may be used. Also activities may be used to improve social relationships or for observation or, when requested by a doctor, as an aid to diagnosis. Many activities achieve more than one end, and the occupational therapist must be able to assess the possibilities of the activities she uses and to consider the *relative importance of each facet* for the patient. Activities can be grouped under the following headings:

(1) *Activities related to work*, either the patient's normal work outside the hospital, or training for a different job, or for sheltered work in the hospital or in the community. Work is an essential part of life and provides status and ability to earn a living. Work situations provide valuable means of assessment for physical capacity, intellectual and manual skills, persistence and reliability. The level of motivation required for work can be judged and working patterns re-established to build confidence and the ability to tolerate working pressures. A wide variety of work opportunities from simple to demanding work should be available to fulfil these requirements, and can include industrial work, office work, gardening, printing, work in hospital departments, and cooking and other domestic routines for women. At each stage the work must be seen as worthwhile by the patient, and meaningful to his particular situation, and should never encourage dependency or institutional patterns. Attitudes to supervision and authority, and relationships with fellow workers are important aspects to assess, and recent research shows that the patients' assessment of their own abilities and prospects is a factor to consider in rehabilitation.

(2) *Activities to improve physical well-being*, including relaxation exercises, 'health and beauty' exercises, outdoor and indoor games, gardening, swimming, walking, etc.

(3) *Activities to enrich interpersonal relationships and socialisation.* The psychiatric patient often has difficulty in living and working satisfactorily as a member of a group. Through his relationship with the therapist, he can be introduced gradually to group events until he can participate fully in an active way, which requires adjustment, cooperation, acceptance and understanding of the other members. Using an activity in a group situation produces interaction related to work and living with other people, and helps patients to identify the therapist as someone who is connected with normal patterns of behaviour. Patients can be helped to feel more socially acceptable

by attention to personal hygiene, care or restyling of the hair, manicuring, and interest in dress and personal behaviour. Selected group activities can cover a wide variety of activities including dancing, cooking, gardening, flower arranging, drama, millinery, etc. Such groups usually comprise six to twelve patients, either chosen by the staff team to work together or as a naturally occurring group with common interests. Activity groups[19] are sometimes held to promote discussion with patients who have difficulty in voicing their feelings, and here activities such as painting, music and drama may be specially planned and used by the therapist for observational and therapeutic purposes. Suitable activities might include preparing a meal, organising an outing, mending furniture or reorganising part of a garden. An activity group can also help patients who have problems in common, so that they can help each other to surmount these. A good example of this is when a small group of housebound housewives go shopping together.

(4) *Activities to encourage personal expression and creative use of leisure time.* These may include music, painting or some craft, photography, gardening, marquetry, billiards, theatre-going, stamp collecting, etc. Classes or individual teaching can often be arranged with the help of teachers, voluntary workers and the patients themselves. Some patients get great satisfaction from pursuing a hobby alone, while others prefer group participation. As participation in such events is voluntary, a great deal can be observed regarding a patient's general capacity to carry out an activity and participate with others in varying conditions.

It is evident from these examples that activities have varied uses. The following points are suggested as a guide to the basic evaluation of them.

Psychological Evaluation of an Activity

(1) *Cognitive.* What demands does the activity make on the patient and/or what could it help to develop, e.g. concentration, judgment, etc.?

(2) *Affective.* In what ways may emotional needs be expressed and/or controlled, e.g. aggression, elation, etc.?

(3) *Conative.* Does this activity enable the patient to satisfy basic needs, e.g. security, acceptance, responsibility for fulfilment and challenge?

(4) *Disabilities.* Which disability would benefit from this activity and during which stages?

(5) *Precautions.* Are any special safety measures essential?

Check List for Determining the Value of an Activity

This list is only of value with a specific patient in mind and will exclude unsuitable activities and prove the need for modification in others.

(1) How long will the activity take to complete?
Is completion of the activity vital to the patient?

(2) Is the activity obviously related to total rehabilitation scheme or should reasons be given?
What incentive is there for the patient to undertake the work?

(3) Does success depend on group effort?
To what extent does the activity involve interaction between other patients and staff?
Will patient need to:

      (i) accept guidance?
      (ii) accept authority?
      (iii) show leadership?
      (iv) collaborate with other patients?

(4) Are many processes involved in the activity?
Is it repetitive?
Is accuracy essential?

(5) To what extent does the activity involve:

      (i) comprehension?   (iv) judgment?
      (ii) concentration?   (v) memory?
      (iii) reasoning?   (vi) alertness?
            (vii) initiative?

(6) Does the activity involve:

      (i) imagination?   (iii) experimentation?
      (ii) creative ability?   (iv) destructive elements?
            (v) outlet for regressive tendencies?

(7) What physical aspects are involved in connection with:

      (i) physical effort required—fine movement, gross movement?
            (ii) sight?   (iv) hearing?
            (iii) touch?   (v) smell?

(8) Are there any special psychological or physical contra-indications?

Check List Regarding Employment of Psychiatric Patients

Department .... Date ....

Period covered by report...

Type of occupation during this period..............................

For each question ring most appropriate word

ATTENDANCE:	Does he always attend unless excused?..	Always	Sometimes	Never
	Does he arrive on time?................	Always	Sometimes	Never
	Does he stay until dismissed?	Always	Sometimes	Never
WORKMANSHIP: (Add details here) QUALITY:		Thorough	Variable	Slipshod
	SPEED:	Fast	Medium	Slow
RELIABILITY:	Grasp of instructions.................	Good	Fair	Poor
	Once shown, does he remember what he has to do?	Yes		No
	Can he see what he should do and do it without being told?	Yes		No
	Attitude to work	Enjoys	Accepts	Dislikes
APPLICATION:	Does he work steadily?...............	Always	Usually	Never
	Does he take unauthorised rests?	Never	Sometimes	Always
	If unsatisfactory, why?			
BEHAVIOUR:	Is he as clean and tidy as he can be?......	Yes	Fairly	No
	Is he good tempered?	Always	Usually	Rarely
	Reaction to authority.................	Good	Fair	Resentful
	Attitude towards staff	Frank		Servile
SOCIABILITY:	Does he make overtures of friendship to other patients?	Mostly	Some	None
	Is he a trouble maker?	Never	Sometimes	Often
ECCENTRICITY:	Would he stand out as odd in an outside work environment?	No	Slightly	Yes
	Have you noticed anything peculiar about his actions? e.g.			

WORK GROUP
SUITABILITY: ....Large one, Small one, Alone

RATING: How much work does he manage to do compared with a paid employee? (e.g., $\frac{1}{8}$, $\frac{1}{4}$, $\frac{1}{2}$, $\frac{2}{3}$, $\frac{7}{8}$, 1)

FURTHER
INFORMATION: If there is anything that you can add about this patient's employability please comment overleaf
(IMPORTANT: can nullify or substantiate findings)

Signature ....

Date.............

Safety Measures

When choosing an appropriate course of treatment, the overriding consideration must be the safety of the patients and any risks must be evaluated and discussed within the treatment team. The referral card, if properly completed, is a means of ensuring the safety of the patient. The symptoms of the case must be known and understood, as well as any particular precautions that are necessary. This applies to patients who may be suicidal and also to those who may have violent outbursts or a serious physical complaint in addition to mental illness. The following safety measures should be noted:

Suicidal Risks

Precautions against suicide are among the most important. The risk is not confined to depressives only: hysterics, psychopaths, addicts and schizophrenics may attempt it. Patients who are overtly intent on suicide will probably be kept on the ward under supervision. Others may have a history of past threats, or their illness may indicate a need for precaution. As many patients now have greater freedom and can obtain matches, scissors and other potentially dangerous items, it is easier for a patient intent on suicide to obtain the means to carry out the act. The therapist must, therefore, be extremely observant of patients in this category. By observing closely individual patients at risk, the majority who are not suicidal need not suffer from restrictions applicable to a minority only, for generally speaking over-protection in hospital makes readjustment to the risks involved in normal life more difficult. The best precautions against suicidal risks are:

> The referral card.
> Observation and understanding.
> Good liaison with doctor and ward staff.

Absconding

Occupational therapists should know the exact number of patients who are under their care at any one time and must keep an adequate register and check the number of patients who arrive and leave. The only exception to this rule is in those units where the treatment is permissive and patients attend the department if they wish to. In this type of régime all the staff should work closely together, so that all are aware of particular problems among patients although patients in such units are usually of *informal status* [20]. Under the Mental Health Act 1959, a patient who is admitted informally may leave at any time and cannot be detained against his wishes unless the responsible medical officer makes an order under section 30, because it is in the interests of the patient's health or safety, or the protection of others, that he remains in hospital. This order expires after 72 hours but gives enough time for other legal arrangements to be made where necessary. If an *informal* patient leaves an occupational group in circumstances which give rise to anxiety, the occupational therapist should take what responsible action she can and let the ward staff know.

Patients may be admitted *formally* to hospital under one of the following sections [21]:

Section 25 (Admission for Observation)
Section 26 (Admission for Treatment)
Section 29 (Admission for Observation in an Emergency)
Section 60 (Court Order for Admission)
Section 72 (Admission from Prison)

These patients should be watched carefully.

Tools and Machinery

Cutting tools, such as razor blades, should be issued with care and a watch kept on them. Loss of a tool in suspicious circumstances should be reported to the ward concerned. The tool check at the end of each session prevents loss of stock and gives the occupational therapist the opportunity to encourage patients to share responsibility with staff for looking after them.

Precautions necessary under the Factories Act to guard dangerous machinery are mentioned in the chapter on industrial work. No patient who is liable to fits should work with or near moving machinery, hot liquids and easily broken glass, i.e. garden cloches, etc.

Dangerous Liquids

All stains and varnishes must be kept in locked cupboards unless in actual use, as should methylated spirits which could be taken by alcoholics.

Departmental Organisation

The department itself should be one in which it is easy for safety measures to be carried out, and in which the absence of a patient can be noticed easily. An observation window between office and department is essential for a single-handed therapist, and the room itself should be light and seen as a whole. Adequate staffing facilitates the unobtrusive observation of patients, and, in addition, periodic rounds of the cloakrooms should be made. The staff should never become so deeply absorbed that they are unable to react immediately to prevent difficulties.

REFERENCES AND RECOMMENDED FURTHER READING

1. Fleming, C. M., *Social Psychology of Education*, chapter iv. London, 1959.
2. Freeman, H. & Farndale, J. (Eds), *Trends in the Mental Health Services*. London, 1963.
3. *Mental Health Act*, 1959. Part 1, Section 4.
4. *Memorandum on Mental Health Act*, Notes 7 and 9. H.M.S.O.*, 1960.
5. Gatherer, A. & Reid, J. J. A., *Public Attitudes and Mental Health Education*. Northamptonshire County Council, 1967.
6. *Mental Health Act*, 1959. Part 1, Section 5.
7. *The Registrar General's Statistical Review of England and Wales*, 1960. *Supplement on Mental Health*. H.M.S.O.*, 1964.
8. Brooke, E. M. *A Census of Patients in Psychiatric Beds*. Table 14. H.M.S.O.* (1963).
9. *Management Arrangements for the Reorganised National Health Service*.* H.M.S.O.*, 1972.
10. Giolann, S. E. & Eisdorfer, C., *Handbook of Community Mental Health*. London, 1972.
11. *Approaches to Action: Services for the Mentally Ill*, 1972, and *Policy for Action: Symposium on Planning of a Comprehensive Psychiatric Service*, 1973, Nuffield Provincial Hospitals Trust.
And see: Kenny, B. & Whitehead, T., *Insight: A Guide to Psychiatry and Psychiatric Services*, London, 1973.
12. Curran, D. & Partridge, M., *Psychological Medicine*, London, 1972.
Merskey, R. H. & Tonge, W. L., *Psychiatric Illness*, London, 1974.
Pollitt, J., *Psychiatry, A Student's Textbook*, London, 1972.
Sim, M., *Guide to Psychiatry*, Edinburgh and London, 1974.
Sim, M. & Gordon, E. B., *Basic Psychiatry*, Section 18, London, 1972.
13. Tooth, G. C. & Newton, M. P. (1961) Leucotomy in England and Wales, 1942–54. *M.O.H. Rep. publ. Hlth. Subs.*, no. 104.
Sargeant, W. (1962) The present indications for leucotomy. *Lancet*.
14. Knight, G. C. (1964) *Brit. J. Surg.*, 51, 114.
Knight, G. C. (1965) *J. Neurol. Psychiat.*, 28, 304.
Knight, G. C. & Stron-Olsen, R. (1969) Stereotactic surgery. *Brit. J. Alc.*, 3.
15. Beech, H., *Changing Man's Behaviour*. Pelican, 1969.
Eysenck, H. J., *Behaviour Therapy and the Neuroses*, London, 1960.
Eysenck, H. J. & Rachman, S., *The Causes and Cures of Neurosis*, London, 1965.
16. Kandel, D., The development of the occupational therapy consultant. Paper read at the 50th Anniversary Congress of the American Occupational Therapy Association, 1967.
17. Huggins, R., The voluntary worker in occupational therapy programmes. *Occ. Ther.*, 30, no. 1.
Volunteers in hospital. *Occ. Ther.*, 35, no. 1, 1972.
And see: Hargrove, A. L., *Guide to the Mental Health Act 1959*, N.A.M.H.*, 1963.
18. Matheney, R. & Topalis, M., *Psychiatric Nursing*, U.S.A., 1970.
Merskey, H. & Tonge, L. W., see ref. 12 above.
19. Jones, M. (1960) Group work in mental hospitals. *Brit. J. Psychiat.*, 112, no. 491.
And see:
Some experiences in socio-drama in a county psychiatric hospital. *Occ. Ther.*, 35, no. 5, 1972.
The value of psychodrama. *Brit. J. occ. Ther.*, 37, no. 8, 1974.
20. Mental Health Act 1959. Part 1, section 5.
21. Mental Health Act 1959. Part IV.
And see:
The significance of illness. *Occ. Ther.*, 35, no. 1, 1972.
Occupational therapy in a modern setting. *Occ. Ther.*, 35, no. 1, 1972.
Principles of rehabilitation of the mentally ill. *Occ. Ther.*, 36, no. 4, 1973.
Rehabilitation in psychiatry. *Occ. Ther.*, 36, no. 4, 1973.
Rehabilitation, clinical and occupational. *Occ. Ther.*, 36, no. 4, 1973.
Hypnosis and relaxation. *Brit. J. occ. Ther.*, 37, no. 8, 1974.

* See *Glossary*, p. 454.

CHAPTER 13

Social Implications in the Application of Occupational Therapy for Psychiatric Conditions

---

Before discussing the prescription and application of occupational therapy for specific psychiatric conditions it is important to consider the location, environment and group situations in which the treatment may be given. In recent years the significance of the social structure of a hospital, ward or unit has been realised. The administration [1], organisation, physical setting and methods of communication may all contribute to the recovery of the patient. If patients are to learn how to improve their social relationships the treatment setting must have a relation to normality. By considering the social aspects of treatment it has been found that convalescent patients make more stable recoveries and leave hospital with a clearer awareness of their problems and better understanding of their anxieties. Disturbed patients are better tolerated and thus improve more quickly in an appropriate setting, and long-stay patients who are not ready for discharge are able to work at varying levels within the hospital [2]. The significance of this kind of integrated approach is seen in those methods of treatment where environmental factors play an important part.

Environmental Influences in Hospital

THE THERAPEUTIC COMMUNITY [3]

Because a therapeutic community involves the entire population of a hospital and is concerned with the maintenance of a supportive environment to assist the emotional maturation of the patient, this aspect of hospital treatment will be dealt with first. Staff and patients are encouraged to take part in a comprehensive treatment programme according to their training and ability. Important features of the system include [4]:

Communication.
Group meetings.
Interpersonal relationships.
Total treatment planning.

Communication

Effective communication between individuals is essential to promote understanding, and is the process by which the views of one person may be made known to another. In a therapeutic community, free communication, whether formal, informal, verbal or non-verbal, is encouraged at all levels between staff, staff and patients, and the patients themselves. In particular the views of patients, concerning themselves and all aspects of hospital life, are welcomed, to stimulate interest and initiative in their daily lives. Material arising from such discussion is then used to help patients understand and resolve their problems. Various group discussions are held and the occupational therapist should be aware of three levels of participation [5] in such meetings:

(1) *Conscious interest, expressed* vocally, and representing what members are feeling at a conscious level.
(2) *Conscious interest, held back,* and representing what members are thinking and feeling but unable to communicate. Looks and behaviour may be some indication of mood.
(3) *Unconscious thoughts and feelings* giving rise to spoken or unspoken words, members being unaware of their cause. This may result in hostility, aggression or even inability to remain in the meeting.

Group Meetings

Patients' ward meetings may be held daily or weekly, to discuss what is happening in the ward situation. The meeting may be limited to the discussion of practical and material problems, but usually progresses to a discussion of what lies behind behaviour. Patients may choose to talk about personal problems, many of which will be shared by others. Every contribution is important and nothing should be considered inappropriate (sometimes what appears to be beside the point has the greatest significance).

The patients usually sit in a circle and the staff should sit among them informally. For all but the more deteriorated patients it is usual to wait for the patients to open the discussion. A long silence may ensue but this does not mean that the patients have nothing to say. If thought necessary the doctor will eventually enquire the reason for it. New staff often find such silences difficult to sustain but should avoid breaking in if possible. The occupational therapist should know the doctors' views regarding staff participation in patients' meetings, as this varies. Matters pertaining to occupational therapy may arise and be discussed by the whole group. The purpose of the meetings is to stimulate discussion, and direct questions from patients should be replied to in terms that will promote further observation. Not infrequently, and particularly with neurotic patients, the occupational therapist may receive a verbal attack from a patient. This should always be viewed objectively as an indication of a patient's unresolved tension and the real reason for it sought. It is common for patients to choose a different person than the one they would really like to address, and a different subject from the problem really bothering them.

Staff meetings, to include ward, department and other personnel, usually follow ward meetings and the interaction of patients is discussed. Staff can describe their feelings and attitudes towards happenings in the patients' meeting, which may vary according to the training and personality of the staff member, and through the examination of these 'role relationships' the true needs of patients can be clarified. Unresolved tension among staff can interfere dramatically with patients' treatment, and in a mature staff meeting difficulties can be brought into the open and discussed constructively. The lead taken by the doctor in these circumstances will vary according to the ability of the group to progress productively. The occupational therapist can contribute by reporting on patients' reactions in occupational therapy, and share other problems and anxieties regarding particular patients.

Interpersonal Relationships

The basic principles in forming a therapeutic relationship are described in chapter 12, p. 253. In a therapeutic community the occupational therapist must be able to assess her own reactions, including her emotions, in her relationship with staff and patients. As in normal life, it is entirely natural to 'like' or 'dislike' people, and as a result, to feel a number of emotions towards them. The therapist must be aware of the difference between a *therapeutic relationship* and *emotional involvement*. The former implies an understanding of emotions which may be evoked between patient and therapist, and lead to greater understanding of the patient's difficulties. Emotional involvement occurs when there is lack of understanding, the therapist seeking emotional satisfaction for herself from the situation. If a patient shows signs of extremes of emotion towards the occupational therapist, i.e. active like or dislike, she should discuss the matter at a staff meeting because it is not easy to sustain such extreme feelings without the support and backing of the doctor and team. Perhaps she resembles someone in the patient's life, in reality or phantasy, and may therefore be able to help him understand the motivating forces behind his emotions, but this deeper approach can only be undertaken with the consent and advice of the doctor.

Particular attention should be paid to the ways in which patients may identify the occupational therapist with other personalities, and try and manipulate her to satisfy immature needs. The therapist must learn to recognise her tendency to identify herself with the role the patient may wish her to play. The most obvious role is that of 'teacher' or 'employer', but can also be 'sister', 'daughter' or, in fact, any role needed by the patient. By discussion with the ward team, the occupational therapist should be helped to define her general role in a particular situation. In an industrial workshop it may be appropriate for her to be viewed as 'employer'. On the other hand, it may be necessary for the minimum of authority to be used, as in the later stages of a domestic rehabilitation scheme. Fundamentally, the therapist's function in the team of specialists is to understand and use the therapeutic relationship within the framework of the activities being used in treatment.

Total Treatment Planning

Through patients' and staff meetings, the occupational therapist will be more aware, and involved in the total life, of each patient in hospital [6], including his medical treatment, psychotherapy, pharmacotherapy, electrotherapy, etc., his social problems in the community, and his reactions to life on his ward. The way in which each patient spends his day is of importance to each member of the team. It follows, therefore, that other members will be interested and concerned in the patient's progress in occupational therapy. The occupational therapist is expected to suggest appropriate activities, but these should be discussed with the ward team first, and then with patients, before being put into operation. Disagreement by staff, conscious or unconscious, over the occupational therapy programme, can prove a serious barrier to its implementation as well as obstruct its therapeutic value for patients [7].

The general aim of occupational therapy within a therapeutic community is to facilitate interaction, communication and insight and to encourage responsibility in all aspects of life. Group activities are valuable and may include realistic work which involves a contribution to the community. Creative activities, such as art, pottery, music and woodwork, can provide new means of expression and achievement. Other activity groups may be more dynamically orientated to encourage discussion between patients, and improve relationships within a group. Psychodrama, art and music have proved successful in this way.

In some therapeutic communities the occupational therapist may participate in small psychotherapy groups, where she will help to promote discussion among patients by reference to reactions in activity groups. Such intensive work depends on medical direction and support and should never be attempted in isolation from the medical team.

The occupational therapist must be familiar with other forms of group treatment which may be carried out by specially trained staff but will have a bearing on her own work. Encounter or Contact groups involve miming or physical contact to encourage non-verbal communication. Acting-out occurs in Dream Groups, which aim to help an individual member by the re-enactment of a dream which is then interpreted by the therapist. Gestalt Groups, developed by Fritz Perls, are a non-interpretive method of treatment, which aims to release emotional feelings in the inhibited and detached person, by the expression of fantasies and the dramatisation of internal conflicts.

PERMISSIVE TREATMENT

This is a different and calculated approach. In its extreme form, the patient is permitted to participate in activities or not, as he feels inclined; he may stay in bed if he wishes, and is not actively encouraged to take any form of responsibility. Routine is practically non-existent.

The specialists who advocate the extreme form of permissive atmosphere in the treatment of patients, particularly the neurotics, maintain that active encouragement to conform to the requirements of the social group encourages regression, in that the patient does not develop independence and initiative. Other specialists feel that a modified form of permissive atmosphere is more satisfactory, as the aim of treatment is to help the patient to become an integrated member of society, and he should therefore be encouraged to conform to the reasonable requirements of the group, at the same time being given every opportunity to use his own initiative and take responsibility for fulfilling his own needs and those of the group, within the framework of the social standards required by that group.

HABIT TRAINING

Habit training [8] is based on the laws of exercise, frequency and recency and is an attempt to restore or maintain those acquired behaviour patterns which enable us to perform many tasks efficiently and with little or no conscious thought. In the psychiatric patient, the breakdown of habits frequently accompanies severe intellectual deficit, when the patient is less concerned with his personal needs, is no longer really interested in his environment or is emotionally unable to feel the effect of his behaviour on others.

No occupational therapist can inaugurate a habit training programme for deteriorating patients except in cooperation with medical, nursing and technical staffs, and should consult the psychologist about possible ratings to be made in her department or with classes in her charge. The patients' day must be so organised that it is filled, and it must follow the same basic routine every day. Nevertheless, care must be taken that the routine is not so exact in inessentials that patients become rigidly unadaptable. Habit training programmes will be fundamentally similar because the methods are related to basic physiological needs, but may vary in detail from one unit to another.

They involve small groups of patients with, usually, one member of staff in charge of varying numbers of patients, but it must be emphasised that the ratio of patients to staff must be kept small, to ensure adequate treatment of the individual patient.

Care of appearance as well as bowel and bladder training are important. The patient may have to be retaught table manners and normal social customs as well as being retrained to occupy himself. Such aims cannot be realised unless the staff are willing to be patient and persevering and the training is made easy and pleasant for the patient. Pleasing appearance should be complimented upon and rewards given for progress. These should relate to the patients' training and needs, e.g. a personal lipstick, a trip to the canteen, a ward tea-party, and they should be given as often as is reasonable. Equally, failure should be met with explanation and guidance, or, if necessary deprivation of privilege. This should not be punitive but used to teach 'cause and effect'. There should be little time lag between the act and its reward or 'punishment', but no patient should ever be criticised in front of others, although reasonable criticism by the other patients may be therapeutic.

It must also be remembered that habits can be lost because they are not easy to maintain. The patient should, therefore, have easy access to lavatories, mirrors, brushes, combs and makeup.

Habit training can be combined with the '*total push*' method of treatment which is the continual active encouragement of a patient to participate and cooperate in a group, necessitating a planned and supervised programme to cover every hour of the day. The aim is to develop social awareness and responsibility, and a sense of being an integral part of a group. It involves the re-education of regressed patients, and, with others, it aims at the establishment of good work habits, development of skills and manual dexterity, and the building of resistance to fatigue. This helps in the exploration of pre-vocational possibilities or, in the case of long-term hospitalisation, in assessment for placement in one of the hospital utility departments or industrial schemes.

Hospital In-patient Treatment

While concern for the patient as an individual is the first consideration, treatment can only be organised efficiently by grouping patients together according to the type of treatment required and the stage of rehabilitation reached. The groups described here emphasise the progressive nature of occupational therapy, and stress the importance of comprehensive treatment, covering hospital and community needs. Psychiatrists today aim to treat and maintain as many patients as possible in their normal domestic and working environments, and in the community to which they belong. Admission to hospital is arranged, if necessary, during the acute phase of an illness, but patients are returned to the community as soon as they are well. In-patient treatment may be necessary for observation, investigation and treatment, because there is a risk of suicide, or disturbed behaviour which cannot be tolerated by the patient's family or in the community. A number of short admissions often take the place of a long stay.

In-patient treatment may be given in a short-stay ward or unit of a psychiatric hospital, or, increasingly, in a general hospital. The Mental Health Act, 1959, recommends:

'A substantial increase in psychiatric facilities in general hospitals . . . both to ensure the better distribution and siting of psychiatric services, and to help ensure that there is the closest possible contact between psychiatric and other hospital services.' [9]

In-patient groups include:

SHORT-STAY MIXED ADMISSION UNITS

These admit men and women patients of all ages, and varied diagnoses, the average length of stay being between three weeks and three months. The occupational therapy programme is planned to meet the requirements of a rapid turnover of patients, but this can only be achieved if the therapist works as an integrated member of the ward team, so that she gets to know the patients as soon and as well as other staff, and is fully involved in treatment planning.

Therapist–Patient Relationship

Here the occupational therapist aims at independence in patients, but must always be ready to give encouragement, support, and security. Where occupational therapy is well established, and particularly where weekly programming meetings are held, new patients will soon become familiar with the organisation. Nevertheless, the importance of the initial and individual approach should never be overlooked, and the therapist should see each patient as soon as possible after his arrival, so that an individual relationship can be formed, and the situation explained. In trying to encourage a satisfactory response, the therapist should make it clear that the patient's views concerning occupational therapy are important and can be expressed either to the therapist, or at ward meetings, if these are held.

Emphasis should be on rehabilitation from the beginning, with the possible exception of very disturbed or disorientated patients who may need a few days of less stimulating activities and time to settle down. Even if most of the activities are held away from the ward or unit, it is a good plan to hold at least a few on the ward for new patients, so that they can get to know each other and the therapist.

General Aims of Occupational Therapy

Earlier diagnosis, advances in chemotherapy, and the general policy of community care, are all important factors in the development of the short-stay unit, and have special bearing on the general aims of occupational therapy which in this setting, include:

(1) *Supporting physical, psychotherapeutic and other treatments* by taking immediate advantage of improvements, and encouraging participation in activities which will help ensure that, on returning home, patients are better equipped to deal with their day-to-day lives. This may be achieved by:

(*a*) Improving actual work techniques.

(*b*) Using activities to broaden insight into emotional difficulties which are lowering efficiency.

(*c*) Improving ability to make good relationships through work and social activities.

(*d*) Emphasising importance of constructive leisure pursuits.

(2) *Helping patients to maintain contact with outside affairs and making the hospital routine as normal as possible.* This can be achieved by encouraging activities related to the patients' usual lives, and, in cooperation with nursing staff, giving them as much responsibility as possible for such personal matters as washing and ironing their own clothes, making their own beds, cooking for some meals, etc. As many patients will return home at weekends, part of the programme can be related to week-end responsibilities and leisure activities, such as preparing meals in advance, making toys for children, talks on car maintenance, etc.

Individual Aims in Occupational Therapy

Through the referral form, and discussion with the rehabilitation team, details of the clinical condition of each patient will be obtained. This must be related to the social and domestic situation before a meaningful individual plan can be formulated. The important features to consider are:

(1) Assessment and observation.

(2) Diagnosis, particularly of degree of insight.

(3) Particular problems in the home situation, for example, a pending divorce, an overbearing father, a very large family, an isolated house. These should be considered from the practical point of view including the type of role problems which may, as a result, be projected on to the therapist.

(4) Whether there has been a long period of work failure, relatively little disturbance to work capacity, or over-conscientious approach to work as a result of illness.

Therapeutic Media

Lengthy projects are inadvisable, and if suggested, can cause real concern to patients, but there are few limits to the variety of activities which can be used to achieve the aforementioned aims (see chapter 12). The skill of the occupational therapist lies in the handling of the situation, as well as in the choice of activity, and in her ability to be flexible but purposeful.

Liaison

The majority of patients will be discharged absolutely, but some may be transferred to the care of the local authority for further support. The therapist should make a report and see that salient features of the patient's rehabilitation in hospital are passed on to appropriate sources, if possible to the occupational therapist working in the community. Some patients may continue to attend as day patients, and, as well as receiving continued rehabilitation themselves can often help in-patients by assuming small responsibilities and helping the occupational therapist.

A small proportion of patients may not improve sufficiently to be discharged and so will pass on to a middle-stay ward in the same, or another hospital. In this instance, the occupational therapist has an important part to play in supporting the patient and encouraging him in an equally positive, although longer, rehabilitation scheme.

PSYCHIATRIC WARDS IN GENERAL HOSPITALS

In some general hospitals, psychiatric patients join the physically disabled patients in a combined occupational therapy department. Here the problem may be one of integration. The psychiatric patients may form themselves into an isolated group, even refusing to mix with the other patients, whose physical ailments, they maintain, upset them. Obviously, the physically ill patients may have similar concern over the psychiatric patients. The therapist must remember that there may be a considerable psychological overlay in physical illness, and the problems of the two groups may not be as separate as they appear. To overcome these difficulties, preparation is needed before patients attend the department. It should be stressed that rehabilitation is the common purpose, and that each patient has individual problems to overcome. Some kind of social event, involving all patients, may promote integration, but there is a danger of this becoming a somewhat superficial way of dealing with a deeper problem. It is usually better for patients to be mixed in smaller groups, and this is possible in industrial or domestic rehabilitatic and similar activities.

Just as some patients with a specific physical disability need individu occupation, some psychiatric patients may need to work alone if their symj toms indicate this, and if they are likely to distress others. It is important have adequate space and facilities for dealing with such needs or emergencie for without these, the occupational therapist would be better advised treat disturbed cases on the ward, or arrange for such patients to attend different times.

NEUROSES UNITS

Because of the nature of neurotic illness, the occupational therapist cann play a significant part in treatment unless she is fully integrated into the war team. Neurotic patients grouped together create a constantly changing an disruptive atmosphere. They make emotional demands on other patients an staff, and generally have an immature and, therefore, unreasonable approac to life. It is obvious that unless the occupational therapist is fully informe and aware of these constant changes of 'climate', and the attitude taken b other staff, she will be manipulated by patients for their own ends, and thu; by becoming incorporated into their emotional pattern, be unable to hel them. The main problem is in overcoming the superficial approach to th employment of such patients. Few neurotic patients have need to improv their work ability: many are intelligent and highly efficient, but their abilit for sustained effort is interrupted by emotional conflict. As most neuroti patients are capable of developing insight, treatment, which may or may no include chemotherapy or other physical treatments, is directed toward developing this faculty. From the occupational therapy standpoint, it is mor profitable for patients to understand and accept the factors which are in hibiting their working at an efficient level, rather than attempt to emplo\ every patient fully. The timetable should be discussed with patients, no only in terms of the activities to be included, but reasons for inclusion o certain activities or for their non-participation in past events, etc.

Special activity groups may be particularly helpful, as patients understanc the significance of them, and feel they are specifically involved. To these car be added groups which aim to help other people, such as making toys for children's home, reading or playing table games with geriatric patients or other wards, etc. Such activities are aimed at developing social responsibilities, as neurotic patients are often unduly self interested. It is useful to consider day to day activities, such as cleaning the unit, preparing meals, gardening, etc., all as possible therapeutic activities. The occupational therapist must be prepared for frequent failure on the part of patients and reasons should be sought either individually or in ward meetings.

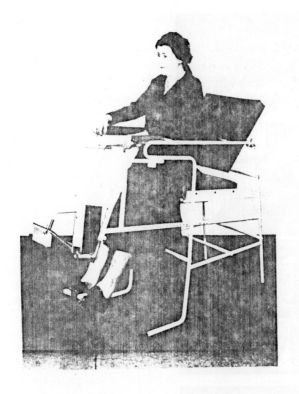

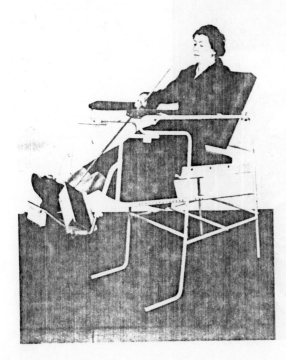

PLATES 1 and 2. Independence for an arthritic patient. The chair designed and made for her in the occupational therapy department.

The arm rests must project beyond the seat, and the corresponding extensions on the floor ensure a secure base when weight is put on them. (See pp. 117, 123)

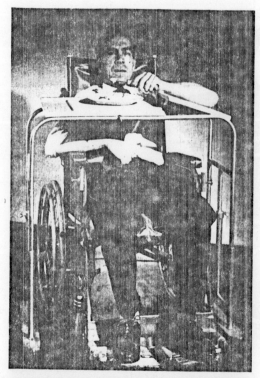

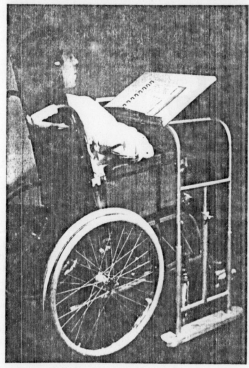

PLATES 3 and 4. Multi-purpose table adjustable in height and angle for a variety of activities. (See p. 125)

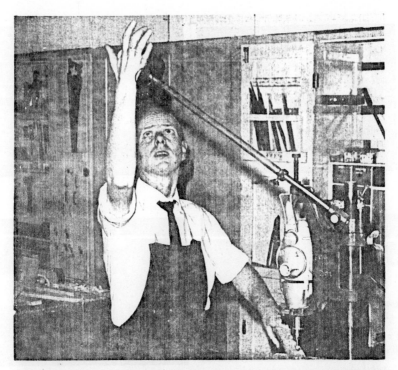

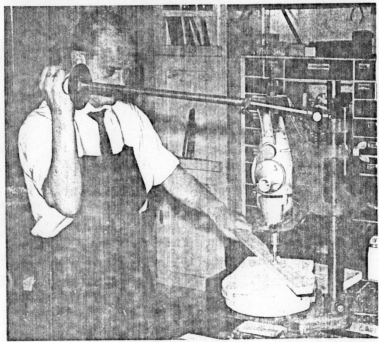

PLATES 5 and 6. Learning to position the hand, grip the lever and then actively release, to improve flexion and extension of oedematous fingers. (See p. 150)

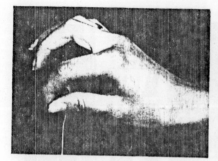

PLATE 7. Precision pinch grip.

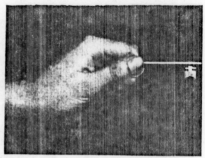

PLATE 8. Key grip.

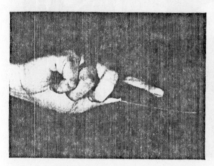

PLATE 9. Small tool grip.

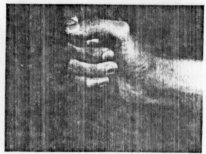

PLATE 10. Cylinder grip.

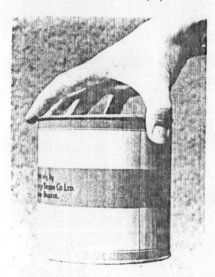

PLATE 11. Span grip.

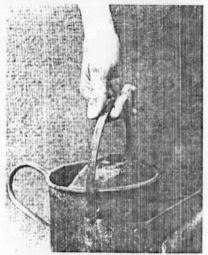

PLATE 12. Hook grip.

(See p. 160)

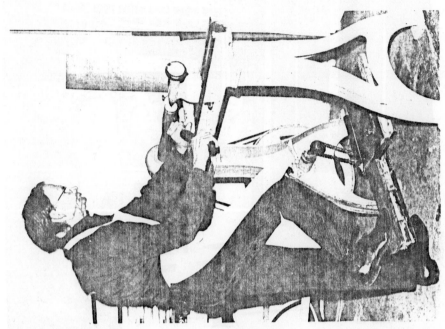

PLATE 14. Extension foot-plate to encourage full range of [...]

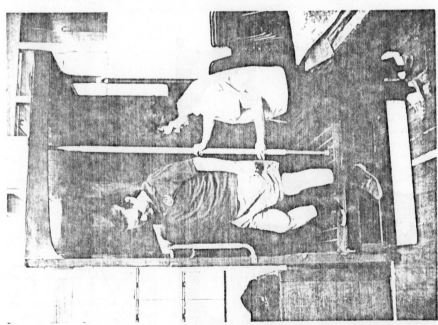

PLATE 15. Training for the use of public transport. Note [...]

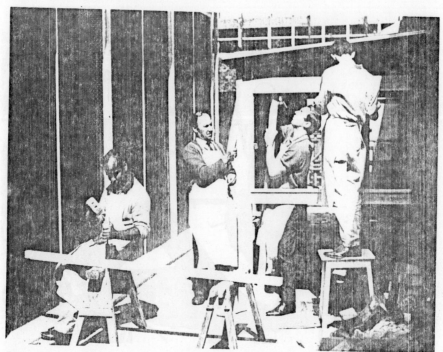

PLATE 15. A realistic work project giving scope for remedial work, group activity, job simulation and assessment. (See p. 190)

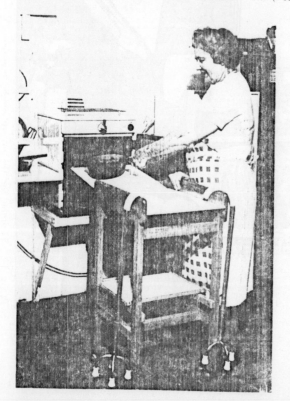

PLATE 16. Walking Trolley. Strong construction to take patient's weight when walking. High sides for comfortable grip and safe carrying of walking aids. Position of low cross bar and design of lower shelf allowing for normal walking action. Adjustable sliding ramp to eliminate lifting. (See p. 190)

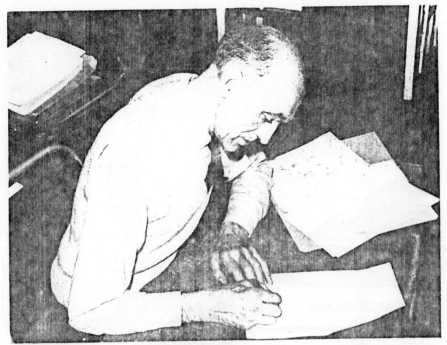

PLATE 17. Practising writing, having progressed from repetitive writing patterns.

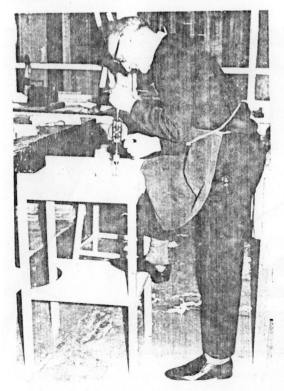

Two facets of treatment for a patient recovering from a right hemiplegia. (See p. 209)

PLATE 18. Woodwork to encourage normal use of affected limbs. Note the spontaneous use of the right leg to steady the stool.

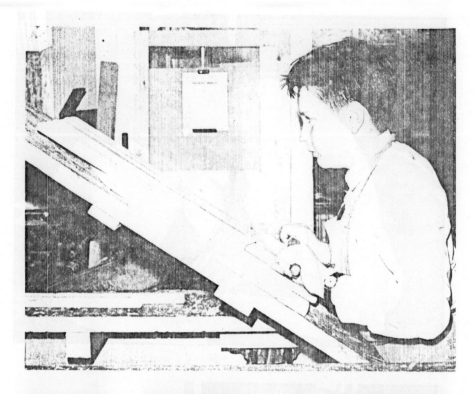

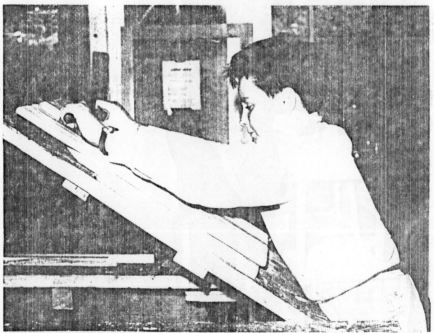

PLATES 19 and 20. Self assisted work after a brachial plexus lesion, using the adjustable inclined section of a woodwork bench. (See p. 210)

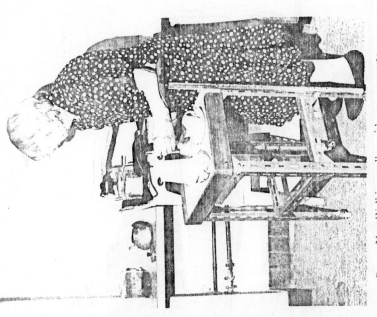

PLATE 22. The same trolley, with the top extended as a table.

PLATE 21. Walking trolley with arm supports.

(See pp. 124-5)

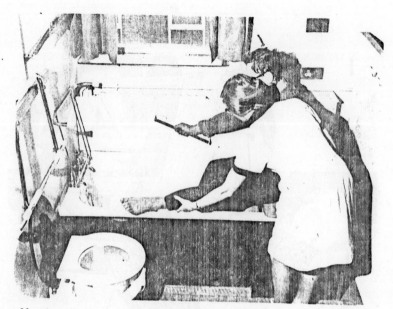

PLATE 23. A patient receiving instruction on getting into the bath using the bath board and handle. (See pp. 24-5)

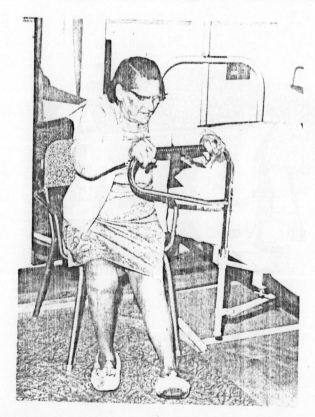

PLATE 24. Hand grip support for moving in and out of bed. (See pp. 24-5)

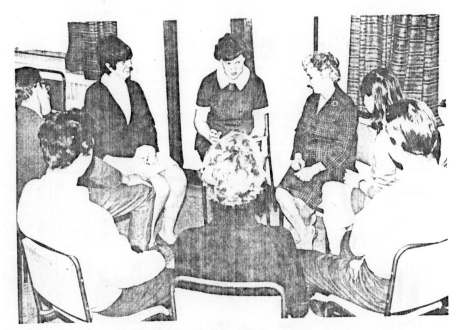

PLATE 25. Discussing the week's programme. (See p. 264)

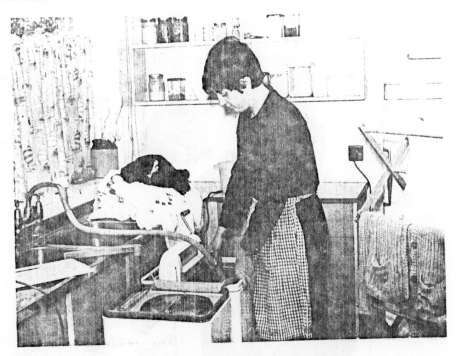

PLATE 26. Domestic rehabilitation. (See p. 264)

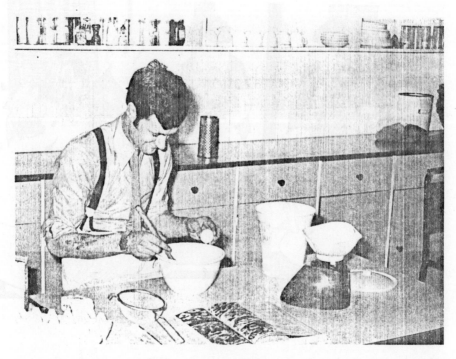

PLATE 27. Domestic rehabilitation. Cookery for a man who will be living alone in a small flat. (See p. 265)

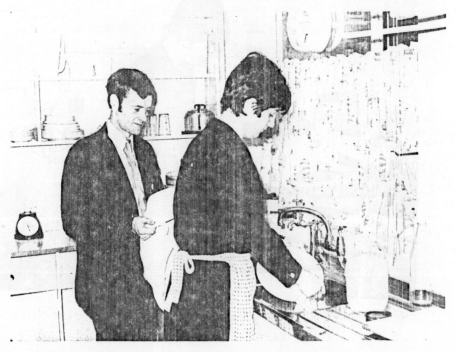

PLATE 28. Domestic rehabilitation. Cleanliness and cooperation. (See p. 265)

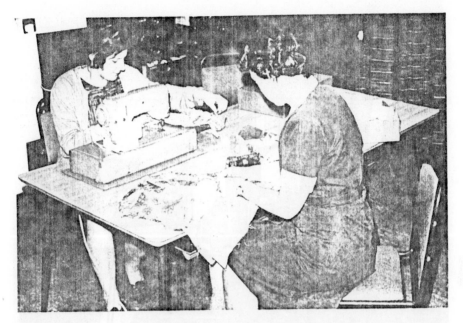

PLATE 29. Dressmaking: personal appearance is an important part of social rehabilitation. (See p. 290)

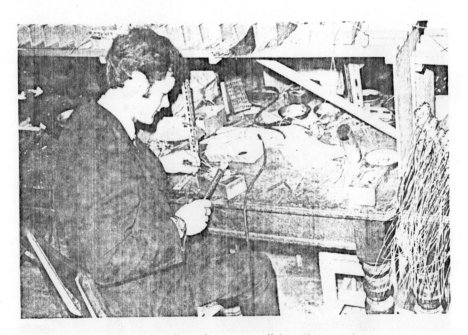

PLATE 30. Preparing to earn a living. (See p. 290)

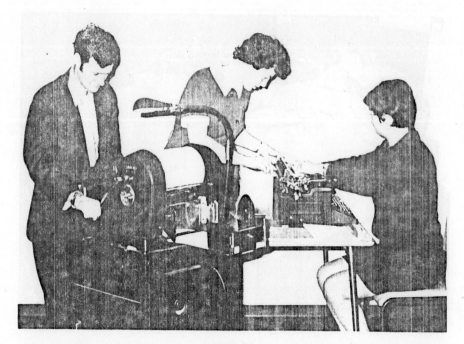

PLATE 31. Social rehabilitation. Producing a magazine. (See p. 291)

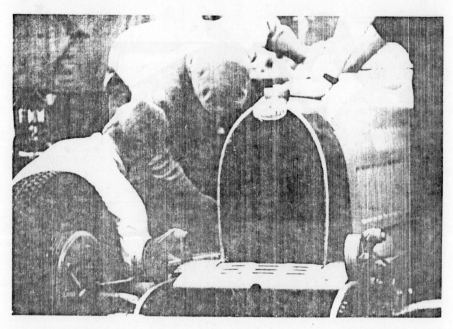

PLATE 32. Hobbies. A patient and voluntary helper share an interest in vintage racing cars.
(See p. 291)

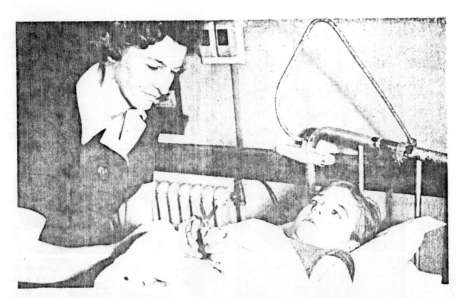

PLATE 33. A child with overhead mirror, starting occupational therapy. (See p. 372)

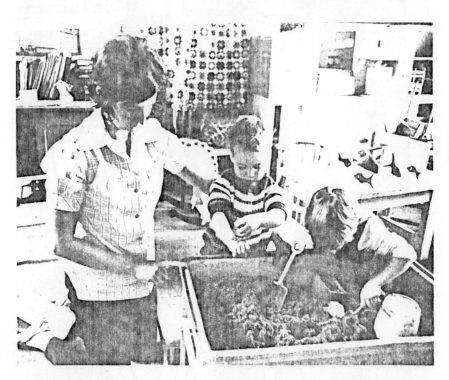

PLATE 34. Children learning balance and limb control through playing with the sand-tray. (See p. 372)

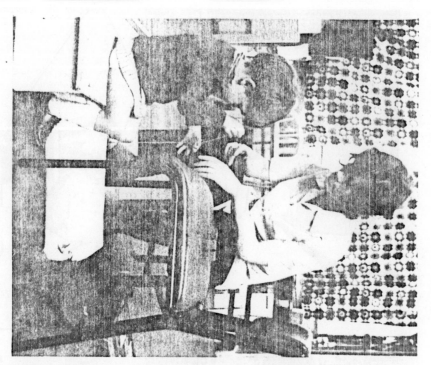

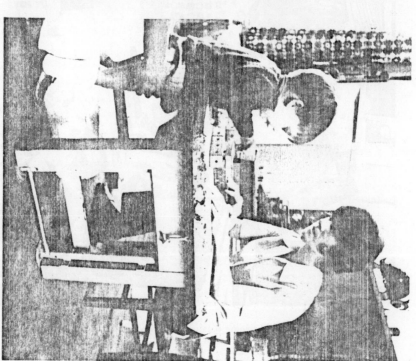

PLATES 35 and 36.   A cerebral palsied child gaining hand and lower limb control. (See p. 372)

MIDDLE-STAY PATIENTS

These are patients who need a longer period of treatment than is possible in a unit catering for acute cases. Their stay may extend approximately from six months to two years, after which they are in danger of becoming long-stay patients. Much has been written recently of the dangers of hospitalisation, and it is now recognised that if a patient remains in hospital over six months he may well lose the incentive to leave. The occupational therapist has an important part to play in preventing these patients becoming institutionalised, by maintaining interests, work habits, links with the community and pride in personal appearance. A high proportion of middle-stay patients are schizophrenics or chronic neurotics. Occupational therapy should aim to maintain all the positive capabilities of these patients, and, in collaboration with the medical team, help them to accept and adjust to limitations.

In hospitals where a graded rehabilitation scheme operates, the middle-stay patient can often be included at the higher levels. Careful initial assessment, and reassessment at frequent intervals, are important, and the patient should be in a stimulating and purposeful environment for the whole of each working day. Women patients should not lose their domestic abilities and, wherever possible, they should be encouraged to help on the ward as well as being included in domestic rehabilitation schemes.

DISTURBED PATIENTS

Despite advances in chemotherapy most large psychiatric hospitals have a group of disturbed patients. Acutely disturbed short-term patients are usually sustained and helped on their own ward, but long-term cases may be housed in a special ward to avoid unnecessary restrictions on other patients. The disturbed ward of any hospital should be a first concern of the occupational therapist. Frequent staff meetings are necessary to plan programmes and share problems regarding particularly difficult patients.

Wherever possible, and in cooperation with nursing staff, it is advisable to split patients into small groups for activities, particularly when it is possible to take a group out of the ward for part of a day. A change of environment can contribute a great deal towards reducing disturbance. A full day's programme should be the aim, split into a number of short activity periods, including physical recreation, creative activities and activities which will appeal to the individual, such as cooking a meal or a visit to the hairdresser. When possible, recreational activities can be organised for men and women patients together, as the presence of the opposite sex often has a good effect on behaviour.

The therapist's relationship with the patient is important. When disruptive behaviour occurs, she should make it clear that this is not approved

10

of, but at the same time the patient must remain assured that she retains her regard for him, and that his poor behaviour has not disrupted the relationship. Patients may feel guilty after a disturbed episode, and the withdrawal of a privilege temporarily may assuage this: it is a far better way of dealing with the situation than letting a patient feel personal disapproval.

LONG-STAY PATIENTS

The term "long-stay" covers a wide range of conditions, particularly regarding the degree of deterioration involved. A large proportion of long-stay patients are schizophrenic, many of whose illnesses appear to have reached a plateau, although some exhibit typical symptoms of institutional neurosis [10]. This population is an ageing one [11], and although schizophrenia still shows a marked tendency to chronicity today, it seems possible that with speedy treatment, continuous after-care and day-hospital facilities, new cases may, in future, be treated successfully in the community [12].

The purpose of occupational therapy for long-stay patients is to provide a comprehensive, graded, rehabilitation scheme, so that patients can achieve the highest level of efficiency of which they are capable, by using facilities both within and without the hospital [13]. In planning treatment the following important factors should be considered:

> Remotivation
> Resocialisation
> Retraining
> Resettlement

Opinions differ as to the amount of time and attention that should be given to occupational and social aspects of treatment, but experience indicates that too much emphasis on work and too little on social adjustment can inhibit progress into the community [14]. Therefore, the main areas in treatment to consider are:

> The provision of activities for a full working day.
> Encouragement of leisure activities.
> Reinstatement of the patient as an individual.

A Full Working Day

In a large psychiatric hospital, it is no easy task to provide a comprehensive graded scheme which will involve all long-stay patients, particularly as much of the work needs to be carried out in small groups of ten or twelve. Industrial work has proved a successful method of dealing with the problem for some patients. It is described in chapter 22.

Careful assessment should precede the organisation of graded work. When patients are grossly lacking in initiative and are considerably deteriorated, work can be started on the ward with a habit-training or similar scheme. The groups can receive concentrated attention from the staff whom they will get to know well. A full timetable of varied, realistic activities is needed, including physical exercise, simple work, visits out of the ward, and ample attention to personal appearance and habits. As work standards and initiative improve, patients can be encouraged to work in one of the utility departments or pass on to an industrial unit. Some hospitals have an employment bureau which is an excellent method of allocating appropriate work available in the hospital.

For women patients, graded domestic rehabilitation schemes may be more useful than industrial rehabilitation. Quite deteriorated patients respond to a domestic environment and can be given graded responsibility, as, for example, in cooking meals:

Stage 1. Food to be cooked is collected from hospital stores by staff and patients.
Stage 2. Food collected by patients.
Stage 3. Patients taken to local shops by staff and buy food together.
Stage 4. Patients go in small groups and buy food.
Stage 5. Individual buys food for herself and then for the group.
Stage 6. Individual budgets allowance for whole week.

A valuable asset in the later stages of rehabilitation is a self-contained flat in which selected patients can live as a small self-supporting group, managing its own household affairs prior to moving into a group home in the community. Houses are now being allocated for these homes by local authorities and some voluntary organisations, and are ideal for patients who would otherwise have to live alone.

Encouragement of Leisure Activities

As all psychiatric illness involves a failure in social adaptation in varying degrees, the encouragement of good social habits is an important aspect of rehabilitation. As many patients find difficulty in making an appropriate adjustment to the opposite sex, leisure activities can provide an excellent means of resocialisation. The therapist can arrange for evening classes to be given, and can include a wide variety of other activities, geared to all levels of accomplishment. Many long-stay patients are capable of a high standard of work and this should be maintained. Many hospitals have a social centre for patients, which they should feel belongs to them. Organised activities may or may not be a part of such a centre, but patients can progress in making good relationships in an unstructured atmosphere, and voluntary participation should be the aim. Excursions to places of interest in the locality are essential if interest in the community outside is to be stimulated.

Reinstatement of the Patient as an Individual [15]

Many long-stay patients are 'emotionally flattened' and have lost some
sense of identity. Activities such as painting and pottery may help to
externalise feelings. Remedial drama, exercises and games will encourage
contact and communication. Psycho-drama can pin-point unsatisfactory
patterns of behaviour. As improvement in relationships appears, increased
responsibilities will give a personal sense of worth.

Voluntary helpers can do much by befriending patients in hospital and
later by taking them out to visit local places of interest or to their own homes.
Long-stay patients desperately need to feel that they can be accepted and
voluntary helpers who are not paid and are occasional visitors to the hospital
only may do a tremendous amount to link patients with the community
again.

In the later stages of rehabilitation, the therapist may need to work
particularly closely with the social worker, who may contact relatives of
patients who have not visited them for many years. Where there is a self-
contained rehabilitation unit or hostel ward, patients can invite and entertain
their friends and relatives themselves. This helps them to feel that they are
able to return hospitality, and can be the beginning of happier community
reintegration.

The money that patients earn during their working week can be used to
stimulate interests. Patients may save for a special holiday or trip to visit a
relative. In the early stages of rehabilitation, patients may need to learn how
to spend, and visits to local shops or cafés can be encouraged, under supervision where necessary. As patients progress and reach the hostel and work
outside hospital, some deduction is usually made for board and food. This is
an important step in their rehabilitation scheme and towards independence.

MOTHER AND CHILD UNITS

In some hospitals there are units where small groups of mothers who need
psychiatric help can receive in-patient treatment, taking their babies with
them. This setting offers opportunity for maintaining or improving the
mother-child relationship and can help in giving security to both.

Treatment Spheres Outside the Residential Hospital

The most difficult period in a patient's rehabilitation is reached on discharge
from hospital when he faces the adversities and rivalries of a normal social
situation [16]. Environmental stress, and the status of the patient in his home
and at work, influence his capacity for work. The sick role accorded him by
relatives may prevent his accepting former responsibilities [17].

Treatment in the community can only succeed if support and advice are available for the patient and his family, and if necessary, some intermediate help to bridge the gap between hospital and home. In some local authority areas, occupational therapists are employed to treat psychiatric patients as a special problem group, but increasingly, the aim is to prevent the isolation of any particular handicapped group, as all disabled persons have many needs and difficulties in common. The aspects of psychiatric occupational therapy are, however, described here separately to emphasise the importance of a comprehensive psychiatric service. The following are some of the spheres in which the occupational therapist may contribute her skills.

IN THE HOME

Visits to patients in their homes can only be successful if planned in consultation with other members of the rehabilitation team, particularly the psychiatric social worker. The role of the occupational therapist in domiciliary work includes making contact to establish a sympathetic relationship for discussing problems related to work or leisure activities. This relationship is all important in helping the person gain insight, confidence and the will to achieve a more satisfying working capacity. This may involve helping other members of the family to develop a less protective attitude, particularly towards those who lack initiative, and can be followed by encouragement to participate in the particular course of rehabilitation required, which may include:

(1) Giving guidance to housewives taking up domestic responsibilities again, particularly where there is a large family, or, alternatively, someone living alone.

(2) Making initial contact to give information and encouragement to those advised to attend a day centre, training centre or social club.

(3) When necessary, to give support to a person starting a new job. (In one area, an occupational therapist called at a home at 8 a.m. each morning to help a husband, who had suffered a schizophrenic breakdown, to start for work on time, until a routine was established and his wife felt confident to support and encourage him.)

(4) Providing employment at home, if there is no alternative because of illness, or other family commitments.

Apart from visiting the family home, the occupational therapist may be asked to visit hostels or lodgings where discharged patients are living.

GROUP HOMES

For patients who have spent a number of years in hospital, it may be impossible or inadvisable to return to their former homes. A home provides accommodation in the community, where companionship is available with a minimum of supervision. In some homes, the residents are expected to run it entirely, some being paid to cook and clean, etc., while others go out to normal or sheltered work. In others a minimum of help is expected, but obviously responsibility for personal cleanliness, general tidiness, and an ability to cooperate generally are required. The occupational therapist may be called in to help residents adjust to this new situation, which may provoke feelings of insecurity and other problems. Her role is to help patients become more independent and responsible. A weekly meeting may be all that is needed to discuss relevant problems such as:

(1) Matters pertaining to the day-to-day running of the home, making up rotas for various duties, etc.
(2) Discussion of problems relating to work, such as difficulties in transport, shift work, etc.
(3) Advice on problems of personal cleanliness; an evening class can be held in hair care, care of the clothes, etc.
(4) Financial and social problems. Queries on, for example, insurance, income tax, etc., should be welcomed as a sign of interest in citizenship. A social worker, or other qualified person can be invited along to give a talk and answer questions.
(5) The use of leisure time. Encouragement should be given to residents to attend events in the locality, such as football matches, concerts, evening classes, etc.

IN LODGINGS

The fact that a patient is in lodgings usually means that he is at work and able to pay his way. Isolation may be the most serious problem here, and the occupational therapist can encourage attendance at a local social club, or pursuit of other leisure interests. In some cases hospital authorities have rented houses and let rooms to discharged patients.

IN TRAINING CENTRES

Training centres provide sheltered work and training facilities for the disabled in the care of a local health authority. To attend a centre may not only benefit the trainee but may be desirable when the psychological health of the family is considered. Many training centres take a proportion of mentally and physically disabled persons, and some include subnormal patients as well. As their organisation varies from one local authority to another, the following account must be interpreted and adapted to particular local conditions and requirements. Training centres may include the following sections:

(1) *A training or industrial unit* with a manager or supervisor in charge with a staff of technicians. This section provides a realistic work situation in sheltered conditions, wherever possible, as a stepping stone to open employment.

(2) *An assessment and selection unit* with an occupational therapist in charge, through which all trainees pass to the training unit or return home after help in home management.

(3) *A social centre or club.*

A Training or Industrial Unit
The value of this is discussed more fully in chapter 22.

A Selection and Assessment Unit for Psychiatric Patients
As the majority of cases will pass through to the training centre, the occupational therapist is concerned with assessing each trainee's potential regarding employment in the unit, and must be familiar with all the work processes involved. The type of work will vary according to the locality, but usually includes light engineering and woodwork, packaging, clerical work and machine work. For psychiatric cases particularly, emotional and interpersonal problems may interfere with working capacities, there may be difficulties in concentration, perseverance, or an inability to get on well with workmates or those in authority. Individual programmes may be drawn up to meet special needs, such as a timetable involving gradually increasing periods of concentration, or a proportion of individual and group work, so that difficulties in cooperation can be discussed and resolved. A section for domestic rehabilitation is essential for housewives or those living alone. Problems of personal hygiene may also be tackled, as in the case of a schizoid man living with his elderly mother who was careless about his appearance and personal cleanliness. Each week he brought a change of clothes to the centre, had a bath, and washed and ironed the clothes he had taken off until a similar routine was established at home.

The particular contribution to be made by the assessment unit can therefore include:

(1) Assessment and initial training.
(2) Domestic rehabilitation, including personal hygiene.
(3) Individual and group activities for specific psychiatric problems.

Social Centres or Clubs
In a social centre attached to a training centre it is usually advisable to encourage members to organise some of the activities, to link them with those in the community on occasion, and encourage the support and participation of relatives.

Role of the Occupational Therapist

The occupational therapist provides the essential therapeutic link in the training programme by:

(a) Being constantly aware of the individual psychiatric problems of each case, and giving help and advice to technical staff when needed.

(b) Making assessments and recommendations concerning the employment of all trainees, working in close liaison with the team of doctors, social workers, D.R.O.*, training manager and his staff.

(c) Keeping records of progress made, making out work reports and serving on the discharge panel when trainees are recommended for outside employment or further training.

IN DAY HOSPITALS AND DAY CENTRES

Terminology

The terms *day hospital* and *day centre* are used differently from one region to another. The term day hospital refers to a unit in which every form of treatment is available as in a psychiatric hospital [18], and to avoid confusion here the term day centre will be used to describe a centre, usually independent of a hospital, for patients who need supportive care through social and occupational services mainly and who require a minimum of medical supervision.

Location

Units for day treatment may be located [19]:

(1) In the grounds of the parent hospital or in a ward or part of a ward which is given over to day patients.

(2) As a separate unit in the community which it serves.

(3) As a part of a community health centre or a mental health centre [20].

Liaison

Apart from the statutory obligations (see chapters 12 and 21), collaboration between local health and hospital authorities is essential. A day hospital or centre may be the joint or sole responsibility of these authorities and the occupational therapist should cooperate with hospital and community personnel, taking every opportunity of attending meetings where the rehabilitation of patients is to be discussed. She should be familiar with the local network of rehabilitation opportunities. If a detailed plan of workshops, units and day centres in the area is not available, then one should be drawn up for reference.

Referrals

Day hospital patients are usually streamed from the usual admission sources. Many day centres take a percentage of patients from local authority sources, who may be introduced by a general practitioner, social worker, mental welfare officer, or relative of the patient, and the rest from a nearby hospital. Others may be used solely for ex-hospital patients. In all cases, referrals are made to the medical officer responsible for the unit, who in turn completes a referral card for occupational therapy which is vital for record purposes. Treatment planning should be at a staff meeting of all concerned for the patients' welfare in order that the clinical and social problems of each patient can be discussed fully.

Attendance

Initially, the doctor will decide, with the patient, the number of days a week that he should attend the unit. Where the problem relates to work, and the patient is to join an industrial or similar work unit, regular attendance is essential, and provides a yardstick by which improvement can be measured. In other cases, for instance for housewives who have children to care for, flexibility is advisable, as long as intended absences are agreed between patient and therapist. Flexibility is certainly important during the period when the patient is managing without the support of the unit. Day-to-day problems arising as a result of variation in numbers attending each day can be solved by spreading part-time attendances evenly throughout the week.

Planning Treatment

There may be schemes for passing patients from a day hospital to a day centre, or from one day centre to another as progress is made. Often there are special factors to consider in relation to location, as for instance on a large housing estate some miles from a shopping area or in a new town where there may be particular difficulties for housebound housewives. It should be remembered that the patient's direct link with his family and home will result in more personal, day-to-day problems being brought to the unit. In a day hospital, particularly, this may result in occasional crises which the occupational therapist must be prepared to handle [21].

Aims of Occupational Therapy

In a day hospital these should be to preserve the individuality and identity of the patient and prevent the development of invalid attitudes; to support physical and psychological treatments and encourage a realistic attitude towards work, helping patients wherever possible to adjust and return to their normal work situation.

In a day centre support should be given to the patient at the highest level of social and occupational efficiency with, wherever possible, upgrading to open employment and to a normal social environment.

Treatment

Day hospital treatment can include individual help through chemotherapy, electroconvulsive therapy, individual psychotherapy, or group treatment through community meetings. These help to promote a therapeutic atmosphere in which patients feel accepted, understood and supported. Smaller group meetings may also be held to encourage the expression of deeper problems, to enable patients to gain insight into their own and others' difficulties, and thus enable them to determine the extent and limits of their own and others' behaviour. Occupational therapy should be an integral part of the total programme and provide the working situation against which progress can be developed and measured. Many day hospitals are centred in converted houses and have a domestic atmosphere which is useful for fostering small groups in more intimate surroundings.

Group work in occupational therapy, carried out in selected or naturally occurring groups arranged around a work project, is considered to have certain advantages [22], providing opportunity for personal reaction and adjustment. Activities should simulate conditions met by patients in their normal work outside hospital, which should require similar concentration, speed and accuracy, and involving working relationships, and realistic methods of reward for output.

Day centre treatments vary. Some aim to help patients discharged from hospital to bridge the gap between hospital, home and work by providing graded work which, at its highest level, will fit the patient for open employment. Some provide long-term, if not permanent, support for patients who are unable to manage open employment but are able to live in the community. A few day centres are concerned with the problem of social isolation and prefer a permissive atmosphere encouraging patients to call in when they feel in need of help or the company of others. For this type of set-up, social, recreational and domestic activities such as cookery, dressmaking and handyman activities for men are preferable.

Many day centres are staffed by supervisors and technicians, and the occupational therapist may be asked to act in consultant capacity in their organisation and treatment planning.

This chapter has shown how the patients' environment can be used as part of treatment, particularly where they are grouped according to their rehabilitation needs. However, in order to understand fully the problem of the individual patient and his rehabilitation, the therapist must be familiar with the course his illness has taken and the inherent problems of his clinical state, and these aspects will be discussed in the following chapters.

REFERENCES

1. Clark, D. H., *Administrative Therapy*. London, 1964.
   Goffman, E., *Asylums*. Pelican, 1968.
2. Clark, D. H., The ward therapeutic community, in *Psychiatric Hospital Care* (H. Freeman, ed.). London, 1965.
3. Jones, Maxwell, *The Therapeutic Community*. New York, 1953.
   Jones, Maxwell & Hollingsworth, S. (1963), Work with large groups in mental hospitals. *J. Ind. Psychol.*, **19**, 61–68.
   Jones, Maxwell, *Social Psychiatry in Practice*. Pelican, 1968.
   Working in a therapeutic community. *Occ. Ther.*, **36**, no. 6, 1973.
4. Moross, H. (1968), A therapeutic community in the setting of a psychiatric teaching hospital. *S.A. Jour. O.T.*, **2**, no. 1.
   And contact Marlborough Day Hospital, London.
5. Milson, F., *Group Work Skill*, London, 1973.
   Ottoway, A. K. C., *Learning Through Group Experience*. Int. Library of Social Reconstruction. London, 1966.
   Thompson, S. & Kahn, J. H., *The Group Process as a Helping Technique*. Oxford, 1972.
6. Martin, D. V., *Adventure in Psychiatry*. London, 1968.
   Martin, D. V. The importance of free communication, in *Psychiatric Hospital Care* (H. Freeman, ed.). London, 1965.
7. Barrett, L. M. (1962), The development of a staff meeting. *Occ. Ther.*, **25**, no. 6.
8. Bennett, D. H., Robertson, J. P. S. (1965), The effects of habit training on chronic schizophrenic patients. *J. Ment. Sci.*, **101**, 664.
9. *Memorandum on the Mental Health Act*, note 7. H.M.S.O.*, 1960.
10. Barton, R., *Institutional Neurosis*. Bristol, 1966.
11. Early, D. F. & Magnus, R. V. (1968), Industrial therapy organisation (*Bristol*) 1960-65. *Brit. J. Psychiat.*, **114**, no. 508.
12. Leyberg, J. T. (1965), A follow-up study on some schizophrenic patients. *Brit. J. Psychiat.*, **111**, no. 476.
13. Wing, J. K., Bennett, D. H. & Denham, J., *The Industrial Rehabilitation of Long-Stay Schizophrenic Patients*. Memorandum no. 42. H.M.S.O.*, 1964.
14. McCormick, W. O. (1964), The work program in research, prognosis and therapy. *Am. J. Orthopsych.*, **5**, 955–959.
15. Morgan, R., Cushing, D. & Manton, N. S. (1965), A regional psychiatric rehabilitation hospital. *Brit. J. Psych.*, **111**, no. 479.
16. May, A. R., Sheldon, A. P. & MacKeith, S. A. (1962), *Lancet* ii, 1319.
17. Sigerist, H. E., *The Sociology of Medicine*. New York, 1960.
18. Bennett, D. H., The Day Hospital. Social Psychiatry. (Ed. N. Petirl Owitsch). *Top. Probl. Psychiat. Neurol.*, vol. 9. Basle/New York, 1969.
19. Farndale, J., *The Day Hospital Movement in Great Britain*. Oxford/London, 1961.
20. Farndale, W. A. (1965), Day hospital or mental health centre. *Paper presented at the Congress of the Royal Society of Health*.
21. Bennett, D. H., *op. cit.*
22. Smith, M. M. & Spear, F. G. (1964), Group treatment in a psychiatric day hospital. *Occ. Ther.*, **27**, no. 10.
   And see:
   Arthur, R. J., *An Introduction to Social Psychiatry*, Penguin, 1971.
   Bion, W. R., *Experiences in Groups*. Wiltshire, 1968.
   Cartwright, D. & Zander, A., *Group Dynamics*. U.S.A., 1968.
   Clark, D., *Social Therapy in Psychiatry*. London, 1974.
   Foulkes, S. H. & Anthony, E. J., *Group Psychotherapy*. Pelican, 1965.
   Rapoport, R. N., *Community as Doctor*. London, 1960.
   Rogers, C. R., *On Becoming a Person*. Boston, 1961.
   Sprott, W. H. J., *Human Groups*. Pelican, 1963.
   Thelen, H. A., *Dynamics of Groups at Work*. U.S.A., 1963.
   * See *Glossary*, p. 454.

Occupational Therapy for Psychiatric Conditions: Part 1

The diagnostic categories referred to in this chapter are in general use but a psychiatrist may not wish to make too definite a diagnosis as often there may be an overlap between one category and another. The psychiatric conditions described here are those which have a particular relevance to the application of occupational therapy. The student should consult a textbook of psychiatry for further clinical details.

The Neuroses

No one neurotic symptom should be taken as indicative of any one type of mental disturbance. It is the combination of a number of symptoms in a recognised syndrome that provides the basis for differential diagnosis. Patients do not always present clear pictures of particular classifications, for a neurosis is one of a group of disorders which manifest themselves in numerous ways. All of them however are concerned with difficulties in the emotional life of the patient.

In considering occupational therapy for neurotic patients, it is important to have some idea of whether the illness is:

> An isolated attack, where the prognosis is good.
> A recurring condition.
> A severe incapacitating chronic condition.

By defining the possibilities for rehabilitation in this way, the occupational therapist can clarify her aims of treatment.

ANXIETY NEUROSIS

Anxiety states usually occur in people subject to general over-anxiety, as a result of hereditary [1] or environmental factors.

Anxiety Reactions Affecting Performance and Personal Relationships

An anxiety neurosis is chiefly characterised by feelings of tension, anxiety, fear or specific phobias, for which the patient can give no adequate reason.

The physical symptoms of tremor and general loss of muscle tone, sweating, and rapid respiration, can affect performance. Loss of weight due to poor appetite leads to poor condition. In severe cases there is danger of collapse.

The psychological symptoms may include irritability, insecurity and feelings of inferiority. Patients are usually over-susceptible and tend to over-react to stress. In occupational therapy, these reactions can result in:

(1) Fear of starting a project, and doubt over powers of achievement.
(2) General lack of interest, slowness, lack of persistence and concentration.
(3) Alternatively, a tendency to aim too high to cover up feelings of inferiority.
(4) Lack of energy and initiative, because of incapacity to turn attention from unpleasant ideas.
(5) Escape into invalidism to avoid stressful situations.

Aims of Occupational Therapy

These will include assisting the patient to adjust to hospital life, helping him to regain self-confidence, lessening tension, influencing him (without pressure) in personal and group relationships, and providing opportunity for the release of energy in activities which will help him to accept or resolve anxieties. Attention may need to be given to improvement of the physical condition. Subsequently, the occupational therapist should assess capabilities in the light of the patient's maximum ability to sustain stress and to meet unexpected difficulties. The patient's interest in the selected rehabilitation programme must be sustained, and should include new interests which can be continued after discharge.

Therapist-Patient Relationship

The occupational therapist should see the patient as soon as possible after admission, but the introduction of an activity should not be hurried, since it is essential that the patient should not be plunged into a new situation before he is ready for it. Serious resistance can otherwise be built up. The therapist should be prepared to adopt any role required by the doctor to support his treatment and should:

(1) Establish confidence.
(2) Be friendly but decisive, not placing too much responsibility on the patient in early stages.

(3) Avoid situations which provoke symptoms, unless deliberately provoked in a group situation.

(4) Give ample encouragement, as self-consciousness is often a serious hindrance to a therapeutic relationship.

(5) As insight increases with psychotherapy, give the patient opportunity to discuss attitudes to work.

Social Relationships

The patient should progressively:

(1) Be placed with a small group of patients.

(2) Be provided with increasing responsibility within the group.

(3) Be introduced to a wider social field, care being taken to prepare him adequately for each new move.

Activities

Activities which take too long or are difficult or isolating should be avoided, nor should the patient be placed in a competitive field until he has improved sufficiently to deal with this situation. In estimating the standard of work within the patient's capabilities, reference should be made to the dominant symptoms of his illness. For instance, a patient might express the wish to review his shorthand, but if slow progress would increase his anxiety, a less demanding activity would be preferable. Because of lack of self-confidence, the patient will often express the wish to do something familiar at first. This may be beneficial, but should be regarded as a first step to a more demanding activity. Muscular tension varies, and on the whole large movements are better than small ones. Games are useful in relieving mental tension, and gardening and other physical exercises are valuable in absorbing energy or improving the physical condition. Relaxation exercises are useful, particularly if the patient is encouraged to continue these at home when discharged. In the early stages, an activity which is finished quickly is advisable, such as making a garment, flower arranging or a visit to the hairdresser. These activities should become progressively more realistic, and finally used as a means of restoring confidence in tasks of daily living, leisure activities and social groups.

Contra-indications

Activities which:

(1) Are beyond the patient's present capacity, even if known previously.

(2) Take a long time to complete.

(3) Result in the isolation of the patient, i.e. on fixed apparatus.

(4) Are too competitive, i.e. working on similar activity alongside a patient with better capacity.

(5) Are too tiring in relation to patient's physical state.

Liaison

It is important that all staff members should be consistent in their handling of the patient. The therapist must be aware of tension-relieving drugs and other treatments being given, which may result in a rapid improvement in the patient's condition so that progression can be planned in the rehabilitative aspects of treatment.

HYSTERIA

Common features of the hysterical reaction are dissociation and conversion symptoms. Preoccupation with physical symptoms presents itself, but these symptoms are secondary and reversible. The causes of hysterical illness are essentially emotional, involving an attempt, heavily disguised, to gain some advantage from the production of symptoms of physical illness.

Hysterical Reactions Affecting Performance and Personal Relationships

(1) The imitation of any form of physical or psychological illness, such as hysterical paralyses, anaesthesias, twilight states, loss of memory, torticollis, etc. Preoccupation with these physical symptoms may result in poor concentration.

(2) A degree of anxiety, if physical symptoms only partly resolve the conflict.

(3) Lack of depth of emotion, sometimes called *la belle indifference*, and egocentricity, in which the patient's total environment is seen in the light of how it affects him and the obligation of others to him. This results in a lack of responsibility.

(4) Highly suggestible, over adaptable, dependent and attention-seeking traits.

Aims of Occupational Therapy

The aims of treatment must be considered in relation to what is attainable practically in the light of the patient's history, and must be correlated with changes brought about through psychotherapy. Alternative and constructive means of satisfying the patient's psychological needs, which are less disturbing physically and socially must be found, so that the need to gain advantage by producing symptoms can be alleviated. Activities should increase confidence and promote a sense of achievement, as well as encourage more responsible attitudes. By assisting the patient to become more socially acceptable, the need to compensate will be diminished. It may be necessary to provide treatment for established physical disabilities, or explore pre-vocational possibilities when there is a residual disability.

Therapist-Patient Relationship

The approach to these patients requires a considerable degree of skill. It is necessary to distinguish between real physical pain and attention-seeking. Too much sympathy tends to provoke rather than relieve symptoms. Although it may be necessary to make some concessions to the physical symptoms in the early stages, these concessions should be withdrawn gradually so that patients do not come to rely on them. In addition the occupational therapist should:

(1) Evaluate the patient's conception of his illness.
(2) Gradually minimise the importance of physical symptoms, as one symptom is easily replaced by another.
(3) Be kind but firm, giving attention where necessary or merited, withdrawing attention if the patient becomes too demanding, for this may provoke further symptoms.
(4) Give praise for achievement and good social behaviour, make use of any improvement to prevent sliding back to easier means of gaining attention.
(5) Be aware of the patient's possessive tendencies and ability to manipulate situations.
(6) Overcome inability to accept explanation and lack of insight by presenting suggestions in an acceptable form.
(7) Observe the patient in varied situations, particularly if there is a problem of accident neurosis.

Social Relationships

It is important that these patients are not placed in a group in which they will become the centre of sympathy, nor in a group consisting largely of similar personalities. The patient should:

(1) Be grouped with patients who can accept any overt hysterical symptoms or behaviour in a matter of fact way.
(2) Be encouraged to undertake responsibilities which will gain attention in an acceptable way.

Activities

A careful assessment needs to be made of the patient's physical capacities, so that graded work, starting with something well within his capacity, may be provided. Achievement is of primary importance so that real satisfaction in an accepted sphere may help to weaken the need for hysterical compensations. Employment which diverts the patient's interest from the symptoms may be achieved by an activity which appeals to egocentric interests, such as dressmaking and cookery for women, or, for men, wooden-toy making, gardening, etc. Activities should be used which take insight and intelligence into account, as the patient may not easily be convinced of his ability to perform tasks assessed to be within his capacity. Opportunity should be given for graded physical exercise, particularly when there is muscular weakness, or long established physical disability; these should include walking, gardening, shopping, sports and dancing. Once improvement takes place, the patient should be given the opportunity to gain attention and confidence by achievement involving individual responsibilities, such as the encouragement of a particular talent, or the management of special jobs of benefit to the group and which will be appreciated by its members. Activities may also be introduced which make constructive use of the occupational advantage the hysterical patient often has in work involving mild showmanship, such as selling hospital magazines, or receiving customers for the hospital's car-wash service. Lastly, wherever possible, a realistic programme to establish the patient in the routine of his former work must be arranged, or pre-vocational exploration undertaken if there is positive indication of a need to acquire a new skill.

Contra-indications

Activities which:

(1) Are below the patient's capacity, permitting boredom and lack of self esteem, i.e. easily learnt, routine activities.

(2) Are beyond the patient's capacity, causing fear of failure and over-compensatory symptoms.

(3) Do not allow the patient to gain the approval of others, i.e. working in an isolated situation.

(4) Reinforce any physical disabilities.

(5) Appeal mainly because of their immediate effect, allowing temporary escape from the planned programme.

Liaison

It is important to correlate treatment with psychotherapy, upgrading the degree of skill and concentration required according to progress. Fatigue and irritability may increase temporarily during psychotherapy, and changes in the patient's condition while taking certain drugs must be anticipated.

REACTIVE DEPRESSION (EXOGENOUS)

This form of depression is usually the result of excessive stress brought on by some clearly defined precipitating circumstance such as a bereavement, an unhappy love affair, or series of frustrations. Many physical illnesses are accompanied by depression too.

The Depressive Reactions Affecting Performance and Personal Relationships

The following reactions will have to be considered in planning treatment:

(1) Feelings of great unhappiness and an inability to face the future.
(2) Insomnia, anorexia and possibly some hysterical symptoms.
(3) Lack of energy and concentration.
(4) Early and excessive fatigue.
(5) Dwelling on endless unhappy thoughts, and in severe cases *danger of suicide*.

Aims of Occupational Therapy

Occupational therapy should aim at diverting the patient from anxieties and assessing individual needs to ensure that the patient is better able to combat future difficulties. For instance, a housewife with limited intelligence may become depressed after years of striving ineffectually to run a home and feed and clothe many children, perhaps with the difficulties of illness or delinquencies. Here, while the psychiatric social worker would work towards improvement in living conditions, occupational therapy could best be directed towards increasing ability to deal with future situations. Instruction in home management, dressmaking, home-nursing, and assistance in hair-dressing and makeup would increase confidence in the woman patient, and for a man with similar depression, home decorating, handyman's work and gardening, as well as self-valeting, might have a similar effect. In addition to increasing ability and confidence, it may be necessary to improve the physical condition. Support will probably be needed while the patient is re-establishing himself outside hospital.

Therapist-Patient Relationship

The therapist should:

(1) Where there is good insight, show understanding by permitting the patient to talk about anxieties and relate them to the work in hand.
(2) Give clear directions, and not require the patient to make decisions until the condition begins to improve.
(3) Gradually withdraw support and encourage independence.

Social Relationships

As a change of milieu is beneficial, the patient should:

(1) Be encouraged in social group activities, where there is a lively interchange of ideas and interests.
(2) Be encouraged to take responsibility within the group as confidence increases.

Activities

In each case the general principle of treatment must be that of relating the activities to the problem facing the patient. While enjoyable, expressive and creative activities may have a relaxing effect at first, they will not wholly satisfy the patient with problems awaiting him on discharge. On the other hand, evidence of successful creative ability may have a stimulating effect and promote lasting interest and assurance. In addition to the practise of skills needed in the patient's normal life, such as cooking, housekeeping, commercial subjects, industrial techniques, etc., opportunity for social development may be encouraged through social club membership, dancing, whist, as well as through group-work projects. Relaxation exercises and other graded physical activities are recommended. Before leaving hospital, the occupational therapist should seek to interest the patient in his local affairs and encourage interests that take him out of the home, perhaps with help from voluntary workers in his area.

Contra-indications

Activities which:

(1) Are too difficult, therefore reinforcing the patient's feeling of failure.
(2) Are unrealistic to the patient.
(3) Permit the patient to work in isolation, particularly where suicidal feelings exist.

Liaison

The occupational therapist will need to work in close liaison with the psychiatric social worker, mental welfare officer and occupational therapist working in the community.

OBSESSIONAL NEUROSES

This illness usually occurs in basically rigid and inflexible personalities, who lack adaptability and are prone to extreme orderliness and discipline.

Obsessional Reactions Affecting Performance and Personal Relationships

The use of ritualistic behaviour is a method of handling the problems of interpersonal relationships, designed to retain control over the environment and keep anxiety at a minimum. Based on a profound sense of inferiority, rituals such as counting and repeating actions or phrases, ruminating on thoughts, and indulging in largely unprofitable speculation, are often accompanied by morbid fears and feelings of guilt. Depression, tension and anxiety are frequently present, sometimes as a result of interference with obsessional acts. There may also be aggressive feelings which cause considerable fear to the patient. These reactions can result in:

(1) Difficulty in starting work, or once started, slowness in doing it due to meticulous, perfectionist attitude, or repeated checking.
(2) Anxiety when faced by new situations, such as making decisions or thinking creatively.
(3) Difficulty in keeping to a timetable, although the patient may be anxious to cooperate.
(4) Distress at being unable to work efficiently, which can result from partial insight into the situation.

Aims of Occupational Therapy

These patients may be in hospital for some time. If psychotherapy is employed it will be fairly deep and protracted, being directed at the underlying anxiety and feelings of guilt. For severe cases, leucotomy may be the treatment of choice, but is rarely carried out until the patient has been under observation for some time, and every other form of treatment has been tried. In such cases, there will be a considerable period of post-operative rehabilitation before the patient is ready for discharge. A true obsessional neurosis is difficult to treat successfully. Although many patients have partial or intellectual insight into their behaviour, it may be a long time before this insight is accepted emotionally and the patient is able to adjust his behaviour. The long term prognosis depends on the development of insight and on factors in the home environment. Occupational therapy should aim to maintain all useful activity and support improvements gained through psychotherapy. Where possible, perfectionist attitudes should be used constructively. In some cases the therapist may be required to assist the patient to overcome his obsessions, in others, to avoid cutting across them in any way.

Therapist-Patient Relationship

Unless the doctor specifies a particular role that he wishes the therapist to use, her relationship with the patient should give security, confidence and reduce anxiety. The compulsive acts should be accepted in a permissive manner unless they are a danger or menace to the patient or others. When a compulsive act has been completed, the patient normally feels relief, and the therapist should use this period to the maximum. Any impatience will increase the patient's feeling of guilt and failure, and the therapist must be tactful and avoid causing undue anxiety. Reference to ritualistic behaviour should be avoided unless initiated by the patient, and such behaviour should be accepted calmly and without comment. The occupational therapist should also:

(1) Seek the full cooperation of the patient by explaining plans for treatment.
(2) Be decisive but not authoritarian.
(3) Avoid unpredictable situations and the need for quick decisions by the patient.
(4) Give ample praise and encouragement when merited.

Social Relationships

The patient should:

(1) Work where there is plenty of room and little likelihood of tools or materials being disturbed, but not in isolation.
(2) Work alongside other considerate patients who will not obtrude too much.
(3) Be encouraged to share in general group activities, without having to take too much responsibility.

Activities

The selection of activities is not easy, and the aims vary considerably with different medical views. Sometimes it is considered that repetitive activities requiring little in the way of decisions, and reducing the chance of failure to a minimum, are desirable; in other cases this may not be so, and activities within a small group, such as play reading and language study may be advised instead. The most important factor in selecting an activity is to avoid work and situations which involve unpredictability and indecisiveness, or self assertion in relationships with others. The neatness, orderliness, high moral standards and, frequently, the high intelligence of these patients are assets which can be put to good use. Patients may be able to help in the department's clerical section or in the store, as long as they are given the right amount of responsibility. The patient will need support in group activities in which his sense of inadequacy may be threatened, and it is advisable to start with an activity in which he already has an interest and skill. Obsessional patients may want to undertake menial tasks, and many doctors think this should be allowed in the earlier stages of treatment as long as they are constructive. A patient may get satisfaction from cleaning the bathrooms daily, or washing cups in the department. As the patient's condition improves progress should be made to a realistic programme, worked out in an acceptable routine, developing flexibility but retaining some definite structure.

Contra-indications

These depend to some extent on the views of the doctor, but generally there should be avoidance of activities which:

(1) Involve the continual making of decisions or contain ambiguities upon which the patient may ruminate.
(2) Cannot be satisfactorily planned in advance.
(3) Involve the element of surprise.

Liaison

The therapist must have full knowledge of the patient's symptomatology and of other treatments in progress, particularly in psychotherapy so that occupational therapy may be developed *pari passu*. Regular reports of the therapist's observations must be made to the doctor. When a leucotomy has been performed a full knowledge of the patient's pre-operative state is necessary in order to assess post-operative changes. Return to activity is required as quickly as possible after the operation, usually within the first week, as the symptoms tend to reassert themselves after an interval, but usually with less emotional effect, so that good habits can be inculcated before they reappear.

Psychosomatic Disorders

There are two main types of psychosomatic disturbance, i.e. those in which the emotional disturbance is thought to be responsible for the production of physical symptoms, and those in which the emotional disturbance plays on physical symptoms already present. This wide group of disorders covers patients who have developed a genuine physical illness as an unconscious method of avoiding anxiety and gaining sympathy and approval, or as an escape from difficult problems. Psychosomatic disorders cover a variety of symptoms, including asthma, migraine, ulcers, urticaria, neurodermatitis and persistent diarrhoea, among countless others. It is therefore difficult to generalise with regard to treatment.

Psychosomatic Reactions Affecting Performance and Personal Relationships

The type of personality most usually involved is the over-anxious, over-conscientious and covertly aggressive. Aggression may be covered by a reaction formation such as timidity. Fear and anxiety are the most usual underlying causes of the physical disturbances, and these may have originated at an early stage of development, being brought into action by stress or strain in the present environment. The occupational therapist must remember that:

(1) The physical illness is real, and complaints of pain, fatigue, etc., are genuine.
(2) Performance in occupational therapy is affected on two levels—the physical disability and the underlying fear and anxiety.

Aims of Occupational Therapy

In view of the diversity of these disorders and their origin, the first aim is to get to know the patient well. The main aim is to help the patient relinquish his defence mechanisms in favour of activities which are not so neurotically motivated. By using constructive work to overcome lack of confidence and feelings of inadequacy, the patient will be less preoccupied with physical symptoms. An outlet for aggression may be needed, and if the physical symptoms have contributed to asocial or antisocial attitudes resocialisation may be an important aim of treatment.

Therapist-Patient Relationship

By the time a patient with psychosomatic illness has arrived at a psychiatric hospital (many have spent long periods in general hospitals undergoing investigations, etc.) his pattern of behaviour is probably deeply ingrained. The patient's past experience with others has usually been firstly to evoke sympathy and attention, followed by impatience, annoyance and finally rejection [2]. This rejection leads to an increase in tension and accentuated physical symptoms. The occupational therapist must accept the patient and his complaints, without indicating pity or concern. Reassurance and encouragement should be given but not in relation to the physical symptoms. As such patients are highly suggestible, the therapist must be careful not to implant further ideas which can be used to produce more symptoms. The patient may wish to pour out details of his complaints: once he has done this the therapist should try and divert his attention. Undue interest in physical details should never be shown, and the therapist should make a point of approaching the patient when he is in a less self-interested mood, so that he feels accepted as a person rather than a physically ill phenomenon. In addition the therapist should:

(1) Give time to understanding the personality involved.
(2) Be gentle but firm, and prepared to accept hostility and irritability.
(3) Recognise and reward positive accomplishments.

(4) Provide reassurance and support which should be withdrawn gradually as the patient's need for this decreases.

Social Relationships

Isolation should be avoided at all costs, as being alone provides opportunity for concentration on body function. An early attempt should be made to introduce the patient to group activities, and gradually he can be given responsibilities within the group. Other patients may well project their own difficulties on to staff by accusing them of callousness and indifference to the patient's ill health. This should be dealt with in a group meeting with the doctor.

Activities

The activities selected must be within the physical capacity of the patient and should involve self expression. Modelling and free painting may be used as an outlet for aggression, also woodwork, metalwork and gardening. Activities which require cooperation within a group should be included in the programme, i.e. cooking a meal, social and recreational activities, etc. As soon as the patient improves, a basic routine of realistic activities should be established, which will give the patient confidence in dealing with every-day responsibilities. Leisure pursuits should also be encouraged in which the patient can meet other people and be accepted through a normal medium.

Contra-indications

Activities which:

(1) Increase dependence on the therapist, i.e. prolonged learning of new techniques.
(2) Are so closely structured that they permit no freedom of expression.
(3) Give so much freedom that the patient has no basic routine to support him.
(4) Aggravate the somatic symptoms thereby drawing attention to these.
(5) Are beyond the patient's physical capacity.

Liaison

Contact with the psychiatric social worker will be necessary in the later stages of treatment to coordinate occupational therapy with conditions at home. Treatment of psychosomatic patients is sometimes carried out in a physical unit, which may pose problems when it is necessary to include the patient in group activities. Whenever the patient's condition permits, it is far better to encourage him to attend a department where he can work alongside patients engaged in a rehabilitation programme.

Psychopathic Disorder

From the definition of a psychopathic disorder given in the Mental Health Act 1959 it will be seen that the criteria for this disability are social rather than medical or psychiatric. Behaviour is characterised by social aggression [3]: there is usually an inability to profit from experience, poor judgment, self-centredness, facile emotional responses, lack of responsibility, aggression under pressure and a tendency to repeat mistakes. Research indicates that signs of physical immaturity are present in a large proportion of those exhibiting psychopathic behaviour, particularly of the aggressive type. It is worth noting that, in certain individuals, psychopathic tendencies diminish in the late twenties or thirties, thus suggesting that delay in maturation is a contributing factor.

It is usual to consider psychopaths under the broad groups of inadequate and aggressive individuals. While the treatment of both present the same fundamental problems, the former obviously are of less immediate danger to those around them, although the results of their inadequacies may have serious repercussions [4].

Psychopathic Reactions Affecting Performance and Personal Relationships

The characteristics described above have a profound effect on the patient's attitude and ability in occupational therapy, including:

(1) An apparent competence which camouflages frequent failures.
(2) Lack of a 'life plan': only the present is significant.
(2) Inability to evaluate himself or his behaviour.
(4) Lack of perseverance and unreliability in every sphere.

Aims of Occupational Therapy

Because the psychopath is unable to learn from experience easily, treatment in a permissive environment can be difficult and disruptive. Some success has been achieved through group psychotherapy [5], and in special units for such cases. The general tendency is to treat by conditioning, based on the principle that if no yardstick of ethics exists whereby a patient can judge whether his behaviour is acceptable or not, certain indications, such as the giving or withdrawing of privileges must be provided for him. The aims of occupational therapy should be towards making the patient aware of his responsibilities to society and building up in him personality assets which may help to combat antisocial impulsiveness. This course is likely to be more suitable for the inadequate individual, rather than the callous aggressive psychopath for whom a conditioning programme may be more therapeutic. The occupational therapist should aim to provide a considerable degree of control but with understanding.

Therapist-Patient Relationship

Psychopathic patients are plausible and usually play on the sympathies of staff and patients, ruthlessly using others for their own advantage. It is not difficult to make contact with most psychopaths, and although this may be superficial, it will ease the introduction of the rehabilitation programme. The therapist, while being friendly, should show that she has a firm grasp of the situation and intends to control it. This attitude indicates to the aggressive individual that bad behaviour will not be tolerated and also gives the inadequate patient a feeling of greater stability. The patient should be told what is expected of him, such as hours of work, place of work, tools to be used and care of these, etc., and any wilful deviation should be corrected immediately. The patient usually resents authority and restraint and any reactions of this nature should be accepted calmly.

Social Relationships

The psychopath often makes a good initial impression in any group, but may soon be rejected by others for causing arguments (without becoming involved himself) or by manipulating them for his own ends. Many psychopaths have intelligence quotients above average and appreciate the ways in which fellow patients are ill, and although they sometimes exhibit some care and concern for others this may be done to gain the approval of staff in the hope that privileges will be granted. The psychopath tends to identify himself with staff rather than patients, and this should be kept under control although it can be used to encourage work. He should be employed constructively in any group situation which does not permit the exploitation of others. This usually means that he should not be given a position of authority.

Activities

Psychopaths are usually physically fit and a full programme of activities should be planned in which work for the community should occupy a large part. Jobs in the utility departments or in sheltered workshops are ideal. Good service and behaviour can be rewarded by more interesting work, more time for recreation (which must also be well planned), or greater prestige. The latter is a powerful incentive for the inadequate psychopath. A social club may provide possibilities for this, perhaps on the committee, although it may be unwise to place him in a position of too much responsibility, e.g. treasurer. Deliberately poor work or bad behaviour may be corrected by immediate demoting or restrictions of liberty and by an increase in working hours or a change to less congenial work. Reward must follow quickly if the position is to be retrieved. Some psychopaths have marked creative and manual ability and may show interest in skilled activities such as art, music, engineering or experimenting with new inventions, and scope for creative expression should be provided.

Contra-Indications

Activities which:

(1) Encourage an unrealistic attitude to life.
(2) Permit the patient to work in an unsupervised situation.
(3) Permit a low standard of work.
(4) Permit him to dabble superficially with a job rather than see it through from beginning to end.
(5) Permit him to exploit others.

Liaison

As psychopaths are such clever manipulators, the occupational therapist must work in close liaison with the whole therapeutic team.

Drug Addiction

Drug addiction is a state of periodic or chronic intoxication produced by the repeated consumption of a drug. It involves an overpowering desire to obtain and to continue taking it. There is a tendency to increase the dose, marked psychological and physical dependence on the drug's effects, and the characteristic withdrawal symptoms when the patient stops taking the drug [6].

Drugs, like alcohol, are taken initially by emotionally unstable persons to lessen the impact of everyday worries, for they have the effect of making life seem more pleasant and the individual more capable of dealing with it. Eventually life becomes unbearable without their support. Such disorders combine functional and organic aspects, and the chronic states which can develop are discussed in the following chapter. At the present time there is a serious increase in drug taking amongst adolescents and young adults, and it is significant to note that because group feelings are strong at this period, a number of relatively normal youngsters now start taking drugs under the influence of more disturbed friends. Recently revised regulations impel registered drug addicts to get their prescriptions from an authorised doctor as a result of which better methods of control are possible. Some centres have been set up, attached to a general hospital for physical or psychiatric cases, and addicts attend these for their prescriptions. These centres are in an early stage of development, but have the advantage of being able to offer help without having to interfere with the work routines of those addicts who have jobs. Drastic methods to prevent drug taking are not usually used, and the problem in such centres is a long-term one dealt with through psycho-therapy. Those addicts without work may tend to loiter outside or stay at the centre, and occupational therapy has a valuable role to play here, in harnessing whatever abilities are available.

In-patient treatment may become necessary if the physical or psychiatric symptoms demand it, or the patient decides to accept withdrawal treatment. The majority of patients are addicted to heroin or cocaine and a smaller number to the amphetamine and barbiturate groups of drugs. Most drug addicts have personality disorders and many come from broken homes or have other difficulties with parents. They are often selfish, plausible and anti-social and have an ambivalent attitude towards treatment, with periods of longing for the drug. Many have unresolved sexual problems and may also suffer from depression. The need to obtain money for drugs before ad-mission to hospital results in many addicts abandoning careers or training courses to seek more lucrative work, or thieving instead of working [7].

Aims of Occupational Therapy

The treatment of drug addiction is based on the withdrawal of the drug, physical rehabilitation, and the difficult task of improving personality attributes which will help in the development of more mature attitudes. The patient experiences physical and psychological discomfort with with-drawal treatment and the occupational therapist should give support and distract the patient's attention from these as soon as possible. Good work habits and interest in the more normal pleasures of life should be encouraged and more satisfactory personal relationships should be developed. As the patient nears discharge the question of employment must be investigated thoroughly, as addicts quickly drift back to old associations and habits.

Therapist-Patient Relationship

Most drug addicts are inadequate persons who have little toleration for the anxieties and frustrations of life. They need relationships which will promote self-respect and confidence so that normal social interaction is worth seeking. As most patients find it difficult to communicate with non-addicts, the occupational therapist may find it difficult to form an under-standing relationship with the patient. She will need to familiarise herself with the jargon used by addicts, and the individual and social problems they have outside hospital. She should not over-sympathise with them, and should accept their behaviour without sanctioning it. Hostility, negativism and aggression may alternate with a demanding and dependent approach, and should all be accepted with equanimity. By having a positive approach her-self to the occupational therapy programme, the therapist will give patients confidence and security.

Activities

In the early stages of treatment activities which show quick results should be used and patients introduced to group activities on a planned basis as soon as possible. Since drug addicts are usually careless about their personal health and hygiene, steps should be taken to encourage a routine which will restore self-respect. The initial establishment of good habits may need constant reinforcement, and individuals or small groups of patients should be given the responsibility of keeping their environment in order. Many addicts are in a very poor state physically, and graded physical activities, such as table-tennis, swimming, gardening, or dancing should be used to improve health. The degree of cooperation will fluctuate tremendously and patients may demand a certain activity one moment and refuse to take part the next. The therapist should try and make constructive use of cooperative periods, particularly when good ideas are put forward by patients, such as cooking a special meal, making a gift for a relative, etc. As treatment progresses emphasis should shift to the kind of work to which the patient will be returning. In the case of students, who have interrupted a course of training, careful discussion within the treatment team will be needed to decide whether this should be continued. The establishment of a good work routine is essential, and sometimes the best results are achieved by placing a drug addict in an environment where there are relatively stable patients, i.e. a sheltered workshop [8].

Contra-indications

Activities which:

(1) Isolate the patient.
(2) Are too sedative and allow disgruntled feelings to predominate.
(3) Are beyond the patients' physical capacity.

Liaison

The occupational therapist must work closely with nursing staff and social workers in the treatment team.

Alcoholism [9]

The prolonged use of a toxin such as alcohol can result in acute or chronic psychoses (see chapter 15). This section is concerned with the compulsive drinker who seeks treatment before his condition has deteriorated too much, perhaps as a result of losing his job or family conflict. The root cause of alcoholism may be a neurotic or psychopathic condition, and the occupational therapist should also refer to these sections of this book. Drinking may start from social pressure or from an inner need, and in persons with strong emotional conflicts may easily develop into a compulsive dependence on alcohol. As alcohol depresses the inhibitory areas of the frontal lobes, judgment is reduced and a false feeling of self-confidence occurs. Deep emotions such as anger, resentment and aggression may then be openly expressed and the alcoholic will feel relieved until he is sober, when remorse is followed by more drinking to reduce tension. Thus a vicious circle is set up; soon drinking is no longer a pleasure but a physiological necessity to restore the alcoholic level to which the body has adjusted.

Aims of Occupational Therapy

It is a relatively simple matter to help an alcoholic abstain from alcohol while in hospital. It is the long term improvement which is difficult to sustain. Various methods of treatment are used, including conditioned reflex methods of intramuscular injection which produces emesis, or drugs such as antabuse which destroy the taste for alcohol. Some doctors feel that these methods are based on fear rather than a genuine attempt to abstain and prefer psychotherapy. Where possible, a group is formed and patients meet regularly to discuss any problems associated with alcoholism so that they feel they are working together on a common problem [10]. When patients continue to attend such meetings after discharge from hospital, considerable success has been achieved. Others find help and support by joining Alcoholics Anonymous.

The basic aim of occupational therapy is to prepare the patient for his return to normal life without his former 'crutch' [11]. As many alcoholics are immature, unstable or inadequate personalities, or have other personality problems and are often lonely too, group work and improvement of social relationships are essential. As insight develops, activities can help the patient resolve feelings of inadequacy through constructive work. Where a patient's previous job has been abandoned, or if he was sacked, reassessment for a new employment is necessary.

Therapist-Patient Relationship

The establishment of a therapeutic relationship with the alcoholic is his greatest need, because of his inability to face his own shortcomings and his often ambivalent attitude towards treatment. The patient may have a false sense of confidence, rationalising his behaviour and minimising his problems. He may have guilt feelings because of suffering caused to others and may also be depressed. Above all, the patient lacks self-respect and needs encouragement.

Social Relationships

Work in groups is considered best, although alcoholics do not find it easy to participate fully, and will need encouragement to accept responsibility. The use of activity groups (described in chapter 12) can help to improve social relationships and the ability to communicate ideas and feelings.

Activities

Individual activities can be used to foster individual talents or to establish the patient in a work routine before discharge. Industrial, clerical and manual work may all be useful, and at this stage of treatment a regular work pattern should be expected. In any specialised unit, patients can become too preoccupied with their common problem, and towards the end of the treatment period, the therapist can encourage activities planned and carried out for the enjoyment of others, such as a children's party, providing pot plants for geriatric patients to look after, etc. Graded physical activities are needed to improve general health.

Contra-indications

Activities which:

(1) Isolate the patient.
(2) Provide the means to obtain alcohol (i.e. money, access to methylated spirits, etc.).

Liaison

As in the case of drug addicts, the staff in an alcoholic unit need to work closely together. If a good therapeutic relationship has been achieved, the patient may well confide particular problems which he has been unable to express to staff he sees less frequently. These problems often concern the home situation or financial position of the patient's family, and all such information should be passed to the doctor and social worker.

Mental Illness and Deafness

Deafness is a term used for hearing impairments of various kinds, presenting different problems according to the degree of deafness and age of onset. Studies show[12] that the incidence of deafness is higher in psychiatric hospitals than in the general population and that such patients present difficult problems of diagnosis and treatment. Personnel are required with facility in manual methods of communication and with knowledge of the psychological problems of the deaf.

Reactions Affecting Performance and Personal Relationships

If a person becomes deaf after language has been acquired, communication is easier as it is possible to retain speech (although this becomes flat and expressionless in tone) and to teach lip reading. However, the congenitally deaf, particularly those whose impairment is profound, may not obtain the necessary experience to develop emotional and social maturity, because it is on language that communication depends in normal society. Apart from the problems of actual psychiatric illness, difficulties in communication may result in:

(1) Poor emotional control, even 'explosive reactions' including physical display of feeling which cannot be verbally communicated.
(2) Isolation.
(3) Apparent lack of intelligence.
(4) Lack of tact or feeling for others.

Aims of Occupational Therapy

These may be considered under the following headings:

(1) *Observation and assessment.* Psychiatric patients who suffer from early profound deafness have language and communication problems that make assessment a difficult problem that can only be overcome by intensive observation. Observation must be carried out by the treatment team over a period of time and in different situations. With adolescents, assessment of talents needs to be made in order that suitable work may be found for them which will allow integration into the community as independent persons with a full social life.
(2) *Communication.* Once the diagnosis has become clear and potential determined, every effort should be made to improve communication. In schizophrenia particularly, withdrawal may be aggravated by poor communication.
(3) *Social awareness.* Problems of adjustment, particularly in the adolescent deaf, may also arise from their general immaturity and inability to integrate into society through lack of social awareness. The therapist has an important role in helping patients acquire social concepts and normal behaviour standards.

Therapist-Patient Relationship

For effective treatment, the therapist must be trained in manual methods of communication. As the lack of communication obviously impedes understanding and may exacerbate the illness, ample time must be given to 'talking' to patients. It is important to explain plans and aims clearly.

Social Relationships

If there is poor command of language deaf patients will have difficulty in integrating into hearing society. Such patients are often isolated and social aspects of treatment are important. Where patients are treated in a special unit, group discussions should be held to encourage the expression of views and difficulties. As progress is made, patients should be helped to mix with others whose hearing is normal.

Activities

In the first instance the patient may need to work individually on any activity which will encourage communication between himself and the therapist. Once good communications have been established, social isolation and immaturity may indicate a need for group activities, such as games, quizzes, work groups, etc. Deaf patients may lose interest in current events, and a daily discussion of 'what's in the news' can stimulate interest. Feelings to which patients are unable to give full expression verbally may be manifested through painting or clay modelling. Miming has been found an excellent way of conveying ideas without the use of manual signs. As social progress is made, excursions into the community can be undertaken.

Contra-indications

Activities which:

(1) Isolate the patient.
(2) Are beyond his comprehension.

Liaison

Without close collaboration between members of the team, which may include social workers and teachers of the deaf, effective treatment is almost an impossibility. Patients can be encouraged to join a local deaf club and mix with deaf patients in the community. As progress is made, some patients may be able to move on to a special residential home, and the therapist can help the patient prepare for the new environment. With such a specialised problem, there may need to be a certain overlapping of roles and the occupational therapist should be familiar with the national [13], regional and local societies which are concerned with the problems of the deaf.

REFERENCES

1. Hoch, P. H. & Zubin, J. Ed., *Anxiety* (1964 reprint). London.
   Rycroft, C., *Anxiety and Neurosis*. Pelican, 1968.
2. Matheney, R. V. & Topalis, M., *Psychiatric Nursing*. St. Louis, 1970.

3. Craft, M., *Psychopathic Disorders*. London, 1966.
4. Craft, M., *Psychopathy and Delinquency*. Bristol, 1965.
5. Smith, B. (1966), Psychopaths—permissiveness or restriction. *Occ. Ther.*, 29, no. 11.
6. *Report on Drug Addiction*. Government White Paper, 1961. Second report, 1965/67.
 And see:
 N.H.S.*, *The Rehabilitation and After-care of Heroin Addicts*.
7. Chein, I. *et al.*, *Narcotics, Delinquency and Social Policy*. London, 1965.
8. Dixon, A. (1968), Drug addiction: some aspects of treatment. *Occ. Ther.*, 31, no. 6.
 An approach to the rehabilitation of drug dependents. *Occ. Ther.*, 36, no. 1, 1973.
9. Kessel, N. & Walton, H., *Alcoholism*. Penguin Books. London, 1965.
 Ritson, B. & Hassau, C., *The Management of Alcoholism*, Edinburgh and London, 1970.
10. Folkson, A., *Drug Addiction and Alcoholism*. Talk given at S.W. Met. Group of O.T.*s. June 1967.
11. Pinto, H. (1963), The role of the occupational therapist in the rehabilitation of alcoholics. *Occ. Ther.*, 26, no. 10.
12. Denmark, J. C. (1966), Mental illness and early profound deafness. *Brit. J. Med. Psychol.*, 39, 117.
13. *Royal National Institute for the Deaf**.
* See *Glossary*, pp. 454-6.

Occupational Therapy for Psychiatric Conditions: Part 2

Manic-depressive Psychoses

There are constitutional and hereditary factors in the aetiology of the affective disorders, and there is a strong relationship between the manic-depressive psychoses and the cycloid personality.

MANIA

Manic Reactions Affecting Performance and Personal Relationships

The occupational therapist is seldom required to treat a patient in an acute state of mania, because of his extreme distractibility. When the patient improves after chemotherapy and electroconvulsive therapy, occupational therapy can be prescribed. Even so, the patient will be highly over-active, incapable of concentration for more than a few minutes, easily irritated or roused to anger, and constantly interfering in the activities of others. He may have a profusion of ideas and make plans with uncritical optimism, more effort being put into a simple job than is required. Self-assertiveness, argumentativeness and a desire to dominate can disrupt the group.

Aims of Occupational Therapy

These will depend on whether the attack is an isolated one or a recurring condition. Immediate aims are to reduce activity, improve concentration, direct domineering tendencies into constructive channels, and improve the social sense. Subsequent aims include the preparation of the patient for his former routine and place in the community, and assessment and pre-vocational help to select work of less responsibility. Although intellect and personality are preserved during normal periods, employers may be reluctant to re-engage a patient in a position of authority when previous attacks have been disruptive.

Therapist-Patient Relationship

Relationships with a manic patient are made difficult by his extreme lack of insight and desire to dominate. Persuasion is better than direction, and self-assertive tendencies should be directed into constructive channels, for example, many such patients are witty and prolific writers, and may react favourably to writing something for the hospital magazine. This offers prestige but will not involve others who might suffer from the patient's overbearing attitude. Direct opposition should be avoided, and diplomacy used when firm handling is required. Argumentativeness must be accepted without becoming involved in it, as must hostility without rancour. By expecting cooperation and a high standard of work, rapport will be strengthened.

Social Relationships

Social obligations should be stressed, particularly consideration of others. In the early stages it may be advisable to isolate the patient during work periods until he can accept criticism. He can then work with the minimum of distraction and be prevented from upsetting others. This can be arranged tactfully by choosing activities which are limited to a certain area. As toleration and ability to accept criticism increases, the patient can be included in normal group activities.

Activities

The use of 'tranquillisers' and the periodic nature of the illness has confined hospital treatment of these patients to comparatively short episodes. Emphasis should therefore be on rehabilitation, as soon as the patient's condition allows it. The patient needs to work in a composed working atmosphere, and narrow and restricted activities should be avoided. Simple, short-term processes involving rhythmical movements are useful at this stage, i.e. industrial work, polishing, hoeing, etc. Noise, speed and argument tend to overstimulate the patient, and should be avoided as fatigue may set in easily. Care should be taken over the choice of tools as, although a manic patient may not use them maliciously, his uncontrolled and energetic movements make the use of heavy and sharp tools inadvisable. Lastly, opportunity should be given to restore confidence in previous work, or adjustment to new work.

Contra-indications

Activities which permit:

(1) Unlimited, uncontrolled movement, i.e. unrestrained dancing, walking, running, throwing, etc.

(2) Frequent switching of processes which increases distractibility.

(3) Unrestrained aggressive outlet, i.e. breaking, smashing and demolition work.

(4) A low standard of work.

(5) Domination of others.

Liaison

On discharge the patient may need support at a day hospital or from visits from a domiciliary occupational therapist in the community, but it must be accepted that re-admission is likely.

DEPRESSIVE PHASE OF MANIC-DEPRESSIVE PSYCHOSES AND INVOLUTIONAL MELANCHOLIA

Depressive Reactions Affecting Performance and Personal Relationships

This illness is characterised by the retardation of physical and mental function described by A. J. Lewis as 'an adaptation of the organism to an intolerable situation'[1]. The features to be considered in occupational therapy are:

(1) Feelings of inadequacy, gloom, self-depreciation, and guilt which may amount to delusions that actual crimes have been committed, together with anxiety and irritability, so that the patient finds concentration on work impossible.

(2) Physical weakness resulting from lack of interest in food, insomnia or insufficient exercise.

(3) Lack of insight. The patient may deny that he is mentally ill, but may have severe hypochondriacal tendencies and complain of bodily ill-health which prevents him from working.

(4) People and social events are avoided.

(5) Speech and thought may be affected, and there may be difficulty in conversing, in following a train of thought, initiating ideas, recollecting or using the imagination.

(6) Loss of 'willpower' may result in neglect of personal appearance.

(7) There is danger of suicide, even when improvement appears to be taking place.

Special Features in Involutional Melancholia

Involutional melancholia is a form of endogenous depression occurring in men and women at the involutional period of life. With the longer expectation of life, depression of later life is becoming more frequent. In many cases the attack may be an isolated one and the prognosis is usually good.

Involutional melancholia can be considered alongside cyclo-thymic depression except in the following features:

(1) Retardation is not so prominent, but anxiety is conspicuous, often shown by severe restlessness and agitation.
(2) The patient may display regret at lost opportunities, or unfulfilled ambitions, or may prove unable to accept increased responsibilities, such as promotion at work which comes after years of waiting.
(3) Delusions may be bizarre and hypochondriacal, and centred around guilt feelings.

Aims of Occupational Therapy

Occupational therapy must be coordinated with electroconvulsive therapy and chemotherapy. Although the condition usually remits spontaneously in time, treatment is aimed at relieving it earlier while guarding against possible suicidal attempts. The immediate aims are to distract the patient from morbid preoccupation by externalising feelings of unworthiness and hostility. Efforts must be made to improve the physical condition. Once improvement is seen, resocialisation can begin.

Careful rehabilitation is necessary as the patient's confidence may be undermined seriously if he is allowed to leave hospital unable to face life and fearing a recurrence. He should be helped to establish a routine associated with his former work, or pre-vocational assessments should be carried out if the frequency or disruptive nature of previous attacks have made return to former work impossible. Patients who have lost husband or wife and have problems of boredom and loneliness at home, may need help in finding a satisfying outlet. Institutionalisation should be prevented in long-standing cases, particularly social isolation and narrowing of interests. Dependence on the hospital between attacks should be avoided where possible.

Therapist-Patient Relationship

The therapist must not be disconcerted by apparent rejection and hostility; extreme retardation inhibits response. The patient's need for affection and social acceptance may go unsatisfied because of his inability to show overt response. The initial approach should make no demands on the patient. A quiet, kind, welcoming manner will give a feeling of security. Explanations and directions should be brief and clear, leaving no decisions to be made. Over-attention must be avoided, but, by choosing activities with which the patient will require help at regular intervals, the therapist will be able to maintain constant contact. As the depression lifts and the patient becomes more responsive, dependence on the therapist should lessen and social contacts be widened.

Social Relationships

As soon as the patient shows signs of interest in other people, he can be grouped with a few quiet and moderately cheerful patients. Hearty, over-active or interfering patients may deepen his depression. As he becomes more communicative, he may begin to express feelings of guilt and unworthi-ness. This may be a necessary form of release and should not be prevented unless it persists or disturbs other patients, when attention must be re-directed along lines of positive achievement. As toleration of others in-creases, the patient should be given small responsibilities within the group.

Activities

Activities chosen for treatment should be interesting enough to hold the patient's attention, while being well within his capabilities, as fear of failure may be prominent. Short-term projects showing quick improvement will help to increase confidence. Failure will provide an argument against further effort. Opportunities to externalise feelings of guilt and obligation can be given, by encouraging service to others. The depressed patient will confine his movements to the minimum, and usually have very poor posture. General physical exercise can be achieved early in treatment by walks combined with an interest, such as collecting flowers for the department. Simple rhythmic exercises to music and old time dancing are beneficial, but care should be taken to avoid extremes of movement until there is real improvement.

With improvement, social activities should be extended. At first attend-ance may be as an observer only, but encouragement to take a minor part should soon be given, and followed by small responsibilities, such as collect-ing subscriptions at a social club, or making tea and washing up. In this way a transition from dependence to independence may be achieved.

Opportunity to take a fresh interest in personal appearance should be arranged without making the patient feel a failure. Nutrition is an important aspect in nursing care, and patients can be encouraged to cook some special delicacies for themselves and a few friends in the domestic unit.

As soon as the patient responds to treatment, and risk of suicide is minimal, he should be encouraged to take an interest in outside affairs. He may need to regain confidence in travelling or shopping. The rehabilitation programme should help him revive skills prior to discharge, so that he can prove his independence to himself. In some cases, sheltered work in the community may be indicated, if the illness is recurrent.

Contra-indications

Activities which:

(1) Permit the patient to experience failure.

(2) Require the patient to work in isolation (precluding social contact and increasing fear of suicide).

(3) Involve speed, noise and confusion of movement.

(4) Involve the use of large, overwhelming or unfamiliar apparatus.

(5) Involve the unsupervised use of sharp tools, ropes or poisonous substances.

Liaison

If treatment is given in hospital, the usual team cooperation is essential. If the patient is not in hospital, it may be advisable to encourage him to attend an out-patient's club or day centre, in which case, the occupational therapist working in the community should be contacted.

Precautions

Continual precautions must be taken against possible suicidal attempts particularly when, during stages of recovery, retardation becomes less marked and volition increases. Patients should be observed carefully, and should not be allowed to wander off into side-rooms or lavatories. In the case of the latter, it is important that, while giving the patient the maximum privacy possible, the therapist should have quick access to them. All the precautions on page 260 should be strictly observed.

Schizophrenic Illnesses

The term schizophrenia is used here for a group of illnesses, leading, in the majority of cases, to a disorganisation of the patient's personality which often results in chronic invalidism and long hospitalisation. This aspect is discussed in chapter 13. Schizophrenia is the commonest mental illness, and occupational therapy is considered an important treatment [2]. The following are general principles of treatment.

Schizophrenic Reactions Affecting Performance and Personal Relationships [3]

The student will be familiar with the characteristic ways in which schizophrenic symptoms interfere with the patient's thinking, emotions, conation and motor behaviour. The predominating symptoms for which occupational therapy is required are:

(1) Withdrawal from society and reality, and an increasing preoccupation with phantasy.

(2) Emotional flattening and consequent indifference to the needs of others, which also causes a deterioration in personal habits.

(3) Poor physical condition due to lack of exercise and poor posture which results in circulatory difficulties, leading in extreme cases to oedema and pathological respiratory conditions.

(4) Reduced activity and volition due to disturbance of volition, which may amount to negativism.

Aims of Occupational Therapy

Treatment will almost certainly include chemotherapy, and electroconvulsive therapy is used for some cases. Insulin is still occasionally used, particularly a modified form where the physical condition is poor. Occupational therapy must aim initially at bringing the patient into contact with reality, preventing withdrawal into phantasy, and improving the physical condition by regular exercise. As the patient becomes more accessible, the area of interest must be widened and social contacts increased. When personal habits are poor, emphasis must be given to self-care, and if necessary, habit training used. The latent schizophrenic often likes regular and routine work, and such tendencies should be directed into realistic and constructive channels. Baker showed that in industrial conditions within the hospital environment, patients were not inferior to unskilled workers in industry, and on these findings widespread use has been made of industrial work (see chapter 22).

Therapist-Patient Relationship

The greatest challenge to the occupational therapist is the acceptance of the indifference shown by the patient. Contact is difficult because of inaccessibility. It is wise to expect no immediate response, but to state one's own case in simple terms. The patient must be left free to respond if he wishes to do so; obvious attempts to gain a response may result in the patient withdrawing further. It is important to try and understand the patient as an individual rather than be side-tracked by bizarre symptoms. The problem of verbal communication is really difficult in some cases, but the patient may have his own meaning for distorted words and phrases, and by showing interest and concern, and observing him closely, an understanding can be built up slowly, even if this is non-verbal. Careful assessment of all activities and social contacts, and observation of their effects on the patient are necessary to ensure that, while progress is maintained, stress is not imposed, nor withdrawal increased. The schizophrenic patient is suggestible, often to an extreme degree. This may be used to advantage by the therapist in promoting work habits at a time when the patient is inaccessible to reason. The therapist should adopt the role of a worker alongside the patient, rather than that of instructor or supervisor, indicating by example what is required.

Social Relationships

By including the schizophrenic in a group of patients, who are in contact with, and enjoying, reality, the concept of healthy social interaction [4] may be suggested, and he should be allowed to absorb the situation slowly and quietly. On the other hand, the withdrawn patient is in danger of verbal attack from aggressive patients, who need an outlet for their aggression and use the withdrawn patient as a 'chopping block'. In this case, the therapist should divert the attention of the aggressive patient, for to draw attention to the schizoid patient may isolate him further from the group. Any move he makes to take an active part must be encouraged gently. The interests of other patients must always be watched, as the lack of self-criticism and self-control of the schizophrenic may have an adverse effect on them. There may be apparent enjoyment of, or indifference to, the difficulties of others. The patient may, for instance, help himself to all the food provided at meals, regardless of other people, unless other patients are served first. Watchfulness for possible impulsive actions in response to hallucinations is also necessary.

Activities

Attention should be given to the value of day-to-day living and the acquisition of good personal and social habits, including a balanced work and recreational programme. Graded schemes which will gradually involve the patient in more active and responsible work is essential. Stimulation is needed, either through the activities themselves, through contact with the therapist, or the other patients. Occupations that are sedative and allow for ruminating are not advisable. Group activities may be used to stimulate interest and activity; gardening, industrial and domestic work are all valuable. For industrial assembly work, [5] careful selection of patients is needed to maintain the speed of work, for the schizophrenic patient may withdraw from a situation which is beyond him.

Regular exercise is important, such as walks, dancing and simple games. In convalescence, when cooperation is gained, physical training or Health and Beauty classes may be beneficial. Trips should be made outside the hospital too, to places of interest, for shopping and to visit friends. Interest should also be fostered in personal appearance. Dressmaking, hairdressing, manicuring and makeup will give confidence to women patients and make them more aware of their effect on others. Insistence on a high standard of personal appearance for men is important, i.e. that they be well-shaven, with clothes brushed and pressed, etc. Facilities for care of the clothes should be available in the department. Mixed social activities often encourage pride in appearance.

Schizophrenic patients tend to dwell in phantasy rather than reality, and cultural activities such as art [6], music, drama [7] and literary work tend, therefore, to hold their interest more readily than manual work. Such activities should be directed and controlled. Painting and modelling, for instance, can be used to help a patient externalise his phantasies and perhaps learn to accept them and conduct his life as if they do not exist, but this type of treatment should only be carried out on the suggestion of the psychiatrist treating the patient. Free expression in art, music or drama, which is required for diagnostic or cathartic purposes should be closely controlled by a psychiatrist as well as the occupational therapist.

Regular occupation is just as important for the patient when discharged as when in hospital, and he may well need some guidance in the choice of a job [8]. Work which requires a high degree of personal responsibility should be avoided.

Contra-indications

Activities which:

(1) Encourage long periods of sitting or standing in the same position, i.e. embroidery, watch-repairing, listening passively to music.
(2) Reinforce phantasy, i.e. undirected indulgence in imaginative activities such as art, music, modelling, writing, etc., unless this is being used specifically by the psychiatrist.
(3) Encourage isolation, i.e. weeding or hoeing, cataloguing books in separate room, etc.

Liaison

Follow-up measures after discharge [9] are most important, as the schizophrenic returning to the narrow domestic circle may lack the stimulation he received in hospital or may drift into the society of eccentrics. Continuity of day-hospital treatment or attendance at a sheltered workshop or day centre will contribute to the management of patients in the community

The following types of schizophrenia may need special consideration because of the predominance of one or more symptoms.

THE HEBEPHRENIC TYPE

This illness, occurring at adolescence or in the early twenties, has an insidious onset and may therefore have become well-established before the patient is received for treatment. Owing to the youth of these patients, the ultimate aim is to resettle them outside hospital. Although in many cases they may never live full social lives, if rightly assessed and placed in jobs which hold interest but do not impose strain, they may live successfully in the community for some years although the ultimate prognosis is poor.

THE CATATONIC TYPE

This form of schizophrenic illness, which occurs generally in the twenties and early thirties, is characterised by either stupor, of varying degrees of severity, or excitement. The onset is more rapid than in hebephrenia and the prognosis is better, although a second or third attack may result in progressive deterioration of intellect and personality.

While general principles of treatment remain the same, great care is necessary in introducing the catatonic patient to a group because of his liability to impulsive behaviour. For this reason the issue of dangerous tools is contra-indicated, and watch must be kept to ensure that he has not easy access to those being used by other patients.

Where stupor is marked, physical exercise may be achieved by guided movements to music, and response may be evoked by simple games involving catching a beanbag or passing an object round a circle of patients, in which the patient automatically performs the required action. *Total push* methods may be indicated for these patients, but care should be taken that forcing does not promote greater withdrawal as a form of self-defence.

PARANOID TYPES

The onset of paranoid conditions occur usually between the ages of 30 and 45. Early symptoms of suspicion and sensitivity develop into delusional ideas of persecution.

Although the clinical forms of paranoid schizophrenia, paraphrenia and paranoid states vary in the extent to which the patient is hallucinated and the degree to which his delusions are systematised, occupational therapy follows the same principles for all these conditions, and they can therefore be considered as a group.

The paranoid patient, because of overt or covert grandiosity and suspicion, finds difficulty in responding to any approach. Friendliness by the therapist may be misinterpreted as 'getting round' him. While letting the patient realise that he is welcome, it is advisable to refrain from efforts to obtain good rapport, letting this develop gradually as the patient becomes familiar with the situation, and more secure in consequence. Satisfactory rapport may be obtained if the patient is given some position of responsibility, thus relieving him of the feeling that he should show gratitude to the therapist.

While overtly expressed delusions should not be opposed, they should not be encouraged. The patient's attention must be diverted towards interesting activities unconnected with his delusions. Endeavours should be made to include the patient in group activities, but hostility may be a barrier and the patient may have to be allowed to work on an individual project until this can be overcome. Repressed hostility may be expended in activities involving force, such as hammering, digging, and work of demolition. It is unwise, however, to allow such patients to use dangerous tools, i.e. axes or picks, as impulsiveness and suspicion may result in homicidal attacks.

As the patient becomes more cooperative he should be helped to encapsulate his symptoms. While acknowledging that he feels persecuted, the therapist must direct his attention to the positive aspects of his problems. He may respond, for instance, to the suggestion that persecutors, if they exist, should not be given the satisfaction of disrupting his life, which he must try to live as normally as possible. A mildly paranoid patient, having accepted this viewpoint, may be resettled outside hospital for a considerable period, if not permanently. Effective follow-up after discharge may present difficulties owing to the suspicious nature of the patient, who may think that contact by the occupational therapist or psychiatric social worker is a prelude to further hospitalisation. Follow-up through the agency of understanding and discreet relations or friends may be the best method. Postoperative rehabilitation, for patients who have undergone leucotomy because of distressing or frightening delusions, may have to be considered.

Senile Dementia

Senile dementia is a pyschotic condition resulting in part from cerebral deterioration. It is often viewed erroneously by the student as a natural progression in the process of ageing, and surprise is expressed that the patient fails to respond to treatment similar to that given to the mentally normal geriatric patient. While many of the symptoms of senile dementia appear to be exaggerations of normal old age, the lack of insight encountered in senility changes the emphasis of treatment. With the normal elderly person the main aim is to encourage a purposeful life with a high degree of independence. In treating the senile patient peace of mind and body are the first considerations [10].

Although these patients may attend the occupational therapy department in the early stages of the condition, as it progresses it is better to treat them in their wards and in homogeneous groups, as confusion, leading to wandering, incontinence, etc., and lack of normal inhibitions may cause difficulties with other patients.

Aims of Occupational Therapy

Treatment must be directed towards alleviating anxiety which is the natural outcome of confusion, and to preserving good habits which still remain. While physical tone should be maintained where possible, senile patients are often too frail for much exertion. If an yttrium implant is given for severe agitated depression, improvement should be harnessed immediately (see chapter 12).

Therapist-Patient Relationship

The occupational therapist must adapt her approach to the patient's degree of understanding and grasp of situations. As the patient may not recognise places or people and may fail to grasp the purpose of events, each treatment session should be viewed as a new experience for him unless signs of recognition are apparent.

Social Relationships

These may be impossible to achieve, owing to the patient's disorientation but group activities should be used where practicable.

Activities

Activities should give opportunity to exercise all remaining faculties, and talents including previously learnt skills or those that have become habitual, are likely to be far more successful than completely new ones. Physical considerations, such as the condition of heart, eyesight and hearing, will also affect the choice. It may be necessary to teach a new process afresh at each subsequent treatment session. Any suggestion that the patient ought to remember it may cause anxiety and strain.

For women, needlework, crochet, knitting, simple raffia work and mending may be practicable; or simple domestic work such as laying tables, preparing vegetables, dusting and polishing may give satisfaction, provided that the patient is not urged to work to a rigid time-schedule. For men, simple woodwork, industrial work, or gardening are usually better than domestic work, unless the latter has been habitual to them earlier in life. If complete operations are not possible a single process may be carried out (i.e. sandpapering, sorting scrap material, etc.). Radio, television, 'sing-songs', can help to stimulate the patient and turn his attention outside the narrow confines of the ward.

Habit training may be necessary, and should aim at establishing for each patient a routine within his capabilities which will give him a feeling of security by reason of familiarity. Much of this will be supervised by the nursing staff but occupational therapy should be a part of, and complement to the scheme. Good habits will be encouraged by the provision of suitable facilities, easy access to lavatories being one of the most important.

As dementia is irreversible and progressive, the patient, in spite of fluctuations, will inevitably become less able and more emotionally labile, and the therapist, while helping him to function at the highest level possible, must observe any decline in mental and physical condition, and modify activities to avoid stress.

Contra-indications

Activities which involve:

    (1) Learning new processes.
    (2) Judgment and initiative.
    (3) The use of dangerous tools, equipment or materials, i.e. boiling water, hot glue or pitch, etc.

Liaison

Collaboration with the ward nursing staff is particularly important because the whole of the patient's day must be planned, including where possible, small tasks undertaken on the ward. Voluntary workers may fulfil a valuable function by offering friendship and bringing in outside interests.

Organic Dementias

In the later stages the treatment of all forms of organic and presenile dementias follows the same principles as that for senile dementia. In the early stages, however, there are certain variations in symptoms which need specific consideration when planning treatment.

Cerebral Arteriosclerosis

The first symptoms of the condition are those of irritability, tiring easily, headache, insomnia, disturbance of memory, giddiness and a tendency to become flustered, and it is characterised by a fluctuating intellectual impairment and possible lapses in responsibility, resulting in deterioration of intellect and personality. Insight is retained for some time and, while it may be an asset, in that patients may be able to understand and profit by advice and precautions, it may cause them considerable distress and anxiety regarding the future.

    The aims of occupational therapy are to help the patients to maintain themselves in the outside community for as long as possible and, when institutional care becomes inevitable, to adjust to the sheltered life with the least possible emotional disturbance.

    While resettlement after confusional episodes is still practicable, the patient's usual job should be assessed to discover if he can continue in it. Sometimes a return may be possible with modification in working methods. Thus confidence may be restored for a time and anxiety relieved. If his previous job is not still open to him alternative work, within his present capacity, may be possible, but vocational training should not be initiated as progressive deterioration will soon render it ineffectual. Exciting or frustrating situations should be avoided as these tend to provoke the symptoms, but the patient should be encouraged to maintain social contacts and intellectual activities. In some cases, hospitalisation can be avoided if the patient can attend a day hospital which provides treatment and relieves the relatives of responsibility for much of the day.

Presenile Dementias and Dementias of Middle Age

The most common of the presenile dementias, Alzheimer's and Pick's diseases, together with Huntington's chorea, which usually occurs early in adult life, present problems for the occupational therapist similar to those of senile and arteriosclerotic dementia. There are variations in the length of time that personality is preserved, and in the associated physical symptoms, which may include stereotyped movements, gross restlessness and choreiform movements (Huntington's), but the ultimate steady deterioration requires the same occupational treatment as that already described.

Encephalitis Lethargica

The mental symptoms which frequently follow this condition fall into two categories:

(1) Personality changes following an encephalitic infection in childhood.
(2) Those which are associated with post-encephalitic parkinsonism.

As the former result in states similar to those of severe psychopathic conditions, treatment will be similar, although personality changes in encephalitis have a more lasting effect.

The symptoms associated with parkinsonism do not constitute true dementia, as many of the basic abilities of the individual are well-preserved. The initial irritability, difficulty in concentration, and fatigue, give place, however, to a general slowing down of the mental processes which results in difficulty in understanding and adapting to situations. This, together with a loss of initiative, presents a problem similar to that of dementia. Insight is retained for a considerable time and the realisation of progressive physical deterioration may cause anxiety and depression which will further complicate the picture. Attempted suicide rather than the direct symptoms of his illness may first bring the patient to hospital, and if he can be helped to overcome anxiety and achieve a constructive attitude to his disabilities, he may return to life outside hospital for a considerable period.

Aims of Occupational Therapy

The first aim of treatment is to alleviate anxiety and encourage confidence. It is important to minimise physical disabilities and alleviation of anxiety will cause the physical symptoms to appear less obtrusive. The extent of ability must be assessed carefully before work is started. Social contacts should be maintained and encouraged.

If resettlement outside the hospital is practicable, efforts must be directed towards making the patient as self-sufficient as possible in regard to daily needs. If necessary, aids must be devised to help him to dress and feed. The patient's retardation must be remembered in teaching their use. It is unlikely that paid employment will be possible outside the hospital once treatment has become necessary, unless in a sheltered condition among understanding people, but a patient may remain a happy and useful member of a domestic circle if he can live within the limits of his disability, and his family can make allowance for slowness and lack of inititative.

Where this is impossible, these patients are usually happier in institutions where social contacts are more numerous and occupation under sheltered conditions is possible.

Therapist-Patient Relationship

The therapist should give the patient time to talk about his problems initially, thus showing a desire to understand him. Speech may be difficult for him, which makes this additionally important. Subsequently, the patient should be diverted from his problems by directing his attention towards topics he can appreciate in spite of his disability, for instance, listening to music, talks, discussions, etc.

Social Relationships

The patient should be encouraged to work with others and join in suitable recreational activities, taking some responsibility of which he is capable. Discussion with others and communication through writing should be encouraged. If rigidity or tremor make writing difficult, large-sized pens and pencils can be used.

Activities

Tremor of the hands and visual difficulties may make fine work impossible; activities involving grosser movements are usually more successful. Tremor may decrease during purposeful activity, and may be controlled considerably by 'anchoring' the patient's hands to fairly stable equipment. Sweeping, mopping, or scrubbing a floor may be possible without the tremor becoming incapacitating, because the broom or brush is resting on the floor. For some patients inability to maintain balance may be a further complicating factor. For these, occupations involving sudden changes of position or direction must be avoided. Such patients are better seated and should never be allowed to climb ladders.

Contra-indications

Activities which:

(1) Require clear sight and fine coordination.
(2) Require good balance and sudden changes of direction.
(3) Encourage 'pill-rolling' tremor.
(4) Involve the use of dangerous tools, equipment or materials.
(5) Cause patient to work in isolated position.
(6) By type or standard of work cause anxiety, thereby increasing patient's physical symptoms.

Liaison

In order to help the patient lead as active a life as possible, physiotherapy and occupational therapy may be prescribed, and links with home, social club, or sheltered workshop may need to be forged.

Epilepsy [11]

It must be realised that a large number of epileptics, whose fits occur infrequently or are satisfactorily controlled by drugs, are able to live successful lives outside hospital. The occupational problem of the epileptic in the community is twofold. Firstly, it is necessary that any job undertaken should be one in which the patient can come to no harm and which is unaffected should a fit occur. Secondly, those with whom he works must be prepared to accept his fits and possible disturbances of mood associated with them.

In-patient treatment becomes necessary only when fits occur so frequently that they cannot be controlled adequately without heavy sedation or when the epilepsy is associated with psychosis or results in dementia. Almost all those requiring hospital care show irritability, perversity and desire for attention which must be considered when treating the patient. While such an attitude may be changed in some cases, by the fulfilment of the patient's need for recognition, in others its persistence presents an obstacle to satisfactory social adjustment.

While excitement and over-stimulation of the epileptic may produce a fit, so equally may idleness. It follows, therefore, that the use of drugs may be reduced if the patient can be occupied throughout his waking hours in relaxing but absorbing activities, and that these should be changed once they no longer claim full attention.

Aims of Occupational Therapy

The ultimate aim will be decided by the possibility or otherwise of the patient being resettled outside hospital. This will depend as much upon social and environmental factors as upon the patient's response to treatment.

If the patient is in hospital for a short period only, while his fits are being stabilised or new treatment is tried, the main efforts of the therapist must be to keep him in touch with outside life, and maintain or improve his standards of social behaviour. Work habits must be preserved and the development of invalid attitudes prevented. The epileptic tends to become morbidly absorbed in the subject of his fits. If it is impossible for the patient to return to his previous occupation it may be necessary to assess his abilities for other employment, and lead up to vocational training. His hopes regarding any alternative work must not be raised until it has been ascertained that employment in that field will be open to him.

Where permanent hospitalisation appears necessary, treatment must be aimed at establishing a full, well-balanced life of work, recreation and social intercourse, within the limits of the institution.

Therapist-Patient Relationship

The therapist's approach to the epileptic must be kindly but firm. Any tendency towards tale bearing or currying favour must be discouraged at the outset, but praise should be given for satisfactory work or behaviour. A desire for attention may be satisfied by giving a patient a particular job for which he is responsible. This may be in the occupational therapy department, ward, or hospital utility workshop. It will usually be carried out with satisfaction and pride, provided it is within the patient's capacity and he is given commendation for it.

Social Relationships

If several epileptics are being treated it is better to place them in different groups in order that the temperamental difficulties of one will not react upon another. An epileptic will settle with comparatively few difficulties into a mixed group of long-stay patients.

When a short-term patient is being treated among acutely ill psychotic or neurotic patients it is advisable to avoid grouping epileptics and hysterical patients together. Both are demanding of attention and the hysteric may simulate fits in order to gain this. Other neurotic patients, retaining their insight, will usually accept the epileptic with sympathy.

If the patient behaves in an antisocial manner the therapist must make him realise that such behaviour is not acceptable. This is best done by drawing the patient aside on some pretext and explaining that he cannot return to the group until he feels well enough to control himself, and act in a more kindly way. His attention should be drawn to the needs of the other patients and his cooperation gained in helping to satisfy these.

Epileptic Fits

The effect of the patient's fits upon the rest of the group depends largely upon the attitude displayed by the staff. If they are dealt with quietly and unemotionally the atmosphere in the department will not be greatly disturbed. Most patients show some distress on the epileptic's behalf on first witnessing a fit, but subsequently are not much affected by the occurrence. The therapist should study each new epileptic patient carefully so that she may know what form his fits take. Some patients have prodromal warnings or auras, but others may fall without warning, in which case great care must be exercised in the choice of activities so that there is a clear space around the patient, free from sharp edged and dangerous equipment. Some patients may have periods of automatic behaviour following a fit, or as the equivalent of a fit, in which they perform actions which usually follow a set pattern. They should be allowed to carry these out as far as possible, control being exercised only if they prove dangerous or cause unpleasantness to other patients. Sufferers from *petit mal* need to be observed constantly as the disturbance of consciousness, being less dramatic than *grand mal*, may easily pass unnoticed in the general activity of the department. If watch is not kept the therapist may be unprepared for the automatic behaviour or confusion which may follow the seizure. A major fit should be treated by placing a cushion under the head of the patient and loosening any tight clothing. If there has been sufficient warning dentures should have been removed and a soft gag, such as a folded handkerchief, placed between the patient's back teeth. During the clonic stage, the patient is less likely to sustain injury if the limbs are supported gently but not restrained. As clonus subsides the patient's head should be turned to one side to allow saliva to drain and any obstruction in the mouth to fall forward. The patient should then be made comfortable and left undisturbed until he recovers.

The patient must not be placed by unguarded fires, dangerous machinery, boiling liquids or open windows, and the use of sharp instruments should be avoided unless under supervision. He should be aware of these precautions so that he may realise how he may cooperate for his own safety, but they should be carried out without fuss, so that he does not develop a hypochondriacal attitude towards his condition. It may be explained that a blind man has to take certain precautions and similarly the epileptic must protect himself from dangers incurred by his own disability.

Activities

Activities for epileptic patients may be drawn from a wide range, as intelligence and aptitudes vary as with normal people. Industrial work, wardwork or work in a hospital utility department will provide situations akin to outside life, and may be the source of pocket-money. Craft activities should be used mainly for recreational purposes. All social and cultural activities should be made available to them, including radio and television (if it has no adverse effects), but these should not be overstimulating. Good habits should be maintained and self-respect increased by interest in, and attention to, appearance. For women anticipating discharge, domestic activities may hold the most interest and methods may be devised whereby household tasks may be carried out with the least possibility of danger should a fit occur.

While the mental hospital can provide an adequate sheltered life for the patient requiring such conditions, a much greater degree of freedom and opportunity is available in *epileptic colonies*. Here patients may live in their own rooms, or houses, often with their families and lead as normal a life as is possible, but with supervision and help at hand. It is to be hoped that more facilities of this kind will be provided in the future, as at present only a limited number of epileptics can be accommodated in the existing colonies.

Contra-indications

Activities which:

(1) Involve constant noise, movement and flashing lights as these may precipitate a fit.

(2) Involve the use of dangerous tools or machinery, working at heights, etc.

(3) Are dull, monotonous and require little concentration, as fits are likely to occur during such situations.

Liaison

Those epileptics who are able to leave hospital and follow a normal career may gain confidence if their capabilities are made clear to prospective employers. The therapist may need to contact the social worker, disablement resettlement officer or employer.

Epileptics needing permanent hospital care, also need regular employment and the therapist must keep informed of patients' progress in a sheltered workshop or utility department.

Alcoholic Psychoses

Although the root cause of alcoholism may be a neurotic or psychopathic condition (see chapter 14) the acute and chronic psychoses are due to organic changes caused by the addiction, covering a wide range of states with their associated symptoms including:

Acute Psychoses

(1) *Mania à potu,* or pathological intoxication, is a state of frenzy or acute excitement occurring after ingestion of often small amounts of

alcohol in susceptible patients who are frequently explosive psychopaths, or have a history of epileptic manifestations.

(2) *Dipsomania* is caused by recurrent drinking attacks in between which the patient often finds alcohol distasteful (see chapter 14).

(3) *Delirium tremens* is an acute toxic confusional psychosis accompanied by terrifying hallucinations which occurs in chronic alcoholism.

Patients suffering from mania *à potu* and delirium tremens are too acutely disturbed for occupational therapy.

Chronic Psychoses

(1) *Chronic alcoholic dementia* is a moral, intellectual and physical deterioration which develops gradually after a long history of steady drinking, and occupational therapy must be related to the degree of deterioration.

(2) *Korsakow's syndrome*. The symptoms here may be:
   (a) Disorder of memory for recent events.
   (b) Confabulation.
   (c) Affective changes.
   (d) Peripheral neuritis.

If this condition follows delirium tremens there may occasionally be confusion and hallucinations.

This syndrome presents problems which are psychological and physical. During the acute stage, care must be taken not to cause fatigue, and work should be light and simple. Polyneuritis and skin conditions limit the choice of activities. As the prognosis is generally poor, and improvement is seldom enough to enable the patient to return to economic independence, sheltered work is usually indicated of a less skilled kind than the patient did prior to his illness. Apart from regular work, the patient should be encouraged to enjoy a full social life.

Other Organic Mental Syndromes

Social and environmental factors may have contributed to these conditions, as in the case of nutritional deficiencies or poisoning by heavy metals. Drug addiction may have been initiated by the administration of drugs for the relief of pain, or by basic fear and insecurity.

Except in the case of intoxication by rare drugs, the mental symptoms produced by the various agents responsible for these states are not in themselves specific and many present similar pictures. The degree of mental disturbance is due to the constitution of the patient and the duration of the intoxications. Mental symptoms range from mild confusion to sub-delirium and delirium. In addition physical symptoms may be present, such as skin conditions in cases of nutritional deficiencies, which will affect the choice of activities. While the treatment of delirium is outside the scope of the occupational therapist, she must be prepared to deal with all other aspects of these states.

Aims of Occupational Therapy

These are firstly, to distract the patient from anxiety caused by disorientation or frightening hallucinations; and secondly, to encourage aspects of his personality which will militate against future breakdown (such as responsibility in nutritional matters, and the establishment of good social, work and personal habits).

Therapist-Patient Relationship

The therapist should provide stability for the patient by being friendly, clear, and firm in giving directions. When appropriate, reassurance should be given by directing the patient's attention towards future healthy achievement outside hospital.

Social Relationships

The patient should be encouraged to take part in group activities as soon as the acute stage of the illness is passed, and as his condition improves, increasing responsibility can be given, such as committee work, organising work groups, recreations, etc.

Activities

The patient should work at a quiet and even tempo. Simple, familiar surroundings help to modify confusion and anxiety. Distraction from anxious thoughts may be obtained by focusing the patient's attention on the job of the moment, and by making no demands on memory while confusion is present. A simple activity, which can be relearned on each attendance, will ensure that the patient is not discouraged by lack of memory nor forced into confabulation. As memory improves more complicated tasks may be attempted and the attention of the patient held for increasing periods of time.

These patients require as much physical exercise and intellectual stimulation as is possible without causing strain, as sedentary or monotonous activities permit attention to wander and the patient to become restless. Gardening is valuable as it can be graded easily, and the fresh air and exercise involved promote a healthy appetite.

Where the patient's history indicates that inability to deal with the problems of life is the basis of an addiction, creative activities may provide an outlet for suppressed drives. Discovery and encouragement of talent may compensate the patient who has been forced into uncongenial work (e.g. the man with administrative ability who has been forced, by lack of educational opportunities, into a routine clerical job).

While the prognosis for most of these conditions is good, it must be realised that future breakdowns are likely to occur where addiction has been the cause of the condition and, if prolonged, this addiction will result in progressive intellectual and personality impairment. Great cunning may be exercised by patients in their efforts to satisfy a craving, and the therapist must take precautions against access to drugs.

As confusion clears, it is essential that the patient's social and work potential should be assessed and the suitability of his past employment considered with a view to his resettlement. Where it is unsuitable (as in the case of a dispenser, nurse or doctor who has become a drug addict) an alternative plan must be made well before the patient leaves hospital, as any tendency to drift into similar situations must be avoided.

Where the patient's intelligence is average or above, responsibility for his future well-being may be encouraged by demonstrations and discussions on nutrition, and in the case of women, by raising an interest in arranging menus and actually preparing well-balanced meals. The young mother suffering from toxic confusion after childbirth may derive benefit from domestic and nursing activities which will give her confidence in her ability to deal with household and family needs. Self-respect should be encouraged by attendance at social events, where a well-groomed appearance and good personal habits and manners are expected. If psychotherapy is prescribed, the occupational therapist may be called upon to collaborate in other specific ways at certain stages of the treatment.

Contra-indications

Activities which by constant change of technique, increase the patient's confusion or disorientation.

Liaison

Fore-knowledge regarding the history and present condition of the patient is essential for the satisfactory planning of treatment.

REFERENCES AND RECOMMENDED FURTHER READING

1. Lewis, A. J. (1934), Melancholia: A clinical survey of depressive states. *J. Ment. Sci.*, 80, 277.
2. Coppen, A. & Walk, A., *Recent Developments in Schizophrenia*. London, 1967.
3. Willis, J. H. & Bannister, D. (1965), The diagnosis and treatment of schizophrenia. *Brit. J. Psych.*, 111, 1165–1171.

Wing, J. K. & Brown, G. W., *Institutionalism and Schizophrenia*, Cambridge, 1970.
4. Brown, G. W., Bone, M., Dalison, B. & Wing, J. K., *Schizophrenia and Social Care*. Oxford, 1966.
5. Baker, A. A. (1956), Factory in a hospital. *Lancet*, i, 278.
6. MacDougall, A. & Bardon, D. T. (1965), The use of art in a psychiatric hospital. *Occ. Ther.*, **28**, no. 6.
7. Krall, M. (1967), Illustrating myths and legends as a group activity. *Occ. Ther.*, **30**, no. 2.
8. Fish, F. J., *Schizophrenia*. Bristol, 1972.
9. Leyberg, J. T. (1965), A follow-up study of some schizophrenic patients. *Brit. J. Psychiat.*, **111**, 617–624.
10. Post, Felix, *The Clinical Psychiatry of Later Life*. Oxford, 1965.
11. Information can be obtained from *The British Epilepsy Association**.

For Further reading:
Crammer, J., *Practical Treatment in Psychiatry*. Oxford, 1969.
Crowcroft, A., *The Psychotic*. Pelican, 1967.
Fidler, G. S. & Fidler, J. W., *Occupational Therapy*. U.S.A., 1963.
Freeman, H., *Psychiatric Hospital Care*. London, 1965.
Griffiths, R. D. P. (1973) A standardized assessment of the work behaviour of psychiatric patients. *Brit. J. Psychiat.*, **123**, 403–408.
Hays, P., *New Horizons in Psychiatry*. Pelican, 1964.
Laing, R. D., *The Divided Self*. Pelican, 1965.
Sim, M. & Gordon, E. B., *Basic Psychiatry*. London, 1972.
Whitehead, J. M., *Psychiatric Disorders in Old Age*, London, 1974.
World Psychiatric Association Report on *Psychiatric Disorders of the Aged*. Manchester, 1965.
* See Glossary, p. 456.

CHAPTER 16

Occupational Therapy for the Mentally Handicapped

Occupational therapy with mentally handicapped patients requires an approach quite different from that used in most other spheres, and the difference between the mentally ill and those who have 'arrested or incomplete development of mind' [1] must be clearly understood before the underlying principles of treatment can be applied properly.

For patients who are mentally ill the main object of treatment is to restore a function which previously existed, and to return the patient to his former employment and familiar surroundings. For mentally subnormal patients the object of treatment is to develop latent potentialities, and capabilities which have never shown themselves before, and to provide social education which will enable them to take their place with confidence in unfamiliar surroundings.

In a bygone age many of these people would have been usefully employed in a menial capacity on large estates where they would have been subject to strict discipline imposed by various upper servants. Working long hours they would have had little leisure for mischief and, in performing simple manual duties, would have been more or less happily absorbed into a niche where the virtue of blind obedience ranked high above qualities of initiative. The present day social system can no longer absorb employees of limited intelligence in this way, and it is therefore necessary to devise systems of training which will help to fit them for employment under modern conditions. Of recent years, local authorities have opened many more day training centres, sheltered workshops and hostels for the mentally subnormal, and an increasing number of the more stable patients are receiving care in these places, and thus remaining in the community.

It is not the purpose of this chapter to detail the many types of mental subnormality nor the various causes from which they may arise. Such information should be obtained from recognised authorities on the subject [2].

The intention of the ensuing pages is to present methods of treatment from a practical standpoint [3].

Important aspects for consideration in the occupational treatment of the mentally handicapped is not the type, but the degree of deficiency and associated physical disabilities. These factors influence the plan of treatment and the prognosis. Following programmes will be discussed in terms of the classifications which became current on the implementation of the Mental Health Act, 1959, i.e. 'severe subnormality' and subnormality [4].

Occupational therapy with these patients must be of a fairly long-term nature: expectation of quick results will bring disappointment. Although the programme of treatment and consideration of problems must be considered for each patient separately, the psychological needs of the patients and practical necessity demand that the greater part of treatment should be carried out in fairly large groups. The mentally handicapped are inclined to be dependent, and too much individual attention may increase their dependence and produce results which are the opposite of those desired.

Individual treatment may be given initially, but should be withdrawn gradually as the patient becomes absorbed into groups where he will develop latent qualities of initiative or even of leadership.

Apart from the specific programmes discussed efforts should be made to make the environment as good, and experiences as varied, as possible, in order to create an atmosphere conducive to mental stimulation.

The Severely Mentally Subnormal

For the purposes of clarification of the treatment by occupation of the severely mentally subnormal this main group has been divided into two subgroups. The treatment for *the very severely subnormal* covers those who usually have an intelligence quotient (in the terms of the Stanford-Binet rating), below 30, but includes those with a slightly higher level as well. Treatment for *the severely subnormal* relates to those in the range of I.Q.s* between 30 and 50.

The Very Severely Subnormal

Most patients in this group are totally unemployable in any constructive capacity, and are almost entirely dependent on nursing care for their continued existence. In appearance they may exhibit many kinds of gross physical abnormality or may appear almost normal. They are stunted in growth, and frequently assume huddled, crouching postures, apparently oblivious of their surroundings. Others may wander, run about aimlessly or persistently injure themselves. Speech is usually non-existent. A word or phrase may be repeated over and over again parrot fashion, or there may be response with apparent understanding, to the stimulus of a well known word such as 'sweet' or 'dinner', but there is no attempt at sentence construction.

Comprehension of speech is limited, but not as limited as verbal expression, and the tone of voice may convey more than actual words. Patients are often noisy, screaming, grunting and croaking, sometimes to a kind of rhythm. These noises may appear to indicate feelings of anger, pleasure, or hunger, but are often without meaning.

Some patients of this group may be extremely excitable, destructive and spiteful, while others are dully passive and impervious to the aggressive attentions of their neighbours. Their appetite for food is usually insatiable and indiscriminate. They will swallow almost anything they can get into their mouths, regardless of taste, texture or form. They are frequently doubly incontinent and have very degraded habits.

At first glance any training programme for such unpromising material may seem valueless, and indeed the many problems associated with each one of these patients present a real challenge to the ingenuity and faith of the occupational therapist. In some cases it may be necessary to resort to the kind of basic training described in the section on mentally subnormal children (see p. 345). Belief in the fact that improvement can be effected—and it *is* a fact—coupled with a common-sense programme based on routine, perseverance and teaching ability will, however, in time produce really worthwhile results.

The ultimate aims in training such patients—apart from the obvious one of helping them to enjoy life—are to:

(1) Prevent deterioration.
(2) Obviate habits harmful to themselves, to property, or destructive (i.e. picking at their skins, pulling out hair, tearing clothes and smashing furniture, etc.).
(3) Assist in habit training routine.
(4) Encourage purposeful activity and lessen dependence on others for personal help.
(5) Direct activities towards constructive channels if possible.

In order to achieve these aims, it is necessary to:

(*a*) Gain their confidence and so attract attention.
(*b*) Obtain their interest so that they may imitate and cooperate.
(*c*) Stimulate purposeful and coordinated activity.
(*d*) Instruct in useful activities.
(*e*) Instruct in constructive activities.

(*a*) *To gain confidence and attract attention.* This may be a simple matter with some patients who are only too anxious for notice and will show off childishly. Others, however, present a much more difficult problem, as they are unresponsive to any kind of personal contact or variation of environment. In most of these patients there seems to be an almost instinctive response to rhythm, so music with a strong beat may be used as an initial means of obtaining their attention. The first sign of awareness of this external stimulation may be a rocking movement and this slight response should immediately be used, and directed to more positive movements, such as clapping or stamping.

(*b*) *To obtain interest and stimulate coordinated movement.* When this first step has been successfully negotiated, simple forms of movement to music may be introduced, and interest and concentration held by variations of tempo, rhythm and depth of sound. Musical games should be persevered with, and may help to induce a competitive spirit. At this stage, which may have taken many weeks or months to reach, other simple movements and exercises can be devised, and by now some degree of interest should have been obtained. Skipping and simple exercises with balls, using them in gradually reduced sizes, form a useful introduction to activities demanding attention and cooperation. It is advisable, however, to continue to use music with these exercises in order to encourage a habit of rhythmical and ordered movement.

(*c*) *To encourage purposeful movements.* Having obtained a reasonable degree of cooperation from the patients by means of rhythmical activities involving large muscle groups, some attention must be paid to increasing their capacity for smaller and more delicate movements. Percussion band work can form a useful bridge between physical activities and the use of smaller equipment, whilst still retaining the essential stimulus of music and rhythm. The various instruments provide a convenient means of developing hand and eye coordination and at the same time the nature of the performance may promote the idea of organised group activity. More purposeful finger movements may be obtained by the threading of cotton reels or beads and the use of educational toys. These should be graduated in size from large to small as sensitivity to touch improves.

(*d*) *Useful activities.* At this point it may be possible to introduce a simple employment of a useful nature, such as sandpapering various articles for the woodwork group, threading off-cuts of chamois leather for window cleaners, or tearing up paper for use in papier maché.

(*e*) *Constructive activities.* When some proficiency has been reached in these and similar types of elementary employment, very simple craft activities may be tried, in order to inculcate good habits of work. It may then be possible to turn to more realistic employment, and absorb some of these patients into teams of others working on simple industrial projects.

The teaching of everyday skills relating to personal independence may be possible with some patients, such as lacing and tying shoes, manipulating hooks and eyes, buttoning clothes, etc. When teaching such skills, the apparatus used for practising them must always be at the same angle to the patient's body, as the item of clothing in question.

The programme of graded activities outlined here, will not be achieved quickly. Each phase may well take weeks or months to teach, and improvement is often so slow as to be almost imperceptible. A dated record of each patient's achievements should be kept, and it will be seen over a period of months or years that progress really is being made.

The occupational therapy programme for very severely subnormal patients should, then, be governed by the following rules:

Adherence to routine both in habit training and occupation.

Daily physical activities.

Carefully graduated occupations.

Persistent individual and group teaching.

The results of protracted training thus outlined will not produce intelligent patients, but will tend to develop the limited potentialities which are there, and should go a long way towards achieving the objectives for which it is designed.

The Severely Subnormal

In appearance these patients are often small in stature and development with poor carriage and a shambling gait. Various stigmata associated with mental subnormality will be obvious, and expressions may be vacant. They can usually dress themselves, but are untidy, with buttons undone and shoe laces dragging. They are fond of personal adornment and will wear several hair slides, brooches, necklaces and ribbons all at the same time. If left without supervision they speedily revert to a dirty and ill-kempt state. Speech is restricted to the most simple words with childish sentence construction of a factual nature. Diction is usually indistinct, but comprehension of language is, as a rule, slightly in advance of their own performance.

The majority of patients in this group are of a placid and happy disposition, suggestible, childishly anxious to please and willing to make the best of their limited capabilities. Some, however, are excitable and aggressive; others, obstinate, spiteful and destructive; a few seem apathetic and depressed. Their temperamental tendencies usually follow a particular pattern and do not fluctuate so much as with subnormal patients. Firm friendships are formed among themselves, which are usually lasting, and seem founded on real feelings of affection.

For patients of this group it is the function of the occupational therapy department to:

(*a*) Stimulate purposeful and coordinated movement.

(*b*) Increase ability to concentrate.

(*c*) Assess potential employment possibilities.

(*d*) Teach some useful employment technique, if possible.

(*e*) Provide opportunity for social development.

These points, which impinge on one another, will be discussed together.

Long term planning and routine are important for this group of patients, to establish good work habits. A systematic timetable should be planned from the outset. Each activity should be broken down to the simplest level so that such concentration as is available is directed to a movement or sequence of movements within their capacity. Verbal instructions are of little use, as speech is imperfectly understood. Demonstration of a technique or activity is the most useful way to start teaching, and this should be followed immediately by the patients' own endeavours. In teaching it will usually be necessary to invoke the tactile sense, which in itself is often dull and requires educating, and to guide their hands and limbs in the required movements. Such movements may have to be repeated many times before they are correctly achieved by the patients' own volition.

When teaching an activity to these patients it is essential to present the same material in the same set of circumstances each time, with as nearly as possible the same key teaching words. A change of place, or even of the patient sitting near to them, may well upset their concentration and working capacity for a disproportionate amount of time. This distractibility may, however, be used with advantage by the therapist in overcoming temperamental disturbances.

Muscular coordination can be improved by all kinds of simple physical activities, and movement to music is again the greatest possible help in obtaining interest and establishing rhythmical and coordinated movement. Ball games may help to improve coordination, while simple games of a competitive nature may stimulate the capacity for individual effort.

The introduction of activities of a more sedentary nature, depends a great deal on the degree of muscular coordination and control attained. If the patient has been allowed to sit about without activity of any kind, the manipulative power of the fingers and hands may be practically nil. In such cases it may be advantageous to use apparatus of the kind mentioned in the section on mentally subnormal children (see p. 346). Such activities should, however, be resorted to only as a means to an end, and work of a more constructive nature should be encouraged as early as possible.

At this point simple forms of craft activity may be introduced with the following objects in view:

(1) To continue to improve concentration.
(2) To increase manual dexterity.
(3) To encourage methodical work habits.
(4) To instil the feeling of confidence and joy of achievement inherent in the completion of a piece of creative work.
(5) To help in the assessment of future employment potentialities.

The next stage of treatment may be:

(f) Training for specific employment within the hospital.

(*g*) Training for processes of an industrial type.

(*h*) Further varied employment within the occupational therapy department for patients who may have good ability, but whose temperaments preclude their employment in utility departments.

(*i*) A programme of intensive training in self help and employment activities for patients who may return home, or be admitted to a local authority hostel.

These points will be taken separately.

(*f*) *Training for specific employment* within the hospital. The present system of employing special staff to undertake most of the domestic work of the hospitals and hostels for the mentally handicapped, has greatly restricted the opportunities for these patients to make a useful contribution, within their capacities, towards their particular communities.

Simple cleaning processes, such as cleaning cutlery and brass, have been eliminated by the use of modern labour-saving materials, and floor polishing by the use of machines. It is therefore more difficult to find means by which these patients can be usefully employed in the domestic situation.

Many patients of this group may be designated 'unemployable' within the hospital because they cannot switch from one work process to another. Nevertheless, it is possible to teach such patients to do one job efficiently. There are still some spheres where domestic skills can be used, i.e. cleaning baths, basins and windows, making beds, laying tables, sweeping and dusting, etc. These last activities can be used or demonstrated in the wards or in the occupational therapy department. In this context it is necessary for the occupational therapist to discover the greatest needs of the local situation, to collaborate with the staff in charge of other departments and so train the patients to fulfill these needs whenever possible.

(*g*) *Training for processes of an industrial type.* Industrial processes form a useful sphere of activity for selected patients, provided that the needs of the patient never become subservient to those of industry. Patients who are unable to participate in more exacting employment may find satisfaction in the continued performance of the same activity, and the repetitive nature of the work may serve a sedative purpose. Employment in industrial processes may also be expedient under the following conditions:

When it is desired to promote conditions for group training such as would be involved in assembly line production.

When there is the possibility of similar work being undertaken in sheltered workshop conditions if the patient went to live in a hostel or at home.

When suitably chosen work can improve coordination or manual dexterity.

(*h*) *Further employment within the occupational therapy department.* In most large communities of the mentally subnormal, there are some who, because of temperamental or physical disability, need to be employed in an environment where close supervision is combined with a variety of activities, planned with reference to their particular difficulties. Such patients should be kept under constant review with the idea of diverting them to a more realistic employment if and when this is possible.

(*i*) *Intensive training in self help.* When it seems possible that the patient may return home or be transferred to a local authority hostel, every effort must be made to see that he is able to deal with life in such altered circumstances. He should be taught to be as independent of personal help as possible, to make the best use of his work potential, and his programme should include such social training as he is able to assimilate.

So far various methods of increasing the working capacity of the patient along the direct line of work processes have been considered. There are, however, indirect methods of increasing their value from the employment point of view, by developing potential initiative. Probably the best way of doing this is by the continued use of physical training and recreational groups. Patients of this group should have at least one physical training class each week, which should be suitably graded according to their physical condition. As a general principle, the lower the intelligence of patients, the greater should be the proportion of time spent in physical activities. All kinds of games and dancing should be encouraged, and where possible social evenings arranged, which may provide opportunities for the display of individual talent.

Shopping walks, too, provide a useful link with normal everyday activities. The patients usually enter into the spirit of such expeditions with great enthusiasm, and often quite surprising capabilities will emerge from personalities which have hitherto seemed merely passive.

Training of the patient will then, from the occupational therapy aspect, consist of physical, employment and recreational activities, all of which should be fitted into a balanced routine, the whole designed for each patient according to his or her potentialities and his stage of development at any one time.

The Mentally Subnormal

To this group belong those patients with an intelligence quotient of 50 or over. Physically they differ little if at all from normal in appearance, but evidence of their immaturity may be manifest in their mode of dress. This will probably be flamboyant in character, with plentiful adornment on special occasions, but uncared for and untidy in the ordinary course of events. The majority have attended ordinary schools, or those for the educationally subnormal, where they may have made poor progress, but have probably grasped the rudiments of reading, writing and making simple calculations. Their speech can be normal, or may be indistinct because of imperfect articulation. Their vocabulary is poor and they have difficulty in expressing ideas, although they can converse adequately on subject matter within their experience. Comprehension of language is usually good within the same limits.

The general intelligence of this group of patients may not be a great deal below the normal, and in a few cases may even be above, but they are unable to make the best use of the intelligence they possess for one or more of the following reasons:

> Temperamental instability
> Social inadequacy
> Psychopathy

Temperamental Instability

This is one of the most important contributory factors to the inability of this group to remain in employment. Many patients have little control over their emotions, become abusive and give way to outbursts of temper and excitability or, alternatively, become morose and sullen for little or no reason, and with complete disregard for their surroundings. Their moods are variable and will alter rapidly for no adequate cause. They lack qualities of perseverance and thoroughness and are often most unreliable. They may nevertheless express ambitious ideas wholly out of keeping with reality or their own capabilities. Good qualities exist, however, and many are capable of great loyalty to people to whom they become attached and, when sufficiently stabilised for employment, will in certain circumstances identify their own lives with those of their employers. Many, too, are kindly disposed towards children, less able patients and animals, but this quality is unreliable and subject to variation of mood.

Social Inadequacy

The quarrelsome natures of some patients, together with their inability to adapt themselves to changing environments and temperamental vagaries of others, make them difficult people with whom to work or live under normal conditions. Their lack of foresight, ability to plan their lives and sense of responsibility, inevitably leads them to economic disaster unless some kind of supportive care is available.

Psychopathy

A small proportion of patients exhibit symptoms of psychopathic overlay, and will commit the same offences repeatedly. The knowledge that such behaviour is unacceptable to society has no more deterrent effect than the inevitability of repeated punishment.

The aims of occupational therapy with mentally subnormal patients must be to:

(*a*) Return to a normal life those who are capable of becoming self-supporting.

(*b*) Return to their homes those who may be taught to adapt to family life, and perhaps make some contribution towards supporting themselves.

(*c*) Help such patients as will always need the supportive care of the hospital or hostel environment to:

(i) Become useful members of the hospital or hostel community.

(ii) Take part in some kind of sheltered workshop scheme.

(iii) Achieve proficiency in craft or other techniques with the object of upgrading to (i) or (ii) above.

General Treatment

Training towards these specific ends must rest on a foundation of:

Security.
Self confidence.
Good work habits.

Security. The instability of these patients is in itself indicative of a real desire for a secure and stable existence. The occupational therapy department should attempt to meet this need by providing firm discipline and a quiet ordered atmosphere. The integration of the individual into a homogeneous group promotes a feeling of security and a desire for acceptance, which is an invaluable aid to resocialisation. These patients have respect and affection for staff who can control them and direct their activities with confidence and leadership. They despise those who are vacillating and indecisive, and will speedily take advantage of such hesitancy by becoming argumentative and unruly. In spite of repeated pleadings, arguments and grumbles in an attempt to get their own way, they instantly lose confidence in those staff who give way to such coercion. With this group a planned and ordered routine combined with quiet firmness and a satisfactory group relationship is probably the most important foundation of their training.

Self-confidence. In spite of a blustering over-confident demeanour, many patients are unsure of their ability to meet life on equal terms, as are the rather diffident and withdrawn ones. Encouragement in care of personal appearance can help to improve self confidence, as can a sense of personal achievement and acceptance of responsibility. The production of any kind of creative work provides an invaluable means of attaining this feeling of achievement, and the completion of a piece of work admired by others, is in itself evidence of ability to do something well.

When behaviour is reasonably stable, some responsibilities should be given. It matters little that they are relatively insignificant, the point of emphasis is that the patient should be conscious that some aspect of group welfare is dependent on his efficiency.

Good work habits. The future success of the patient in his employment may well depend on the habits of work inculcated during training. The key teaching points are:

> Concentration.
> Perseverance.
> Consistency.

Concentration is dependent in the first place on the degree of interest present, and in the second, upon lack of distraction. It is important, therefore, to take some trouble in finding an activity which is sufficiently unusual to be intriguing but is at the same time in harmony with the patient's interests. Such an activity should be initially presented in circumstances which do not contain distracting or irritating factors, but at a later stage, more distracting conditions may be introduced in order to approximate more closely to a normal working environment. Limited concentration may necessitate alternating periods of active and sedentary occupations, the period of time devoted to one or the other being gradually increased according to the type of employment ultimately envisaged for the patient. There should be specified periods of time allocated to each activity, and the patient should not be allowed to change his occupation except at these times.

Perseverance is a very difficult quality to instil and depends largely on the incentive of a satisfactory goal. In the first instance the activity should be such that the initial step and the ultimate goal are not too far apart. By this means the patient may quickly realise the satisfaction of achievement. The difficulty of the work should be increased gradually, and with it the degree of perseverance necessary for its completion. In many cases the only effective incentive is the personal one of making an article for a relative or friend. No patient should be allowed to leave work unfinished, because enthusiasm has evaporated. Thoughtful planning of a timetable should ensure that the completion of a project, and the start of a further stage in training, should coincide.

A consistently good standard of workmanship is perhaps the most important of all. Concentration and perseverance are useless if the result is work of poor quality. With patients of this group the standard of work produced will be precisely that demanded by the occupational therapist. These patients have the capacity to produce excellent results, but if slovenly and careless work is accepted, only slovenly and careless work will be presented. Work may be simple, but the standard can still be high. It cannot be too strongly emphasised that poor workmanship is indicative of inefficient teaching.

Patients should be encouraged to be critical of their own work and should be taught to strive for improvement. They will appreciate an attitude of discrimination and will respond all the more to praise which is not too easily earned. Criticism must be given tactfully, however, and not in such a way as to discourage further effort. For instance the remark, 'You have done this and this so nicely, it seems a pity to leave this in to spoil it', will usually have the desired effect.

Specific Training

It sounds paradoxical to say that specific training can be outlined only in general terms, but in fact, a specific programme can be compiled for each patient only with regard to his particular potential ability, degree of intelligence and initiative, temperament, and home circumstances. The combination of these factors is infinite, and so it is best to consider a programme of rehabilitation which can be applied to the high grade group in three stages.

The initial stage. Occupational therapy should play the chief role in rehabilitation at this stage and should be a period of observation and assessment. It is necessary to get to know the patient as an individual, and forecast his employment potentialities and social capabilities. Activities used can be any available within the resources of the department, the more varied the scope the better. They should cater for work, social and recreational needs.

The intermediate stage. Here occupational therapy should be considered as supportive and recreational in character. A degree of stability should now be present which will allow for work in less sheltered conditions. Patients should work part-time in the wards and utility departments of the hospital, but should return to the occupational therapy department for continuation classes such as cookery and dressmaking for the girls, or woodwork and general utility classes for boys. Educational classes should also be available where academic possibilities are present. The feeling that they are learning something which will be of use when they leave the hospital does much to keep alive ambition and combat the stagnation of institutional life. Some of the educational programmes on television form a useful basis for discussion groups.

The final stage. Occupational therapy should now take an educational and social form. This should be a period of preparation for a normal mode of living, and employment may be in the utility departments or on a daily basis outside the hospital.

From the educational aspect patients should be prepared for the ordinary problems of day to day living in an entirely practical manner. Most patients at this stage are capable of standards of work which are acceptable to outside employers. Many, however, are far less able to organise their own lives satisfactorily in unfamiliar surroundings, and the transition from hospital care and supervision to personal independence entails many pitfalls.

In the case of female patients particularly, special training in household management is necessary. These patients should be taught to plan their own meals with some regard for a balanced diet and a limited budget. They should be allowed to purchase the raw materials for such meals from the local shops, taught to prepare and cook these, and to understand the perishable nature of some foodstuffs and the correct methods of storing others.

Instruction should be given in ordinary household cleaning operations, and in the use of modern labour saving equipment, such as electric polishers and vacuum cleaners.

Personal appearance and the care of clothes is another important subject, and time should be given to methods of laundering and mending clothes, and again, in the use of washing machines and spin driers. Visits to the local launderette may take place, and instructions given on the types of material to be taken to be dry-cleaned, and those which can be drip-dried.

Advice and demonstrations can be given on hair styling, makeup and other forms of personal care, and attempts made to divert rather exaggerated tastes into less flamboyant- but not necessarily less fashionable-channels.

Many patients are unused to travel on public transport and need practice in making bus and train journeys. It is helpful to provide them with various commissions which will necessitate making journeys by public transport into unfamiliar territory, so that they may gain confidence in finding their way about.

It is useful, too, to teach them to use public telephones, as the knowledge that they can, if necessary, communicate quite quickly with the hospital, gives them added confidence when they leave.

Some instruction may be given in methods of obtaining employment, and in making the best of themselves when being interviewed for a job. Guidance may also be given on the management of their financial affairs, including such items as methods of saving, the uses of insurance, and the uses and dangers of hire purchase.

It is often an advantage to arrange a series of talks, perhaps on such subjects as beauty care or floral decoration, as apart from the actual content of the talk, a visitor from outside the hospital will always have a stimulating effect. Interest and discussion will also be stimulated by the showing of films and filmstrips applicable to the content of the training programme outlined above.

The scope of such training is enormous, and the point at which it should start, and the length to which it should go, can be determined only on a strictly individual basis according to the degree of intelligence present and the length of time that has been spent in what may have been an over sheltered environment.

Social activities should demand something more than mere participation in dancing or visits to a cinema, and should require some effort on the part of the patients themselves in preparing and organising various informal functions. Community life inevitably results in a dimming of originality and initiative, and social occasions should provide an opportunity for resuscitating these qualities. Recreational activities should be available on a voluntary basis, and may merge with the social programme, although opportunity should always exist for more individual forms of recreation, such as reading, gardening and personal hobbies, should these be required. The formation and development of a social club for this type of patient, would be a project well worth the consideration of the occupational therapist, and would present numerous opportunities for indicating various points of behaviour expected on social occasions.

From the foregoing, it may be seen that occupational therapy with the mentally subnormal will depend for its success largely on the teaching skill and personal drive of the therapist. It may therefore be appropriate to conclude by emphasising certain fundamental points.

(1) Every activity should be assigned to a patient as part of a plan of treatment, with a definite objective in view.

(2) Each activity should be just within the patient's capacity, so that he is neither bored by its simplicity nor discouraged by its difficulty. On the whole it is better that it should be a little too easy than a little too difficult. A discouraged patient loses confidence in himself *and* the therapist.

(3) Prepare activities for every patient before they arrive at the department so that they can start work with a minimum of fuss. An unemployed patient is a potentially troublesome one.

(4) Avoid lengthy explanations when teaching a new activity—speech is imperfectly understood. Directions should be brief and simple.

(5) Use demonstration as a main method of teaching; things seen are remembered much longer than those heard.

(6) Allow plenty of opportunity for gaining the feel of the medium in which the patient is to work.

(7) Progression should be planned in a series of carefully graded steps.

Conscientious and energetic teaching, positive enthusiasm and a thoughtful choice of activity, can produce results in the rehabilitation of these patients which are most satisfying, and sometimes quite surprising.

A considerable amount of research has been done in recent years in the training of the mentally subnormal by Drs O'Conner and Tizard, and members of the social psychiatry unit of the Medical Research Council, and by Drs A. D. B. and A. Clarke at the Manor Hospital, Epsom. Dr H. C. Gunzburg at Monyhull Hall has also done some work on education and social rehabilitation of the mentally subnormal. For references to useful publications, see below.

REFERENCES

1. *Mental Health Act*, 1959, 4 (2), p. 2.
2. See:
   Bender, C. E., *Mongolism and Cretinism*. New York, 1949.
   Burt, C., *The Subnormal Mind*. London/Oxford, 1955.
   Burt, C., *The Backward Child*. London, 1958.
   Curran, D. & Partridge, M., *Psychological Medicine*. Edinburgh and London, 1972.
   Hilliard, L. T. & Kirman, B. H., *Mental Deficiency*. London, 1957.
   O'Conner, N. & Tizard, J., *The Social Problem of Mental Deficiency*. London, 1956.
   Penrose, L. S., *The Biology of Mental Defect*. London, 1972.
   Tredgold, R. F. & Soddy, K., *Textbook of Mental Deficiency*. London, 1963.
3. And see:
   Gibson, J. & French, T., *Nursing the Mentally Retarded*. London, 1974.
   Gunzburg, H. C., *Social Rehabilitation of the Subnormal*. London, 1960.
   Gunzburg, H. C., *Social Competence and Mental Handicap*. London, 1968.
   Hallas, C. H., *The Care and Training of the Mentally Subnormal*. Bristol, 1974.
   Morgenstern, M., Low-Beer, H. & Morgenstern, F., *Practical Training for the Severely Handicapped Child*. London, 1966.
   Segal, S. S., *No Child is Ineducable*. Oxford, 1967.
   Stevens, M., *Observing Children who are Severely Subnormal*. London, 1968.
4. *Mental Health Act*, 1959, pp. 2 and 3, 4 (2), and (3).
   And see:
   Better Services for the Mentally Handicapped, Department of Health and Social Security*, H.M.S.O.*, 1971.
   The Team Approach, National Society for Mentally Handicapped Children*, London, 1971.
   Holland can show us how to care for the subnormal. *Occ. Ther.*, 35, no. 9, 1972.
   Role of the occupational therapist in the field of mental handicap. *Occ. Ther.*, 36, no. 9, 1973.
   Occupational therapy at a school for the retarded. *Occ. Ther.*, 37, no. 8, 1974.
* See *Glossary*, pp. 454-6.

Part Four

CHAPTER 17

Occupational Therapy for Children and Adolescents with Psychological Disorders

---

The occupational therapist can play a vital role in the treatment of children and adolescents with psychological disorders. The selection of suitable therapists to undertake this specialised work is of prime importance. The criteria for selection are:

(*a*) A warm person who has had a stable and happy upbringing.
(*b*) A real understanding of and experience with children and adolescents.

As the variety of psychiatric illness in young people is wide, it is proposed here to divide the types of disability into five main groups:

(1) Subnormal and severely subnormal children.
(2) Children with brain damage.
(3) Psychotic children.
(4) Emotionally disturbed children.
(5) Emotionally disturbed adolescents.

Subnormal and Severely Subnormal Children [1]

The statutory definition of subnormality is given on p. 246. Since April 1971 the Department of Education has been legally responsible for the education of all children, including the severely subnormal who were previously catered for by the Health Service or Mental Health Department of the Local Authority. There are, however, children who are too disturbed or handicapped, among them those suffering from spasticity, autism, etc., who are not able to benefit from the teaching environment, and may well be referred to hospitals or special centres, and will require treatment from an occupational therapist.

In estimating the future of subnormal children from the social and employment aspects, a child with an intelligence quotient of 40 and a stable and equable temperament, is likely to be more successful in life than one with a much higher I.Q.* who is restless, unstable, and exhibits anti-social behaviour.

Severely subnormal children present problems based on innate or acquired defects, possibly exacerbated by lack of awareness and understanding on the part of parents or teachers. They manifest themselves in:

(1) Reduced sensory awareness.
(2) Extreme slowness in learning.
(3) Poor muscular coordination.
(4) Speech difficulties.
(5) Complete inertia or extreme over-activity.
(6) Behaviour difficulties, often in an exaggerated form.

A common cause of lack of success with these children is an inability to 'get down to their level'. The physically well-developed boy of about ten years of age, who persistently throws everything on the floor, has, in reality, a mental age of, perhaps only one year old, and is reacting in a way which is *normal for his mental age*.

Treatment must begin at the very roots of learning[2]: there are no short cuts, and no substitute for dogged persistence. The aims of treatment are:

(1) To prevent deterioration.
(2) To help the children to become less of a nursing problem.
(3) To train them to make the best use of the ability they possess.

TREATMENT AND TRAINING OF SEVERELY SUBNORMAL CHILDREN[3]

This corresponds to that part of the child's life where, if normal, he would be gathering experiences on which to base further learning. The initial training includes development of:

> Play
> Manual dexterity
> Sensory perceptions
> Response to stimuli

Organisation of Treatment

Repetition of a known pattern provides the child with an essential feeling of security. Treatment should take place within a framework which does not vary, but with enough flexibility to allow for individual interests and variations in concentration. Physically active and sedentary occupations should alternate, and the length of each session be determined by the interest and concentration shown.

Individual attention may be necessary where instruction in some particular skill is the aim, but it is the group situation which contributes most to the development of such essential attributes as self-confidence and social competence. Too much individual attention may encourage the child to lean too heavily on the therapist, and thus limit his own initiative and personal effort. Competing with other children at the same level, and finding his own niche in a community geared to his own rate of progress, provides a social climate in which he can realise his particular potential to the full.

Play

The capacity for play is inherent in normal children, but often needs active encouragement in severely subnormal children. First toys should be large, and include wheel toys, building bricks, large balls, push and pull, and cuddly toys.

Although jealously guarded, there will be no real attempt at play. Often mere possession of a toy is all-sufficient. Imagination will be non-existent, or poorly developed. Children must be encouraged to handle different kinds of toys so as to experience variations in the quality of their 'feel', and by manipulating moving toys, begin to make a relationship between themselves and space. This fundamental ability commonly develops very slowly. Sand and water play should be encouraged, as much may be learned in terms of quantity and volume from using various pouring vessels and sand tools. Contrasting textures stimulate an almost irresistible urge to play in most children.

Manual Dexterity

Educational toys. The function of these toys, which are extensions of those developed by Montessori, are twofold:

(1) *To provide interesting and manipulative exercises*, encouraging muscular control and coordination. This includes hammer pegs, screwing toys and bead threading, which, when graded in size, can produce a delicate scale of finger movements.
(2) *To present, in concrete form, abstract thought processes*, by presenting opportunities for exercising powers of discrimination. This includes a variety of toys in which colours, shapes, sizes, quantity and volume must be compared, like ones sorted out, and differences noted.

Sensory Perception

Although in these children the special sense organs are apparently physically sound, the impact of sensory sensation seems to be dulled. Practice in the use of their senses is given, in order to make them more aware of their potential, particularly of touch, hearing and sight.

Touch. The ultimate degree of independence will depend on the child's ability to handle materials. Dressing, for instance, requires a combination of muscular coordination, control and delicacy of touch. Practice may be given in feeling different substances by putting various objects in a bag and asking a child to pick one out while blindfolded. Other exercises of this kind may be devised.

Hearing. Increased incidence of true deafness is unlikely but the poverty of these children's vocabulary and imperfect diction suggests that the impact of sounds they hear is greatly reduced. They must, therefore, be taught to listen. This can be done in a variety of ways, by use of the percussion band and discrimination between instruments, by a blindfolded child trying to catch another who is ringing a bell, and by listening for some tiny sound in complete silence, etc.

Sight. The use of colour provides the most convenient method of exercising this sense. Most toys are painted in primary colours. Other colours are introduced gradually, and progression is made by matching shades and tones. Peg boards can be used for colour matching in the early stages, and, later, coloured papers, crayons and paints introduced.

Taste and smell, are senses of rather less importance in the training programme, but can be discriminated with food at meal times.

Response to Stimuli

The rate of response of these children is in direct ratio to their degree of intelligence. They may be encouraged to respond more quickly by the use of certain exercises. The initial stimulus may be loud and sudden, a blast on a whistle or the beat of a drum, at which signal the children should perform some simple action quickly. This may be made into a game. Later, there may be exercises with speech as the stimulus, and the children required to act quickly on instructions such as 'Hands on heads', 'Stand up', etc., each instruction to be given in quick succession, in a brisk tone of voice. These exercises can also be given to chairbound patients.

Development of Abstract Thought Processes

The child, having been given a background of experience which encourages him to appreciate the scope of his sensory organs, and to gain some idea of spatial relationships, needs then to develop abstract thought processes, on which learning ability will later depend. In order to learn, one must be able to develop:

Concentration
Observation
Memorisation
Use Imagination
Draw reasonable conclusions from given facts

(1) *Concentration.* The span of attention of the severely subnormal child may be only momentary, and these moments should be extended by appealing to his interests. Play with a chosen toy should be encouraged and the length of play increased daily. The toy should be changed occasionally so that play does not become a meaningless habit. Jig-saw puzzles can improve concentration.

(2) *Observation.* Nature walks and demonstrations of growing plants, watching bird tables, discussions on recent outings or a new wall picture, etc., encourage this habit.

(3) *Memorisation.* Here the subject learned should be understood, and for the hospital-based child, care must be taken to talk about things he can understand or see. Simple memory games, with frequent repetition of material already learned, helps to train the memory.

(4) *Use of imagination.* Apart from rote learning, the intelligent application of learning processes is largely dependent on imaginative ability. With few exceptions, the mentally subnormal child exhibits little evidence of active imagination, preferring to reproduce ideas presented by others. To stimulate imagination and encourage initiative in an active way, such activities as dressing-up, acting out stories, puppetry and music to movement are useful, while on a more passive plane, painting, modelling and other art forms may help to bring about imaginative and original thought.

(5) *Reasoning and judgment.* The use of constructive toys demonstrates the need for forethought. The child learns that if he is assembling a toy successfully the pieces must be put together in a certain order. Here he is beginning to use powers of judgment and reasoning, and until this stage has been reached, he cannot benefit from more formal methods of teaching.

The foregoing plan of treatment must be supplemented and reinforced by many other activities of a nursery school character. Physical education is most important. The more severely subnormal the child, the greater the need for stimulation by physical activity. Gross movements are encouraged at first and when some degree of muscular control has been achieved, more precise and coordinated movements are expected.

The provision of attractive equipment such as steps, slides, stilts, climbing and balancing apparatus, appeals to the sense of adventure, which, often due to over-protection, is apt to be dulled. Scooters, pedal cars, and bicycles provide further incentives towards achieving a sense of balance and coordinated movement.

The use of music is a great stimulus to movement, and may be used to increase or decrease activity by changes in mood and rhythm. Singing games introduce the idea of cooperative play, while simple dances are an extension of the cooperative aspect and require efforts of concentration, memory and control. Team games are usually more suitable for older children.

Self-help and Self-expression

Personal independence should be encouraged as early as possible. As soon as sufficient muscular control and coordination has developed the child should be taught to dress and undress himself and manipulate various fastenings. The use of buttoning and tying frames should be avoided: it is always best to use his own clothes, or a garment specially made for teaching purposes, with different types of fastenings in appropriate places. Toilet training can be helped by adherence to strict routine, and it is essential that there should be cooperation with any existing habit training programme.

Most severely subnormal patients enjoy helping with ordinary household tasks, and should be encouraged to do so. Further treatment, and training of more able children, will proceed on simple educational lines and must provide for social development and increase of contact with the outside world. Experiences must be as rich and varied as circumstances will permit, and should include excursions to local towns and villages, travel by public transport, visits to places of interest and shopping expeditions.

Speech may be non-existent or confined to one or two ill-pronounced words. Even if referred to a speech therapist, speech therapy may be supplemented by exercises planned in consultation with the speech therapist and designed to strengthen the lips and soft palate, and facilitate tongue movement. Such exercises involve the use of blowing games with bubble pipes or table-tennis balls, while suction may be instigated with the aid of drinking straws. Tongue movements can be stimulated by the use of mirrors, but such exercises should be of short duration. Above all, the therapist's own speech should be clearly and deliberately articulated. It sometimes happens that a child is able to speak, but shows a marked reluctance to do so. Puppetry may help here, the child identifying himself with the puppet character, and losing his own self-consciousness in the process. Play acting may have the same effect.

Behaviour Problems

Behaviour difficulties are numerous, but more difficult to deal with than in normal children, because severely subnormal children are self centred and have no sense of right or wrong, unless this is conditioned. A year old baby in a tantrum can be put into a cot until he recovers, but a physically well-developed twelve year old, showing similar reaction to frustration, can be a real danger to other children.

The most effective method of dealing with outbursts of uncontrollable temper is to isolate the child for a short time. He then ceases to be the centre of interest, and his frustrations can burn themselves out without damage to others. He will soon begin to feel isolated, and wish to return to the group. He can then be given some occupation within his scope, which will earn him praise at a suitable moment, underlining the point that socially acceptable behaviour brings its own reward. Anti-social behaviour such as window breaking, furniture smashing, stone throwing and persistent running away, can reach epidemic proportions if not checked at the outset. Further information on treatment for temperamental instability and social inadequacy of the mentally subnormal is given in chapter 16.

Children with Brain Damage

Brain damage may be connected with epilepsy, tuberculous meningitis, encephalitis and other rare conditions, or traumata such as accidents to the head or birth injuries. Children with brain damage may manifest severe behaviour or intellectual problems which will obviously vary with the location and extent of the damage. They may also have epileptic attacks with abnormal encephalogram findings, or show such findings without fits. Severe and permanent personality change is not uncommon, and normal social development may be arrested by general excitability, and uncontrollable temper outbursts during which such children may be most aggressive and destructive. There is often a hypersensitivity in personal relationships; and a lack of emotional control which makes them unable to resist provoking other children until they are themselves attacked in retaliation. They may show poor self-awareness and a lack of muscular coordination which makes them not only clumsy but accident prone. In relation to their educational development they are handicapped by marked distractibility and perseveration in speech and activity; as well as showing very severe visuo-perceptual difficulties.

A large proportion of severely brain damaged children suffer intellectual defect and are treated in hospitals or centres for the subnormal, and the student should refer to this section for details of occupational therapy. It is of the utmost importance that the degree of impairment be assessed so that suitable rehabilitation may be planned; the children may need more individual attention than is usually recommended for subnormal or severely subnormal patients [4].

Post-encephalitic states in children may result in restraint being in complete abeyance resulting in wayward or criminal behaviour such as thieving and sexual assaults. Such children are difficult to control and many are eventually confined to hospital, where a full occupational therapy programme is essential, to include plenty of exercise.

Cases with minimal injury [5] may be presented as behaviour problems and much care and skill may be required in differential diagnosis. In dealing with such cases the occupational therapist trained in observation can be of great assistance through her special knowledge of child development and patterns of play. These children may show apparently psychotic features in their behaviour, particularly where cerebral injury causing visual disturbance leads to abnormalities of visual behaviour.

As the treatment of brain damaged children is a highly complex and specialised sphere of work, an occupational therapist is advised to have had, if possible, experience of working with normal, psychotic, emotionally disturbed and subnormal children, first.

Psychotic Children

The term 'childhood psychosis' includes a variety of psychotic conditions, and opinions differ as to whether child psychotics are a homogenous group or include cases arising from varied aetiologies. To avoid confusion here, the term 'childhood psychosis' is used to indicate schizophrenic-like states found in childhood, and the term 'infantile autism' is used to describe the syndrome first recorded by Leo Kanner. Two aspects of occupational therapy are described here:

(1) General treatment of the psychotic child.
(2) Specialised treatment in early infantile autism.

GENERAL TREATMENT OF THE PSYCHOTIC CHILD

Many theories are advanced as to the cause of childhood psychosis, and lack of certainty means that treatment must continue in the light of known symptoms and the problems experienced. Its purpose is to improve behaviour and allay mental deterioration. The occupational therapist may be asked to treat psychotic children who are too young for admission to the hospital school, or those in need of special treatment because of a high degree of disturbance.

Difficulties of Psychotic Children

Psychotic children may have the following difficulties in varying degrees and combinations:

(1) *Disturbed relationships with people.* These children are aloof, exhibiting visual avoidance, and finding difficulty in forming attachments and mixing with other children. They appear preoccupied, stare into space, and do not exhibit their feelings.

(2) *Speech*, may be retarded through delay or regression. Echolalia may be present among children who do speak and prenominal reversal is common. Non-speaking psychotic children often make their needs known by taking the person to the desired object.

(3) *Ritualistic and compulsive phenomena.* Psychotic children are often ritualistic and appear to be striving to keep the environment or situations the same. The children form abnormal attachments for a particular object and become intensely upset if it is mislaid. They perform repetitive acts, e.g. dangling shoe laces, threads, etc. This appears to be some attempt to block out reality.

(4) *Motor phenomena.* These children may be hyperkinetic and show marked stereotyped repetitive movements, exhibiting complicated hand and finger mannerisms.

(5) *Perceptual difficulties.* The most striking feature is an apparent lack of response to sounds: children are often referred because of apparent deafness. They frequently show a failure to respond to pain appropriately.

(6) *Concentration* is poor, showing a marked lack of persistence and a short attention span.

(7) *Temper tantrums* may be precipitated by interruption of obsessive and other stereotyped behaviour. The children are easily frustrated by failure to communicate and understand, and are prone to self-injury through head banging, pulling out hair and tearing at their faces.

(8) *Intelligence.* As these children may function as mentally retarded it is difficult to measure the intelligence quotient, and there may be a variation in the results of different tests. The child is often untestable on verbal tests but does well in those requiring manipulative or visuo-spatial skills. The pattern of intellectual function suggests that there is a defect in the use and comprehension of language.

The Aim of Treatment

This is to stimulate social, intellectual and emotional progress, to help the child become happier, to overcome his difficulties and to develop his potential to the highest possible point. The environment must be sufficiently attractive to the child to keep him in contact with reality long enough to learn from it, and to want to be part of it. This needs time, skill, ingenuity and patience on the part of the therapist, and progress may be slow and frustrating. At first, there may be no response from the child but the therapist must persist until a warm relationship is formed and the child does things to please and be praised.

It is desirable that the psychotic child should receive both individual and group occupational therapy, the former taking precedence in the initial stages with a gradual introduction into a small homogenous group. At first, the child has no desire to please and tends to use people as tools or as 'cuddle machines'. He does not seem to notice or comprehend things in his environment as normal children do, and he picks on objects which are useful to him in his preoccupations, to the exclusion of other useful material, although tactile and kinaesthetic senses seem well developed. The child experiences many teaching difficulties because of perceptual problems, a 'built in' resistance to learning and the habit of opting out of difficult situations.

Perceptual abnormalities necessitate special methods. The environment must be structured and organised, for psychotic children do not progress in the permissive atmosphere of a normal nursery school. They must not be overwhelmed with stimulative materials for they do not know how to play or to learn through play and store experience for future use. It may be necessary to help a child learn basic everyday skills such as dressing himself, tying shoe laces, taking himself to the toilet and washing himself. Practice in these skills prepares him for more complex procedures. The therapist must use simple, clear speech, giving uncomplicated single instructions, often teaching the meaning of 'sit down', 'shut the door', etc. Ingenuity and patience are needed to break down instructions and techniques to fundamentals, repeating them at frequent intervals. Often, too, the finer movements must be educated and much of the Montessori apparatus is useful and brings many senses into play, combining touch, sound and vision (see also p. 347).

Group Treatment with Psychotic Children

A useful method has been devised using a programme which can be followed through each week, as these children appear to benefit from a structured routine and environment. They should be divided into small groups with a high staff/patient ratio. The programme includes activities such as habit training, music, including percussion band, physical training, music and movement, clay, sand and water play, painting, cookery, gardening, pet-keeping, craft subjects, and work with apparatus designed to develop muscular dexterity, improve visuo-perceptual powers and to give a conception of size, colour, shape and quantity. The following facilities are required in the department:

(1) A work or teaching area.
(2) A section for messy activities.
(3) A quiet room, devoid of too many extraneous stimuli, to which a child can retreat at times from a rather puzzling, chaotic world, or where he can be given some 'cuddle therapy'.

As in all branches of occupational therapy, it is essential to work as a member of a team under medical supervision, discussing problems of handling, treatment and progress. Work in conjunction with the hospital school would call for the exchange of ideas and information so as to maintain a consistency of approach. Careful and detailed reports should be kept of the progress made and methods used, for scientific evaluation of the work done. The following points are useful to consider when reporting on progress:

    (1) *Social relationships.*

        (*a*) To other adults.

        (*b*) To other children.

Note whether the child responds better alone or in a group and observe difficulties created by group stress.

    (2) *Affective state* as shown by either emotional flattening, emotional lability, temper tantrums or aggressive behaviour.

    (3) *Intelligence.*

        (*a*) Ability to learn new skills.

        (*b*) Ability to overcome difficulties.

        (*c*) Memory.

    (4) *Interests and concentration span*; also relation with reality.

    (5) *Motor abilities* and any special aptitudes.

    (6) *Range of activities* and fluctuations of fitness for work or play.

Note the work habits and approach to material, i.e. whether unduly destructive, meticulous or constructive.

    (7) *Sensory development.* Note any visual or auditory avoidance and speech patterns; mannerisms or stereotopies; whether habit training has been established or whether regressive behaviour such as incontinence of faeces or urine is present.

SPECIALISED TREATMENT IN EARLY INFANTILE AUTISM

A great many children are referred under the diagnosis of autism when, in fact, they are brain-damaged, subnormal or have other handicaps associated with 'autistic' behaviour. A difficult task is the initial assessment as to whether or not the child has 'Kanner's syndrome', and might benefit from the type of treatment outlined below, which is specific to one occupational therapy department, factors of which may, however, also be used elsewhere.

Nature of Disease

In 1943 Leo Kanner first described the syndrome of early infantile autism [6]. He listed five characteristics, namely:

    (1) The inability to relate to people from the beginning of life.

    (2) Failure to use language in order to communicate.

    (3) An obsession for maintaining sameness.

    (4) Preoccupation with bits of objects.

    (5) Evidence of good cognitive potentialities.

Later, he cut it down to two:

- (1) An extreme isolation.
- (2) An obsessive insistence on preservation of sameness.

Principles of Treatment

The aim of treatment is to establish a warm relationship with the isolated child, and through this, to encourage the development of speech [7], social skills, and purposeful activity. The child is brought into the hospital for up to one year and has daily intensive therapy for one hour each day, in the setting of a total therapeutic programme.

Pre-assessment and Selection

The following should be considered:

- (1) Age (under five for a better prognosis).
- (2) Behaviour which appears primarily withdrawn rather than bizarre.
- (3) Stereotypes, which should decrease in intensity and frequency when the child is in isolation [8]. The reverse is true in brain damage.
- (4) Agility, and ethereal physical beauty.
- (5) Gaze aversion: they do not look into peoples' eyes and reciprocally, dislike being looked at.
- (6) Obsessionality and dexterity in manipulating objects.

Recording of Progress

Daily notes should be kept so that trends of progress can be assessed. It is also helpful if other therapists can observe treatment sessions through a two-way screen, to monitor progress objectively. The therapist should include the mother of the autistic child as much as possible by describing in detail to her what is happening in each session. The mother is generally extremely distressed and feels guilty in being unable to establish a primary relationship with her own child. She wishes to learn the skills of the therapist so that she may be the therapist but it must be explained to her that the child needs to form a unique and new relationship with a stranger.

Treatment

Autistic children are believed to be in a continual state of high cortical arousal [9] despite the paradoxical indifference of their behaviour. They are mute and are often thought to be deaf, probably because this state limits sensory input most of the time to a single sense modality, predominantly that of vision. Treatment is therefore carried out in a quiet, small room, devoid of excess stimuli, furnished only with a soft grey mattress, carpet, wall mirror, foam cubes and a sac-chair. Toys are carefully selected to cover the developmental stages from birth to the present age of the child and placed in a box with a feeding bottle, filled with orange juice.

These children are resistant to change. The therapist therefore encounters the child at precisely the same time each day. The sessions are ritualised. The therapist wears the same overall, shoes and hair-style each day and the room and toys are arranged in the same way. The therapist sits well behind the child, opposite the wall mirror: in this way both can observe each other indirectly, in their reflections. The therapist makes no attempt to 'gaze fixate' [10] or speak unnecessarily, so the child is introduced to what would seem to be an ideal situation which make no demands on him.

The child is allowed to investigate the room, the therapist, the toys and the feeding bottle, in his own time, and the therapist responds only when asked to interact by the child, either by:

(1) Playing with the toys and simple games which require some sort of physical contact.
(2) Echoing any verbalisation, or adding simple, further explanation or stress to any vocabulary used by the child.

In the second month of treatment the feeding bottle becomes of primary importance in establishing the relationship:

(1) It is something the therapist can give the child, who, until now, has seemed totally aloof and to have no need of other people.
(2) It is comforting and relaxing to the child who cuddles up to the breast.

The child may also be in nappies, as autistic children are particularly slow to become toilet trained. After a period of regression back to the bottle the child can gradually be 'potty trained' by the nursing staff, alongside his progression in treatment.

Having established some contact with the child, 'rough and tumble' play becomes important. Contrary to what one would think, autistic children like being tickled, 'rough-housed', and growled at. The child spends less of the session with the bottle and can be weaned onto a cup. The child begins to 'gaze fixate' the therapist and she, in turn, with reciprocal shyness, can begin to 'gaze fixate' him, as a means of communication.

A child who has been totally mute will go through pre-speech noises. When speech comes it is slow and echolalic.

When the child feels secure with his therapist he will venture outside the treatment room for increasing periods of exploration before running back to her. It is convenient if a small group of nursery age children can be playing outside the treatment room so that the autistic child can gradually join them with his therapist. Other therapists are present so that the autistic child can be weaned from his therapist upon whom he has become dependent. When he has established more relationships with adults he is able to join in with other children. Simultaneously with progress with his therapist runs improvement, in his daily interactions with other people and his mother.

Simple nursery activities are encouraged, such as painting, sand and water play, cooking, feeding rabbits, etc., to stimulate speech and enable the child to progress to a normal nursery playgroup on discharge. Success is achieved when the child positively rejects the therapist in preference for his parents.

Conclusion. Because one is anxious for the child to have made as much progress as possible before leaving hospital, it is a temptation to put pressure on him to achieve as much as possible both in verbal and social attainments. However, if one has managed to establish one warm relationship, then one has done something towards putting his basic emotions in order. Upon this he can build other attainments at his own pace, and somewhat more independently, provided there is no undue pressure, which might counteract the improvement achieved.

Emotionally Disturbed Children

The occupational therapist's work in this field is closely interrelated with that of the psychiatrist, psychologist, and social worker. The emphasis is on the treatment of the whole family in the widest possible way, drawing when necessary upon all the available facilities within the community. This is *family psychiatry* [11].

Symptoms of Emotional Disturbance in Children

A useful classification of symptoms of emotional disturbance in children considers them under three main headings:

(1) *Mood changes:* anxiety, apathy, lack of concentration, shyness, phobias, compulsions, etc.
(2) *Psychosomatic (i.e. physical) symptoms:* enuresis, encopresis, skin troubles, asthma, etc.
(3) *Behaviour symptoms; temper tantrums:* delinquency, inability to concentrate, etc.

Inevitably, on investigation there will always be more symptoms beside the original presenting ones.

The Function of Occupational Therapy in Family Psychiatry

Investigation. The practice of family psychiatry requires an initial investigation into the psychodynamics of the whole family. This involves an understanding of the adult point of view, and an appreciation of the 'child's eye' view of family relationships. The occupational therapist endeavours to obtain this view, by using the techniques of *play observation* and *play diagnosis*.

(1) *Play observation* consists in observing the child systematically in a free play situation. An objective assessment is obtained by which the parent's report on his behaviour can be evaluated. With small children it is sometimes advisable to have both mother and child together in the playroom, as a vivid first-hand picture of the mother-child relationship can thus be obtained.

(2) *Play diagnosis* has a twofold aim:

(*a*) To encourage the child to reveal what he knows about himself, and his relationship with family, school and neighbourhood.

(*b*) To encourage him to reveal his problems as he sees them.

In diagnostic interviews the following types of play are useful:

(1) Wendy house and doll play.
(2) Grecon people used in conjunction with a doll's house and furniture.
(3) Glove puppets.
(4) Water and sand play.
(5) Dressing up.
(6) Drawing and painting.

It is usual to check the information disclosed through one medium, by that disclosed through another, since emphasis is placed upon the child's general pattern of response towards the figures around him, rather than upon a specific reaction.

Long Term Therapy

When a child is referred to the occupational therapist for long term therapy the psychiatrist gives her a brief outline of the case, the symptoms and the aims of treatment, and progress is discussed in weekly sessions. The occupational therapist's first aim is to establish rapport with the child. The initial approach varies with each case, but throughout the treatment with young children, play is the medium through which a relationship is built up. Within the security of this relationship the child can talk freely about himself and his problems. With older children a similar relationship is effected through craftwork, music, keeping of pets, stamp collecting, painting, etc. There are four main aims in using long term therapy:

(1) To support the child while the parents receive treatment.
(2) To support the child when the environment cannot be changed, or when he cannot be separated from it.

(3) To help separate the child from his parents, e.g. in preparation for placement in a boarding school or foster home.

(4) To influence a change in the child's personality.

The last aim requires a particularly strong relationship with the therapist. This allows the child to express his phantasies, fears and guilt, enabling him to share his feelings with the therapist, who offers him encouragement and help to resolve his problems.

Illustration of Play Therapy

In order to illustrate what actually happens in long term therapy, through play, there follows a brief description of the series of play therapy interviews, undertaken by the occupational therapist with an eight-year-old boy.

J was referred by his general practitioner because of:

(1) Attacks of breath holding, several causing him to become blue in the face and even to pass out completely.

(2) Backwardness at school, although he was of average intelligence.

J had a middle-class background. Father, hardworking successful business man, only able to give limited attention to his children. Basically a warm and affectionate person. Mother anxious and insecure with marked emotional difficulties.

J the 'middle child' having an older brother and younger sister. Mother always had a Nanny for the children, but felt a special responsibility for J who was more sensitive and difficult than the others. She therefore tried to give more time and attention to him with disastrous results.

Rapport building interviews. At the initial interview J, although tense and shy, accompanied the therapist willingly to the playroom. The therapist concentrated on putting J at ease. J mentioned some of his toys at home. He wanted to paint a picture. The therapist suggested that he should paint a picture of his home and the people who lived there. J accepted and spoke quite vividly about his home and family. Then J wanted to play with the water tray; he enjoyed pouring and squirting the water. He needed considerable assurance from the therapist to deal with each new situation. It was comparatively easy to make a relationship with J; with many children it is much harder and may take a number of sessions to win the child's confidence.

'Trying out' interviews. The next few interviews were essentially 'trying out' ones. As J became more secure he indulged in more messy play, using water, sand and clay. Occasionally J became over-excited, particularly while playing with the water. The therapist quietened him down by putting her arm round him, remaining calm herself. J found this physical contact reassuring. He tried various methods of prolonging the interviews, but the therapist was definite about stopping at the end of an hour. If J were engrossed in his play, she would warn him ten minutes before the end.

Steps in therapy. The therapist saw J for 42 individual one hour interviews. He became increasingly at ease with the therapist and was able to express, through play and through direct verbal communication, how he felt about his life experiences.

Description of early interview. J selected a large teddy bear, with whom he seemed to identify. The bear had a tough time of it, and was ordered about by J. He next used the bear as a model for a series of paintings. He painted a picture of the bear alone, and then a number of illustrations of the bear and his family. These were bright, happy pictures—Father and Mother bear, with a number of young bears prancing around them. J was meticulous in the execution of these paintings, setting himself a high standard. J also did two very gloomy oppressive pictures of the bear, in a greeny-brown colour.

He did a clay model of the bear: and made liberal use of a rolling pin and knife in constructing him, showing a considerable amount of aggression. The therapist was expected to act the part of the bear. J would say, 'There, how does *that* feel?' and the therapist would call out, 'Ouch, Ouch, it hurts.' When completed, the bear had a very aggressive look about him! Towards the end of another session, J picked up an armful of dolls and toy animals, stuffed them into the toy oven and shut the door. Once again he became aggressive. He asked the therapist whether it would be possible to leave them shut in the oven until he came the following week. At the next interview, he went straight to the oven, and opened the door, saying, 'There, what did it feel like being shut in there for the whole week'.

Interpretation of early interviews. It seemed that J identified with the bear. The cheerful bear family paintings seemed to indicate that basically his was a fairly happy and united family. The fact that the pictures tended to be crowded and full of activity probably indicated that J (who is a sensitive and rather shy child) often found life at home too hectic. The gloomy pictures probably indicated how J felt when the intense relationship he had with his mother became too much for him and he developed one of his breath holding attacks, or a severe sick headache. The strong aggressive feeling shown when J was making the clay bear was probably an indication of the emotional battering he had received from his mother. The incident of stuffing the toys in the oven was, perhaps, a form of retribution to the world around him, for making him feel as if he were going to suffocate.

Description of more interviews. For several consecutive interviews J used nearly the whole of the time for making models of his own inventing out of a wooden constructional set. Some of these were most ingenious. J concentrated hard while making the models; the therapist encouraged and praised him. Several times J stated that he felt he was slow at working things out. The therapist replied that this did not matter because he got there in the end. Also, he set himself a high standard. J was also able to apply this concept to discussing his achievement at school, and also how he felt in competition with his brother.

Interpretation of interviews. It became apparent that J's parents expected a very high standard of achievement from their children. At times they probably applied considerable pressure. J tended to become anxious over this and lacked confidence in his ability. The therapist was able to use her good relationship with J in order to encourage him and increase his confidence in himself.

Description of later interviews. In the final, carefree and happy interviews J spent the whole time making some delightful clay animals. Each was carefully finished off, painted and varnished. J took them home to a special place in his bedroom.

Interpretation of later interviews. J and the therapist both realised that this was the final stage of therapy. (J was shortly going to join his brother at a boarding preparatory school.) The clay animals had no significance in themselves but the activity of clay modelling was something of mutual interest to J and the therapist. Undertaken within the positive context of their relationship, the completed clay models were precious to J as a reminder of this friendship.

Progress. Gradually there had been an improvement in J and his ability to deal with life. It was fortunate that J was to go away to boarding school. Undoubtedly it was advisable that he should have a break from his home. At the start of therapy, it was thought unlikely that J would manage life at the fairly rigid and conventional boarding school. However, probably mainly as a result of therapy, J adjusted to his new environment reasonably quickly. Gradually his school work improved; he is popular with staff and children and has a number of friends.

J continues to correspond with the therapist and asks for an appointment to attend the institute during the school holidays.

Summary. The aim of this illustration has been to show:

(1) The key importance of the relationship built up between the patient and the therapist.
(2) How this relationship is used in the therapeutic process.
(3) Although the therapist is treating one member of the family, she is continually thinking of him in relationship to the other members of his family, and the community.

During the time that the therapist saw J the psychiatrist in charge of the case had regular interviews with the parents. This was an important part of the therapy for this family. The therapist worked closely with the psychiatrist, throughout, writing regular reports for him, discussing progress and setting new therapeutic aims.

Therapeutic Group Treatment for Emotionally Disturbed Children

The treatment of emotionally disturbed children, in small groups, undertaken by occupational therapists with student or suitable voluntary help, can be of great value. If a disturbed child is able to relate to other people satisfactorily, within a small therapeutic group, it is a positive step in helping him to relate adequately in other group situations in his everyday life. Group therapy of this kind may be considered under the following headings:

(*a*) Group structure.
(*b*) Group environment.
(*c*) Group handling.
(*d*) The role of the occupational therapist as part of the group.
(*e*) Activity in relation to the group.

Group structure. From experience it has been proved that a ratio of 8 or 10 children with 2 therapists or 1 therapist and 1 student or voluntary helper; or 4 or 5 children with 1 therapist, are the ideal numbers for a group. In most groups one gets a combination of shy withdrawn children, balanced by over active aggressive ones. Skilfully handled by the therapist, this mixture is a definite advantage, as the different children will help each other. It is an advantage for the therapist to have at least one individual play session with a child, before attempting to introduce him into a group. She is then able to start making a relationship with the child which will give him security in meeting the group situation. It will also give the therapist an opportunity to make an assessment of the way in which the child is likely to react to the group.

Group environment. Indoor and outdoor facilities are required for this type of group. Common sense safety precautions should be taken, so that the maximum amount of freedom can be permitted safely. In practice careful observation obviates the need for many restrictions.

Group handling. The therapist behaves in as natural a way as possible. It is her responsibility to create an understanding, tolerant atmosphere in which the children feel secure and able to express themselves freely. On the other hand, all children need boundaries and limits. It is vital that these should be established and maintained consistently. At times this will inevitably require a considerable amount of skill and patience. If there are two adults in control of the group it is obvious that they must agree beforehand upon the basic principles of group handling. Any difficult situations that arise should be discussed in detail, if possible immediately after the group therapy session.

The role of the therapist as part of the group. The therapist has to be constantly adapting herself to the needs of the moment. A high degree of observation and perception is required if the group is to function effectively, and if the maximum therapeutic value is to be gained from situations that arise. In one group session the therapist may be required to play a variety of roles.

Activity in relation to groups. Many types of play and activity can be utilised successfully in a group situation. Those of most value are:

(1) *Material and equipment to encourage free expression:*
   Water, sand, clay, drawing and painting equipment. Record player and percussion band.

(2) *Equipment to encourage acting out:*
   Wendy house, doll's house and grecon people, dressing-up clothes, glove puppets.

(3) *Activities and equipment for indoor group-play:*
   Large blocks, constructional toys (connector, particularly good) games, e.g. skittles, darts, bagatelle, snakes and ladders, pic-up-styx, happy families, etc.

(4) *Activities and equipment suitable for outdoor group-play:*
   Balls, bats, wigwam, stilts, climbing trees, swimming.

Emotionally Disturbed Adolescents

In an adolescent unit the occupational therapist will be cooperating with the psychiatrist, psychologist, social worker, nursing staff and teacher. The occupational therapist will be asked to undertake:

(*a*) *Long term therapy* with individual adolescent patients. A wide range of activities are employed to establish a therapeutic relationship with the adolescent, within which the resolution of his problems can take place.

(*b*) *Group therapy* with small groups of adolescent patients, again using activities which are likely to interest young people, but always remembering that it is the positive relationships which are being built up within the group that are of prime importance. The daily programme may include a school programme as well.

Long Term Therapy for Individual Patients

When working with individual adolescent patients, an atmosphere must be created in which the boy or girl feels relaxed, and in which to establish a relationship in which they feel secure and able to express themselves. It should be remembered that for many, the transition from childhood to adulthood has its problems; how much more so for the already unhappy and disturbed child.

Treatment in long term therapy is concerned with relationships so, to illustrate what actually happens during treatment, there follows a brief description of a series of interviews, undertaken by an occupational therapist with a 14-year-old boy. B was referred by his general practitioner because of:

(1) School phobia.
(2) A severe stammer.
(3) Clinging behaviour with his parents.
(4) Fears of entering a large building or going into a crowd.

Background. B comes from a rural area. Parents have lived in the same small community all their lives. Father employed on a large estate in the neighbourhood; mother tends to nag: says that she was shy as a child and had difficulty in going to school. B is an only child. The family live in an isolated cottage.

Rapport building interviews. In the initial interview B was tense and anxious, with the result that his stammer was bad and he was unable to get a word out beyond saying 'umm' in answer to questions. Having ascertained that B enjoyed drawing and modelling, for the second session the therapist suggested that he should make a clay model. He quickly and surely shaped the lump of clay into a fox's head; as soon as he had completed the mouth he was able to talk for the fox. Next he shaped a duck which the fox gobbled up. Then another lump of clay became the farmer with his gun, but before he had a chance to shoot, the fox jumped on top of the farmer and squashed him flat. By this stage, B was talking in an animated and vivid way and was quite at ease. The therapist was able to direct the conversation on to his family and everyday life at home.

Interpretation of initial interviews. Because of B's severe stammer and initial feeling of shyness and insecurity with the therapist, clay modelling was a definite aid to communication. B became absorbed in the modelling project, then relaxed and was able to talk quite easily. The man with the gun was found to be the subject of a constantly recurring dream, which could have been significant.

Steps in therapy. The therapist saw B for 50 individual one-hour interviews. The relationship between B and the therapist continued to grow; he became increasingly at ease with her and was able to express his deeper feelings related to his life experiences.

Description of early interviews. Glove puppetry was found to be another aid to communication. B always selected the same three puppets: father, mother and boy. He made the puppets speak in a lively and animated manner and there was practically no sign of his stammer. The therapist was expected to take the part of a verbal and responsive audience. Simple table games, such as halma, which required a minimum of concentration, were also found to be a useful aid to communication.

Interpretation of early interviews. Much of B's play with the puppets was obviously based on his life experiences, and a vivid picture of family relationships emerged. The table games were used partly as something to do together, whilst establishing a deeper relationship and partly as something to do while talking about his difficulties.

Description of further interviews. B was still sharing the only bedroom with his parents so the social worker and occupational therapist worked together to remedy this. The social worker discussed with the mother the practical arrangements for making a bedroom on the landing for B. The therapist was able to discuss the move with B. In a few weeks the change was successfully accomplished and B was sleeping on his own. For two interviews which took place at this stage B arrived in a very upset state. In the first of these sessions B told the therapist about a re-occurring nightmare he had been having for some time. In this dream he was either walking or riding his bicycle in the country near his home, and a man with a gun was chasing him. Sometimes he could see the man, at others he just knew that he was there: he had a terrible feeling of panic and fear. He would try and get away from the man by running or bicycling fast, but he could never go fast enough, and a suffocating feeling of panic built up inside him. At this stage he always woke up. B communicated most of this information by writing it down, as his stammer was severe because he was so upset.

In the second of these interviews, B told the therapist that there were some days when he was overwhelmed by a feeling of depression, without any apparent cause. B went on to tell the therapist about two incidents in his childhood which had triggered off very strong feelings of fear. They were as follows:

(a) When he was about three years old he had pulled the tablecloth causing the teapot to fall over. B had been quite badly scalded, and had to be admitted to hospital as an in-patient.

(b) When he was about six years old he was playing in the playground when he fell over and knocked his nose which bled profusely. The other children all stood round and stared.

Interpretation of further interviews. B now had a sufficiently strong relationship with the therapist to be able to confide in her about his feelings of fear and panic. He had been unable to explain these feelings to his parents.

Description of final interviews. The interviews continued to follow a similar

pattern with various activities being used an an aid to communication. Initially
· it had been hoped that B would be able to return to school, but this was not
possible. After some time, the local education authority arranged for him to
have individual teaching at home, on two mornings a week. In some cases of
school phobia it is possible for the occupational therapist to work in cooperation
with the social worker and teacher in assisting the child to return to school.

Progress. B is now less afraid to go out on his own. He will go on errands to
the local shop, but not if there is a crowd there. He is playing football and
going for bicycle rides with other boys in the village. He joins in some of the
activities of the local youth club, but only when the meetings are held outside.
He is interested in pop music and motor bicycles. The therapist encourages B
to talk about these activities and interests. B is now coming up to school leaving
age and is talking in quite a realistic way about obtaining a job on a farm. The
therapist will continue to give him support until this is achieved.

Conclusion

(1) The aim of this illustration has been to show:
   (*a*) The key importance of the relationship built up between patient and
        therapist.
   (*b*) How this relationship is used in the therapeutic process.
   (*c*) Although the therapist is treating one member of the family, she is
        continually relating the situation to the other members of his family and
        community.
   (*d*) The importance of working in close cooperation with other members of
        the treatment team—in this case, psychiatrist and social worker.
(2) If the family concerned had lived in a less isolated area, it would have been
    possible for the therapist to have worked out a wider treatment programme,
    introducing the patient into an adolescent club group being organised by the
    occupational therapist.
(3) A different approach could have been used by the psychiatrist in charge
    of the case. This would have involved removing the patient from his home
    to an in-patient adolescent unit.

Group Therapy for Emotionally Disturbed Adolescents

The treatment of emotionally disturbed adolescents in small groups, is a
worthwhile part of the occupational therapist's contribution to a family
psychiatry programme. These groups can take the form of a therapeutic
youth club, an essential condition of membership being that, because of his
emotional difficulties, the adolescent is unable to fit into or benefit from an
ordinary club. An atmosphere is created in which it is possible for the
members to feel secure. Through club activities the therapist supplies the
adolescent with positive emotional experiences, that counter adverse home
relationships.

Group structure. From experience it has been found that if the group is to
function effectively it should not have more than eight members with one
therapist and one student or helper. The age range can vary from 12 to
16 years. (Adolescents over 16 years old may require a different type of
group, possibly using discussion techniques without activities. This will

probably be conducted most effectively by a psychiatrist and may include the social worker and other team members.) The groups may be mixed, or separate for boys and girls. The therapist should have at least one interview with each member before attempting to integrate the individual into the group. It is also essential that she should have background knowledge of each adolescent and his family.

Group environment. Surroundings should be congenial, ideally a spacious, bright, warm room with easy chairs, which would be conducive to spontaneous and relaxed discussion. There should also be space for games and dancing; facilities for simple cooking or mechanical handwork for the boys would be additional assets.

Group handling. The therapist should behave in a natural and relaxed manner. It is her responsibility to create a friendly, understanding and tolerant atmosphere. Boundaries, limits and rules, should, as far as possible, be made by the group.

Role of the therapist as part of the group. Carefully selected young occupational therapists are ideal to deal with adolescent groups; providing that they have adequate support from an older person when required. The young therapist will predominately take an 'elder sister' role within the group.

Activity in relation to the group. The better the relationships within the group, the less important does the activity become. Quite often when a group is well established most of the session is spent in spontaneous discussion, using simple games and activities as something to do at the same time, but many kinds of activity in which young people are interested have their place in this type of flexible group.

REFERENCES AND RECOMMENDED FURTHER READING

1. Ellis, N. R., *Handbook of Mental Deficiency*. New York, 1963.
2. McDowall, E. B., *Teaching the Severely Subnormal*. London, 1964.
3. See chapter 16, this book and *Proceedings of the First Congress of the Int. Assn for the Scientific Study of Mental Deficiency*. Surrey, 1968.
4. Strauss & Lehtinen, *Psychopathology and Education of the Brain Injured Child*. New York, vol I (1947), vol. II (1955).
5. Gessell, A. & Amatruda, C. S., *Developmental Diagnosis*. New York, 1960.
6. Kanner, L. (1944) Early infantile autism. *Paediatrics*.
   O'Gorman, G., *The Nature of Childhood Autism*, London, 1967.
   Rutter, M., *Infantile Autism—Concepts, Characteristics and Treatment* (Study Group No. 1., Inst. for Research into Mental Retardation), London, 1971.
7. Ounsted, C. (1965) A behavioural and electroencephalographic study of autistic children. *J. Psychiat. Res.*
   Ounsted, C., Autistic children, Excerpta Medica International Congress, 1966.
   Ounsted, C. (1967) Autistic children, *Occ. Ther.*, **30**, no. 9.
   Weston, P. T. B., *Some Approaches to Teaching Autistic Children*, Oxford, 1965.
8. A *stereotypy* is repetitious, idiosyncratic behaviour which acts as a safety device by preventing further sensory input from the environment and protecting the brain from further excitation, e.g. finger play, spinning, rocking, tapping and swinging doors.

9. Hutt, S. J., Hutt, C., Lee, D. & Ounsted, C., *Arousal and Childhood Autism*, London, 1964.
10. Hutt, C. & Ounsted, C., The biological significance of gaze aversion with particular reference to syndrome of infantile autism *Behav. Sci.*, 1966.
11. Howells, J. G., *Theory and Practice of Family Psychiatry*. With edited contributions. London, 1968.
    Howells, J. G., *Modern Perspectives in Child Psychiatry*. Oliver and Boyd.
    Howells, J. G. & Anderson, R. (1960), Family psychiatry and occupational therapy. *Occ. Ther.* vol. 3, No. 11.

The following books will be found useful by the occupational therapist treating children with psychiatric problems.

Allen, F., *Psychotherapy with Children*. London, 1964.
Axline, V., *Dibs In Search of Self*. U.S.A., 1964.
Bender, L., *Child Psychiatric Techniques*. U.S.A., 1952.
Copeland, J., *For the Love of Ann*, London, 1973.
Corbett, J., *How do you do Cookery*. London, 1966.
Dentsch, H., *Selected Problems of Adolescence*. London, 1968.
Eppel, E. M. & M., *Adolescents and Morality*. London, 1966.
Erikson, E. H., *Childhood and Society*. Pelican, 1963.
Freud, A., *Technical Lectures and Essays*.
Gessell, A. & Ilg, F. L., *Infant and Child in the Culture of To-day*. London, 1942.
Grey, J., *Party Games for Young Children*. London, 1963.
Hadfield, J. A., *Childhood and Adolescence*. Pelican, 1962.
Hartley, R., Lawrence, F. & Golderson, R., *Understanding Children's Play*. London, 1952.
Haworth, M., *Child Psychotherapy*. London, 1964.
Jackson, L., *Child Treatment and the Therapy of Play*. London, 1948.
Kanner, L., *Child Psychiatry*. Oxford, 1957.
Klein, M., *The Psycho-Analysis of Children*. London, 1950.
Lambert, J., *Adventure*, London, 1974.
Matterson, E. M., *Play with a Purpose for the Under Sevens*. Penguin, 1965.
Millar, S., *The Psychology of Play*. Pelican, 1968.
          The Psychology of Adolescence. Univ. of Swansea, 1966.
Monstakas, C. E., *Psychotherapy with Children: The Living Relationship*. London, 1959.
Pearson, J., *Playgrounds*, Penguin Books, London, 1974.
Rich, J., *Interviewing Children and Adolescents*. London, 1968.
Rutter, M., *Maternal Deprivation Reassessed*, London, 1973.
Savage, R. D., *Psychometric Assessment of the Individual Child.*, Penguin, 1971.
Wing, J. K., *Early Childhood Autism: Clinical, Educational and Social Aspects*. Oxford, 1966.
Winnicott, D. W., *Playing a Reality*, Pelican, London, 1974.
Wood, M., *Children: The Development of Personality and Behaviour*, London, 1973.
And see:
Occupational therapy groups for maladjusted children. *Occ. Ther.*, **35**, no. 10, 1972.
    The development of a day autistic unit. *Occ. Ther.*, 36, no. 5, 1973.
    Child psychiatry, the need for occupational therapy, *Occ. Ther.*, 36, no. 8, 1973.
    Occupational therapy staffing and facilities for a child psychiatry unit. *Occ. Ther.*, 36, no. 8, 1973.
    The Children's and Young Persons' Act 1968. London, H.M.S.O.*
And see Reading References for chapter 18, this book.
* See Glossaay, p. 454.

Occupational Therapy for Children with Physical Disorders

Occupational therapy is an integral part of treatment for children and adolescents in acute and chronic stages of disease and disability as found in hospital wards, out-patient clinics, schools for handicapped or retarded children and special centres such as a spastics' centre.

This chapter is mainly concerned with the hospitalised child in a general children's hospital or in a children's ward of an adult hospital and with the out-patient child attending such hospitals [1].

The Approach to the Child Patient

A consistent and secure relationship needs to be built up between the child and one therapist. An immediate response cannot be expected and the child must be given time to keep pace emotionally with what he is required to do or accept. The therapist must be able to communicate understanding and acceptance and give support and reassurance. Her approach should be friendly but positive, especially when handling aggression or withdrawal behaviour patterns.

She must remain objective throughout, and realise that unacceptable responses are expressions of the child's inability to manage; she must then adjust her approach accordingly, anticipating his responses and helping him to channel these into acceptable behaviour. Sometimes she can help to foster a more positive attitude amongst harassed staff to what are regarded as 'naughty' or 'difficult' children. Regular treatment sessions give a sense of security; warning should be given before the session is to end and the child told when the next is to come. Explanations, simplified if necessary, can be given for reasons for treatment. It is important to remember that treatment is carried out firstly through the therapist's relationship with the child and secondly through the activity used.

Assessment [2]

The therapist must assess the child's needs before planning treatment. In doing this she must take into account the particular child's developmental level, his past and present medical history, and his home and school background. She must be perceptive of lack of motivation and of signs of stress and be observant of his behaviour and ability to communicate with family, staff and other children.

In order to make adequate assessment and to plan and carry out treatment, the therapist must have a knowledge of the following:

(1) *Normal development* from birth to adolescence. The emotional, physical and social needs of the normal child, how these are expressed, and the results if they are not satisfied.

(2) *The effects of hospitalisation.* The behavioural patterns which may result from separation from home and family, and of how to meet the child's emotional needs, especially those of the child who has to be physically immobilised.

(3) *The diseases of childhood* and the effects of these on mental development and behaviour and on physical growth and well being.

(4) *Play and play materials:* how a normal child uses these and how they can be adapted for the sick or disabled child.

(5) *The importance of her relationship with the child* as a therapeutic medium and techniques of approach, handling and methods of kindly but appropriate discipline.

Treatment [3]

Positive measures may be needed to counteract the effects of hospitalisation and the conditions dictated by sickness or disability. Particular considerations in planning a treatment programme are as follows:

Separation from Home

This is especially traumatic for the child whose mother is unable to spend time with him during the day, as is now common practice with unrestricted visiting hours. He may feel rejected or that he is being punished for something he does not understand. Reassurance is badly needed in either case and if possible several short periods of treatment should be given daily, preferably by the same therapist, until a sense of security has been established. Activities associated with home are helpful and parents or relatives should be encouraged to show special appreciation of anything the child may make for them. A favourite possession from home may also be comforting to handle—a soft toy perhaps or a collection of ribbons. As occupational treatment something could be made in which such treasures could be kept safely. Where accommodation is available and the mother is able to stay in the hospital with the child the need for reassurance will not arise in the same way, but definite treatment sessions given by the occupational therapist may still be necessary.

Physical Restraint

This may be by plaster cast, frame or bandages. An outlet for energy by acceptable means should be given and also an outlet for self-expression within restriction. It is wise for a therapist to supervise release of restraint, as, for instance, the untying of the hands of a child with a skin condition.

Restriction of Activity

This may be necessary for the sick child. Some may have no inclination to be active; for others inactivity may be irksome and the reason for it not understood. Constructive, creative and imaginative play can be used. Correct positioning must be ensured to minimise fatigue and to control energy.

Pain and Discomfort

A child experiencing this may be helped by being given opportunity for self expression and dramatic play, as an outlet for frustration. Reassurance and explanation of the discomfort can lessen tension and help to overcome fear.

Isolation

Visual and auditory aids can be used to make this situation more tolerable. Regular visits and treatment are particularly important, as is the provision of some interest for the child when he is alone.

Remedial Measures to Overcome Physical Disability

A graded treatment programme may be needed to encourage restoration of function and a return to normal, physically and psychologically. Toys and other play materials offer endless possibilities for remedial use for the young child. Those of seven years and over enjoy making things. Imaginative or mechanical construction and craft work are all of value. An adult is usually interested in his treatment because it is 'doing him good', but a child needs something that he will enjoy doing for its own sake. The therapist should try to get to know the child before specific treatment is required, and this can be helped by early referral.

Methods of treatment will be based on the several principles of re-education of function described in chapters 5, 6 and 7, and the treatment timing, content, and progression will be coordinated with that of the physiotherapist. Training in activities of daily living, appropriate to the age of the child, should be included. Close cooperation with the nursing staff is essential.

Special Measures to Overcome Emotional and Behaviour Disturbances

It may be necessary for the therapist to provide a non-directive play situation and a supportive programme. The child's disturbances are likely to be secondary to his disease or handicap and can be helped by opportunity to use his initiative constructively, thereby increasing his self confidence. Methods of treatment for more serious forms of disturbance are discussed in chapter 17.

Observation of Performance and Behaviour

While engrossed in play a child will be more relaxed and less self-conscious, and the true level of ability and disability can be assessed more reliably than in a formal test situation. The findings may contribute to diagnosis and better planning of treatment.

Providing Opportunities for Normal Development

Occupational therapy provides opportunity for the development of skills appropriate to the age and level of attainment of the child. Many such children are not ill, and their daily programme includes schooling, in addition to appropriate treatment. The occupational therapist will work in close co-operation with the teacher. The therapist, for example, may give the child help in controlling his pencil and other implements: the teacher can give the therapist information on his potential for learning and his concentration. Formal schooling should be supplemented by group activities, as well as time allocated for individual 'ploys'. Because hospitalisation often imposes dependence, and this may be a serious handicap when the child returns home, independence and inititative should be encouraged by every means possible through activities which help to develop motor and sensory skills, powers of communication, socialisation and a sense of responsibility.

Children undergoing long-stay treatment may be permanently disabled, and problems of personal independence may, therefore, be difficult to overcome. Many congenitally disabled children are young for their age and this will affect the time at which they can be taught to do things for themselves. Their first incentive may be to learn to feed: other activities such as washing and dressing may be resisted until later.

Cooperation with other Specialists and Parents during Treatment

The necessity for cooperation is emphasised in every section of this book, but it is particularly essential for anyone taking responsibility for any part of the care and treatment of the child. The hospital team will consist of the nursing staff, physio-, occupational and speech therapists, dietitians and medical social workers, the school teacher, voluntary or paid aides, and the parents, and, where the child is older, perhaps the youth employment officer. The doctor guides all treatment and resettlement plans.

In admitting a child, the help of a good mother may be the key to satisfactory adjustment and treatment, and in preparing a child for discharge, his mother is again all important. If, having watched, she understands about the treatment and will encourage similar activity at home, earlier discharge may be possible. In the case of a heavily handicapped child, both the physio- and occupational therapists may have something special to teach the mother, so she must attend for certain treatment sessions and be present when plans and 'follow up' are discussed.

Over the whole treatment period there must be frequent consultation, and, if necessary, definite changes of plan, and for the child, a feeling of security must be engendered by an atmosphere of cooperation.

Activities Used in the Treatment of Children

Activities must be selected according to the child's developmental level as well as according to their therapeutic value. Toys and other play materials have many possibilities for adaptation for therapeutic use, and one activity may fulfil more than one aim of treatment, as for example the use of a hammer pegboard as an outlet for energy and controlled aggression, for shoulder and elbow movement and for sustained grasp and eye-hand coordination.

Because it is not possible to give a full account of useful activities, and indeed hardly necessary in view of the many excellent books, catalogues and demonstrations in this field, only brief mention is made here of certain categories, their purpose and precautions necessary in using them.

Sand-water play. Facilities for this are essential in an occupational therapy department, and an added asset is an outdoor sandpit.

Toys. These can be manipulative and constructive, helping to develop skill, spatial perception, and awareness of colour, size and shape, etc. They should be sturdy, easily cleaned and sterilised, and without poisonous paint, sharp edges or splintering wood.

Games and educational activities. These can be used individually or in groups, to stimulate concentration, coordination, education, interest and re-socialisation, and to counteract isolation. Active outdoor games can encourage mobility, and specific exercise, and can be used for ambulant as well as wheel-chair patients. They may offer outlets for aggression and hostility, or opportunity for acceptance.

Art and craft work. As an extension of games and educational activities these give opportunity for originality and achievement, as well as for specific exercise. They should be uncomplicated and show quick results.

Adult and home activities. These, adapted to the child's capacities, can bring pride and pleasure and help in the preparation for return to home. They would include play with dolls and dolls houses, dolls hospitals with dolls beds; feeding bottles, telephones for 'pretence conversations,' etc.; cooking, machine and handsewing, typing, printing, carpentry and gardening (indoors and out).

Music and drama. Most children respond to these and they can be adapted to provide either sedation or stimulation, or to encourage movement and self expression.

Facilities and Basic Equipment [4]

Facilities needed include a large play area, a small individual treatment area with a one way window, office storage space, floor and wall space and garden and outdoor play area. *Basic equipment* needed, other than that mentioned previously, includes adjustable tables and chairs, shelves and cupboards, wash basins, mirror, toilet facilities, bed or couch, mats, a sandpit, a doll's house area, easels, bed trays, boards and adjustable bed tables.

Precautions

The following are indicated:

General Precautions

(1) Care in choice of media:
    (*a*) When open wounds are present, for example, do not use sand.
    (*b*) When a respiratory or skin condition is present, avoid irritating substances.
(2) Sharp equipment should be supervised when young children are present.
(3) Tools and all parts of equipment should be checked after use.
(4) Equipment should be sterilised and cleaned to avoid cross infection.
(5) Barrier nursing precautions should be observed.
(6) Care should be taken in replacing cot sides and arm stays.
(7) Dietary and fluid balance regulations must be observed.

Specific Considerations in Regard to Specific Conditions

The treatment of illness or disability in children will, to a great degree, follow the recommendations given in preceding chapters, but there are certain special points to remember in certain cases.

Children in hospital for observation can be helped by occupational therapy, alleviating fear and offering an alternative for direction of emotional energy.

Children with infectious or contagious diseases may need barrier nursing. Materials used should be introduced in small quantities and be appropriate for sterilisation.

Children with disorders of metabolism. The most common of these is diabetes mellitus. The child may be admitted to hospital so that his insulin, diet and energy expenditure can be stabilised. The occupational therapist may be asked to help in devising a programme for him which will achieve this.

Short term surgical cases may need interest and occupation to prevent fear and, later, overactivity.

Children with disorders of the respiratory system may be in hospital for short or long periods. Those with spasmodic asthma may be nervous and excitable, and can be helped by an appropriately reassuring approach. Those with extensive pulmonary troubles, fibrosis or bronchiectasis, need treatment to maintain general health, improve posture and create diversion.

Diseases of circulation fall into two main categories, congenital heart disease and rheumatic heart disease. In the former occupational therapy is used to determine activity tolerance, to allay fear and to improve circulation and appetite. Post-operative treatment contributes to improvement by graded activity. For rheumatic heart disease, during the period of complete rest, occupational therapy is needed to keep the child occupied and contented, and progress must be most carefully graded.

Diseases of the blood and lymphatic systems do not call for specific treatment, but a valuable contribution can be made to the contentment of the child by suitable occupation.

Disorders of the endocrine system, such as cretinism and myxoedema call for stimulation of the child's development and progressive training for normal life.

Diseases of the nervous system cover a wide variety. In the post-acute stages of meningitis occupational therapy can offer reassurance and the re-arousal of interests and skills. After the acute stages of poliomyelitis graded occupations may be given, avoiding strain and fatigue but helping to develop coordination and muscle strength, as indicated by medical instruction. The approach to a child with chorea is similar to that for the one who has had meningitis. Occupational therapy is also of value in treating hemiplegic children, and those suffering from disturbances of coordination (see chapter 10).

Diseases of bones, joints and muscles. Treatment for these, to include rheumatic fever, rheumatoid arthritis, osteomyelitis, muscular dystrophies, fractures and dislocations, undue fragility of bone (osteogenesis imperfector) and congenital abnormalities follows the general principles that are described in preceding chapters. There will be special emphasis, for the growing child, on prevention of contractures and deformities.

Eye treatment including eye surgery. This may call for reassurance, prevention of fear of having eyes covered, distraction from discomfort and prevention of crying and, later, control of eyes when bandages are removed.

A regular timetable for visits of the therapist is important here, and ingenuity is needed in devising appropriate occupations.

Burns. Early referral is important so as to create a satisfactory child-therapist relationship for what will be a long and distressing period of treatment. The psychological effects of burns are marked, and if possible it is advisable for one therapist to undertake the treatment.

Treatment, which is also referred to in chapter 11, often involves non-active participation by the child at first, and treatment periods may need to be brief, a sense of security being built up by their regularity and by reassurance and explanation to the child. During the non-active stages, pictures pinned to the wall each day, goldfish, radio and recorded music, weather charts and growing seeds are useful. If the patient has to lie prone it may be helpful to have the top of the bed turned so that the child can see into the centre of the ward.

As soon as permissible the programme is upgraded and if necessary remedial exercises to prevent contractures are commenced. It may help the child if the therapist remains with him during dressings as a supportive figure. Maintenance of correct position is important in the prevention of contractures in severe cases.

The therapist may need to work in close liaison with the parents, possibly arranging treatments to coincide with their departure. At times the psychological trauma and guilt feelings associated with the accident may limit their ability to give the necessary support to the child. The therapist, because of her close association with the child, may be able to suggest ways of overcoming their difficulties.

Care must be taken to observe strict barrier nursing precautions when these apply.

No special reference has been made in this chapter, as in the preceding one, to occupational therapy specifically for adolescents. In physical diseases and disabilities treatment for adolescents will follow the methods and progression given in chapters 5 to 11. Where special attention needs to be given to emotional problems or behaviour deviations reference can be made to chapter 17.

REFERENCES AND RECOMMENDED FURTHER READING

1. Role of an occupational therapist in a children's treatment unit. *Occ. Ther.*, 35, no. 3, 1972.
2. Children's functional assessment. *Occ. Ther.*, 37, no. 10, 1974.
   An assessment playgroup. *Occ. Ther.*, 36, no. 2, 1973.
   Aspects of developmental screening. *Occ. Ther.*, 36, no. 10, 1973.
3. Equipment for children in plaster. *Occ. Ther.*, 35, no. 10, 1972.
   Starting a toy library for handicapped children. *Occ. Ther.*, 36, no. 1, 1973.
   Technology, toys and therapy. *Occ. Ther.*, 37, no. 10, 1974.

4. Assessment of handicapped child for most suitable type of chair. *Occ. Ther.*, **36**, no. 10, 1973.

And see:
Apley, J. & MacKeith, R., *The Child and His Symptoms*. Oxford, 1968.
Bowlby, J., *Child Care and the Growth of Love*. Pelican, 1953.
Bowley, A., *Natural Development of the Child*. Edinburgh, 1960.
Bowley, A., *The Psychological Care of the Child in Hospital*. Edinburgh, 1961.
Gessell, A. & Ilg, F. L., *The Child from 5 to 10*. London, 1956.
Gessell, A., Ilg, F. L. & Ames, L. B., *Youth: The Years from 10 to 16*. London, 1965.
Hostler, P., *The Child's World*. Penguin, 1959.
Illingworth, R. S., *The Development of the Infant and Young Child*, London, 1970.
Kahn, J. H., *Human Growth and the Development of Personality*. Oxford, 1971.
McMullin, M. D., *Indoor Games and Amusements for Children*. Hutchinson, London.
Matterson, E. M., *Play with a Purpose for Under-Sevens*. Penguin, 1965.
Noble, E., *Play and the Sick Child*. London, 1967.
Parsons, Sir L., *Modern Trends in Paediatrics*. London, 1951.
Plank, E. N., *Working with Children in Hospitals*. Tavistock Publications. London, 1964.
Sandström, C. I., *The Psychology of Childhood and Adolescence*. Pelican, London, 1968–69.
Schad, C. J. & Dally, A. T., *Occupational Therapy in Paediatrics*. Univ. of Illinois, Iowa, 1959.
Todd, K. M., *Child Treatment and the Therapy of Play*. London, 1948.
Valentine, C. W., *The Normal Child and Some of his Abnormalities*. Pelican, 1956.
Wall, N. D., *The Adolescent Child*. London, 1955.
West, W. L., *Occupational Therapy for the Multiply Handicapped Child*. U.S.A., 1965.
Winnicott, D. W., *The Child, the Family and the Outside World*. Pelican, 1964.
Yudkin, S. & Holme, A., *Working Mothers and Their Children*. Sphere Library, London, 1969.

Part Five

CHAPTER 19

Occupational Therapy for the
Cerebral Palsied

Cerebral Palsy is the term used to describe the group of disorders caused by a non-progressive brain lesion occurring before, during or soon after birth. The condition is complex involving impairment of neuromuscular function with or without sensory defects, learning difficulties with or without intellectual defect, emotional problems, and sometimes speech defect. Because the treatment for different types of cerebral palsy does not differ greatly and in so many cases the conditions are mixed, they are not described separately. The terms however should be understood. *Spasticity* is characterised by extreme activity of the muscle stretch-reflex and inability to relax, so blocking the action of the antagonists. *Athetosis* is distinguished by involuntary, purposeless movements. *Ataxia* is the term applied to incoordination which is not produced by spasticity, athetosis or muscle weakness. Balance is affected.

For obvious reasons the special schools, special units in hospitals and the residential and assessment centres screen and select the candidates most likely to benefit from the facilities offered. Some receive treatment, usually physiotherapy, in their local schools for the handicapped. Requests for vocational assessment for school leavers by the Spastics Society* can be made by parents, friends, doctors, therapists or social workers.

Whether the therapist is concerned with the treatment of children or adults, she must have knowledge of normal physical and mental, perceptual and intellectual development, and be able to understand the significance of mental rating. These factors are the bases of all treatment. Much of what is recommended for the treatment of children could also apply to the adolescent, with appropriate modification. This chapter has a section for each. The first deals with therapeutic progression from an early age, the second with problems of vocational assessment.

CHILDREN

The Treatment Team

The team consists of the doctor, physio-, occupational and speech therapists and, where applicable, the teacher and educational psychologist. Pre-school training is best given by the occupational therapists. Every member of the team should have special training for the work.

On admission each child, and a parent, should be seen by the team, and his programme should be reviewed every three months at a conference of everyone who deals with him. The parent should remain in close contact, understanding the treatment and training and, where possible, carrying certain aspects of these on at home. The occupational therapist should be prepared to visit the home to ensure that the prescribed treatment is appropriate.

The Aims of Treatment

Treatment begins as soon as the diagnosis is made, possibly as early as at six months old. In most cases it should be given daily and certainly not less often than twice a week. The occupational therapist aims to assist development and to improve function in both physical and perceptual tasks. If the patient is treated early, considerably improved physical function may be achieved by the age of seven. The child will need training in applying abilities he has learnt to different tasks in his environment and for his future placement in life. However, although a child may appear to have reached his full potential physically, experience shows that with further treatment he may show progress at any stage of life. Concentration, willingness to try, and a change of environment may lead to improvements and the patient may become more persistent when older, and progress developmentally even when adult.

From six or seven onwards schooling is important for most children. Time taken from school work should be minimal, the therapist preferably working closely with the teachers in the class room. She will advise on the choice between handwriting and typing, and on provision of specially devised equipment. She will also be closely concerned with those children who show specific learning difficulties and are in need of individual perceptual training.

From the age of fifteen or earlier the role of the therapist is directed towards pre-vocational training and assessment. For those with well above average academic ability the normal school curriculum should be satisfactory, provided they have enough mobility to get to and from a place of work. For others, training to meet the basic demands of life should have priority; personal care, mobility indoors and out, and simple domestic tasks. These all presuppose some degree of functional use of hands and this must be assessed from an A.D.L.* and a work point of view. Personality factors, powers of concentration and educational standards, for example, ability to read simple notices, are equally important.

Assessment

The progress assessment charts of Gunzburg (see References), which are primarily for the mentally retarded, are a great help in evaluating objectively the degree of independence and ability of each child. They are also a help in planning treatment and measuring progress. The therapist should assess the abilities of a child and his potential. The latter is difficult and can only be judged through experience. It is wrong to expect a child to struggle to feed or dress himself if there is really no hope of success: continuous failure brings disillusionment and saps endeavour. Assessment is difficult. It is as easy to underestimate as it is to overestimate prospects and some children may achieve a surprising amount if a lot is expected of them. Assessment charts are valuable but they can never provide the whole answer. Because it is difficult to chart how each task is performed the chart itself should be directed solely towards what the child can or cannot do in functional tasks. It should however be noted whether the task was achieved normally or abnormally. Progress in tasks such as dressing, feeding, toiletting and writing should be graded, as should the development of normal grasp in each hand.

Treatment Methods

Positioning and Chairs

Positioning has an effect on function and each child should have a suitable chair. The best positions will be decided with the physiotherapist. A chair individually designed and made by a carpenter under the direction of a therapist is best. Where this is not possible chairs are available commercially although, because of their adaptability, they tend to be bulky. Many adaptations can be made to a normal child's wooden chair such as the fitting of arms, side supports, head pieces, thigh straps, and pommels on the seat to prevent adduction.

The main points to consider in the design of the chair are:

(1) The child must feel secure and should have adequate support but not so much that he will not progress to the next stage of independent sitting.

(2) It should fit exactly from hip to knee, and knee to foot rest. Chair arms, if needed, should be at a height which gives support but does not hunch the shoulders.

Prolonged sitting is not good for any child and mobility and variety of position should be encouraged. Activities can be done in prone lying over wedges, or sitting on floor seats. Good positioning can encourage manual dexterity and improve head control and trunk stability.

Development of Manipulation

The occupational therapist is particularly concerned with the improvement of physical function in regard to manipulative skills. Ability charts have shown that the cerebral palsied child follows the normal sequence of development more closely in manipulation than in other spheres, such as locomotion or speech. Arm and shoulder control contribute to hand control, so does accurate reach. The athetoid lacks control and the spastic must increase his range. Grasp is developed along normal lines, but whereas the normal baby will have a grasp reflex only up to two or three months, the cerebral palsied child may retain this, and normal grasp may not develop. Stimulation to the palm of the hand will usually diminish the grasp reflex. The child first attempts voluntary grasp on the ulnar side of the hand but normally this soon changes to a radial grasp and later to holding small things between finger and thumb. In the spastic child efforts to grasp are hampered by the thumb being adducted across the palm, the result being an inadequate grasp on the ulnar side of the hand. A leather thumb splint which allows some mobility can be helpful; after a year or two it may be removed without the thumb going into adduction. At one stage a normal baby leads in with the index finger when reaching for things, isolating it from movement of the others. This leads on to the fine pincer grasp at about forty weeks. The cerebral palsied child will find pincer grasp easier if first taught to point. To encourage this the therapist can place her hand over the child's, holding down the ring and little fingers. Alternatively she can bandage them towards the palm thus forcing him to use his thumb and forefingers. Intentional release is normally developed at the same time as the pincer grasp.

Many spastics grasp and release with their wrists in ulnar deviation. Before trying to correct this it is important to assess whether it is due to spasticity or is simply a mechanical way of getting an adducted thumb out of the palm of the hand. The child is taught to release, first by placing cubes into large containers and gradually through training he will acquire more precision until he can place one cube on top of another. Hand splints may be helpful but, apart from the thumb splint, they are of more use in older children. An athetoid child may have more control if his wrist is stabilised by a splint on the dorsum of the wrist. The manipulative skill which the child has acquired must be applied to activities such as writing and typing. Pencils may need individual adaptation. Pencil control is taught through carefully graded exercises. For the child who will never write, typing should be taught. This is an excellent finger exercise and leads to improvement in hand control as well as giving a means of communication. Reconditioned electric typewriters are available for cerebral palsied children at a small cost. Some children may not be able to manage even on an electric typewriter with a keyboard guard and for these a typewriter with an enlarged keyboard or, for the intelligent child, the Possum* typewriter may be available.

Eye movements are closely associated with manipulation. If a child is unable to follow an object normally with his eyes he should be given treatment to improve his visuo-motor coordination. A marble race is a toy which is used for this.

Perceptual Training

Many children have perceptual handicaps, which may show as a difficulty of recognition (agnosia), in performance (apraxia) or in both. Agnosia may be related to any of the senses but the occupational therapist is most concerned with the tactile, kinaesthetic and visual senses. A child may have poor sense of the position of his body in space and he should be helped to an awareness of this at an early age. Later he can build up concepts of position; first, of things in relation to himself, and later, in relation to each other. He is also taught to appreciate shape, size and texture, both tactually and visually.

It is necessary to assess where a child's main difficulties lie so that training can be applied to these problems. Too much valuable time can, however, be spent on assessing the child's abilities in individual tasks. It is important that training should start early and that the child himself experiences both sensation and movement. Body image may be improved by his manipulating a doll into certain positions or by constructing cut-outs to make a face or figure. This will be meaningless, however, unless he applies it to himself. He must first learn, through the movements of his own body, how his arms and legs move. If necessary the sensation of these movements can be reinforced by doing them against resistance. He must also be taught concepts of position, such as under and over, through moving into these situations, thereby learning not only the words but the concepts, so that he can apply them in different circumstances. Recognition by touch is trained by placing objects and shapes in the child's hand and asking him to identify them without looking. He is also taught to distinguish textures, temperatures and weights.

The child with perceptual difficulties will often be distractible, being unable to pick out, and keep his attention on, the prominent stimulus in any situation. He must learn ultimately to be in a group and be able to deal with distractions. If at first he is treated in a 'quiet' room, toys and distractions should be introduced gradually.

When a child can appreciate size, shape and relationships, using three dimensional objects, he must learn to recognise the same situations in two dimensional pictorial representation. At this stage the Frostig Program can be used profitably. This covers the development of visual perception in five main areas. It can be used for children of any age, being particularly valuable for older children who may find other forms of perceptual training childish. *Dyslexic* children should be mentioned here as their perceptual problems are similar to the cerebral palsied and they too, can be helped by the *Frostig Program* (see References). For older children games can be used in perceptual training: ball games train eye–hand coordination; more static games such as draughts and chinese chequers teach spatial relationships.

The therapist treating perceptual disorders should study the work of Marianne Frostig, Jean Ayres and Newell Kephart (see References). The *Montessori Sensorial Apparatus* has been found to be particularly useful with young cerebral palsied children as it isolates specific factors thereby enabling the child to concentrate on size only or on shape only. It is also a good size to handle and encourage accurate movements.

Activities of Daily Living

Feeding. Because of the physiological link between speech and feeding, the occupational therapist works closely with the speech therapist. Both face problems of impaired respiration and of incoordination of lips, tongue, jaw and palate.

Some children can be helped to feed themselves with simple adaptations such as enlarged spoon handles. Angling the handles of spoons should not be done unless the child is unable to feed independently without this. An angled spoon encourages a flexed and ulnar deviated wrist. The child needs to achieve a reasonable amount of head control for feeding. He must bring his head forward to take the food off the spoon with his lips. Many children will need guidance of the arm but only minimal support should be given.

The two main movements patterns used in feeding are based on *Temple Fay* or *Peto* methods. In the Temple Fay patterns the elbow is supported level with the shoulder and movements are on a horizontal plane. In Professor Peto's method the child stabilises himself by leaning on his elbows; he drinks from a mug with two handles which he grasps with both hands. It is important that the method used at a centre or school should also be carried out at home. The therapist should therefore show the mother the method and indicate how much assistance to give.

Dressing. The mental age and the physical handicap of the child must be considered, and compared with normal development. A normal child learns to undress himself before he can dress himself. The mother is advised on the easiest clothes to manage. Simple adaptations may help, such as replacing press studs by *velcro*. Dressing can be preceded by other simpler activities using the same movements: for example, the child is taught to place a quoit over his hand and to pull it up to his shoulder as practice for pulling his sleeves on. Undressing and dressing should always be for a purpose and often the best time is before and after physiotherapy or pool treatment. Each child should be taught to dress himself in a position in which he feels completely stable. Some children will manage best sitting in a chair, others in a floor seat.

As well as the physical difficulties involved there may be perceptual difficulties. The apraxic child will find dressing especially difficult and his clothes (night and day) should be as similar as possible to avoid confusion.

The Chart A (see pp. 393-4) is used to record a child's progress by the occupational therapist. Similar charts on relevant points are kept by the physiotherapist and speech therapist, and a summary is made from these on Chart B (see p. 395).

ADOLESCENTS AND ADULTS

While at school the cerebral palsied child is unrealistic about his abilities and his future. It is unlikely that he has had to take responsibility commensurate with his age group, to make decisions or to compete with others. This is especially true of those at schools for the physically handicapped or other special schools where there is no opportunity to compare their abilities with those of their normal contemporaries. Athetoids in particular are often over optimistic about the future. It is not until they try to find a job, see the youth employment officer or later the disablement resettlement officer that they begin to see their abilities in perspective. The emotional problems, normal in adolescence, such as relationships with parents and with the opposite sex, are all the more complex when life as a child has been restricted by disability.

Assessment

This must inevitably include assessment in activities of daily living including travelling (see chapters 6 and 7), and then the all-important assessment for work. This can be done under four headings:

(1) Perceptual ability.
(2) Physical ability.
(3) Concentration, speed and endurance.
(4) Social and emotional adjustment.

Perceptual Ability

Sensory perception tests are carried out to isolate the patient's defects. Some perform badly on all tests and others only in one. The findings will have a bearing on work potential and ability to train.

Visual fields. Many C.P.s* do not have the normal 180° of vision and so need to turn their heads in compensation. The degree of limitation must be checked and recorded.

Superficial and deep sensation in the hands can be tested by checking two point discrimination and by drawing letters on the dorsum of the hand for identification. Such faults as breaking bits by drilling too hard, jamming machines, fumbling with small assembly work or cross threading screws may be symptomatic of loss of sensation rather than muscular incoordination or stupidity.

Stereognosis. Inability to recognise objects by feeling them is a grave disability in handling materials.

Weight discrimination. Five blocks varying from $\frac{1}{4}$ lb. to $1\frac{1}{4}$ lb. are to be placed in order of weight. Those who find this difficult will also have handling problems at work, for power must be proportionate to the resistance offered.

Tests Related to Work Situations

The following are examples of tests directly related to work situations:

Location test. Twenty 6-inch rods must be put through a concealed hole, (see Fig. 29 (i)) in a time varying from 1 to 8 minutes. This will necessitate both stereognostic and kinaesthetic sense. Those who are slow at this test find it difficult to handle objects which are out of sight.

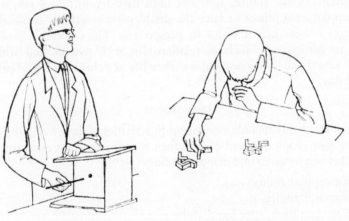

FIG. 29.   (i) Location test.   (ii) Copying patterns.

Judging size and measurement. Four metal right angles, $1\frac{1}{2}$ inches long are laid out in a pattern. The patient must copy this with four similar pieces. Those who find this hard will have difficulty in accurate measurement, recognising mistakes and placing work in a jig. (See Fig. 29 (ii)).

Drilling test. To check the ability to operate a drill and manipulate the jig and components.

Rotary convertor plane-o-graph. This machine gives an indication of control and speed of movement. A handle comparable with that on a milling machine has a pencil attached. The lead is in contact with paper which moves sideways at a constant speed. By turning the handle sine waves are drawn on the paper. The quicker it is turned the more frequent the waves.

Concentration, Speed and Endurance

A conveyer belt is ideal for training in picking up and placing pieces rapidly. The belt speed is increased as the worker becomes more adept. This provides an objective assessment of speed of working. Industrial outwork is usually timed in order to assess a fair price with the factory. This 'norm' can be used as a standard with which to compare performance.

Competitive games, both as part of treatment and as recreation, will provide opportunity for assessing both concentration and speed.

Social and Emotional Adjustment

In a residential centre such as Sherrard's Industrial Rehabilitation Unit* there are ample opportunities to observe behaviour and identify problems of individuals both in social and work situations. This is more difficult to do for out-patients in a general hospital as it is rarely possible to provide a realistic industrial environment in a hospital. The special centres try to provide an environment as near normal as is possible with opportunities for teamwork, for taking decisions and for showing initiative and leadership potential. But communal living will inevitably create and perpetuate difficult situations; personality clashes with fellow residents or with staff and acceptance of a structured régime may be hard to tolerate. Self discipline and a sense of responsibility towards, and social integration with, the community may take time to develop. To compete in employment both are essential.

Treatment Methods

Work, if necessary adapted to the individual's needs, is one of the best methods of treating the adolescent or adult cerebral palsied. Before being mentally and physically ready for sheltered or open employment, up to a year may have to be spent in a special centre adapting to work requirements. Where the patient has special remedial needs, half hour daily sessions of individual treatment should be given. The aims will be the same as those for children but the media should be more sophisticated. Competitive games are excellent, both for specific remedial movement and for developing a sense of fair play and the right attitudes towards winning and losing.

Physical Ability

Grades of functional achievement can be assessed under the following headings:

Hand function—right or left hand

(1) Arm use with (*a*) arm extended (*b*) arm flexed.
(2) Ability to hold down work with hemiplegic or most affected hand.
(3) Grip and hold down work.
(4) Grip with some finger control.
(5) Gross finger movement, grasp and release.
(6) Fine finger movement and good hand function.

Mobility

(1) Sitting only.
(2) Standing, occasionally for very short periods.
(3) Balancing and standing part of the day.
(4) Mobile between benches; standing all day.
(5) Standing all day and carrying work between benches.
(6) Standing all day and carrying work.

It is important for the therapist to have an accurate system of measuring function and ability, and it will be encouraging for the patient to see records of his improvement in control and range of movement. Improvement is cumulative and can go on throughout the patient's life.

Hemiplegia

These patients will not only have little or no functional use in the affected hand; there will be limitation of movement in all joints of the upper limb. To be employable, use of one hand is seldom enough and for this hand to be functional it is necessary to have reasonable control of shoulder, elbow, hand and fingers. Fifteen per cent usage of the affected hand may make the difference between earning and not earning a living. Treatment must aim at mobilising the shoulder, at increasing elbow and wrist extension and at improving supination, grip, and release (see chapter 10).

Some Treatment Techniques

Turning a large handle as on a mangle, attached for example to a brush making machine, encourages shoulder movement, elbow and wrist extension and grip. If necessary the hand can be bandaged in position.

Playing with large draughts made from scrap metal (round pieces play square pieces). These can be pushed if they cannot be lifted. Progression will be to solitaire played with lead pieces, followed by pegotty, first picking up with the unaffected hand and transferring to the affected hand, then using the latter alone.

Turning large screws 2 inches in diameter, first learning to grip and then to turn the screw. This helps develop pronation and supination, flexion and extension of the wrist and finger movements. Progression for finger dexterity will be screwing and unscrewing increasingly smaller nuts and bolts.

Dropping discs on to a draughts board and throwing quoits provide release of grip and, with the latter shoulder movement, wrist and elbow extension.

Although such a high degree of control and fine finger movement will not be required in the patient's eventual work, the greater dexterity they achieve, the better their general functional ability.

Athetosis

Athetoids need the help of weighted resistance to increase control over their movements. With improvement the resistance can be decreased gradually until they can do finer work. As coordination improves weighted draughts lead to turning screws and finally to putting matchsticks into cribbage boards. Machine work using levers and handles is more suitable for athetoids than assembly work.

Epilepsy

It is hoped that the patient will be stabilised on drugs before assessment is expected. Epilepsy presents special problems of personality and careful choice of work must be made. If there is any liability to fits the epileptic C.P.* patient should not work on machines (see chapters 6 and 15).

Resettlement

Open Industry

Experience at Sherrard's I.R.U.* has shown that some cerebral palsied are employable after training, especially in light engineering, and that they can live independently in lodgings.

Sheltered Workshops

The type of work in Remploy* factories varies geographically and that available locally may not be suitable. In addition entrance standards are high. The Spastics Society* has a sheltered workshop and hostel in Birmingham where a basic wage is earned and in which those with 50–75 per cent capacity for normal work output can be accepted.

Day Centres

When output is less than 50 per cent regular attendance at a day centre is recommended, with a view to upgrading should work abilities improve. Even those who are severely incapacitated will benefit from the stimulation of joining in a group. The Spastics Society* runs work centres, some residential, which provide industrial work with payment for the work done. Local authorities also have centres, some with transport facilities, where the emphasis may be on industrial work, craft work or socialising activities.

Residential Centres for the Unemployable

There are many of these in the country run by the Spastics Society*, its local branches and other organisations. They vary in character and purpose. Some are able to develop active schemes, others are predominantly to provide care. It is important to choose the centre in which the individual will fit best intellectually and emotionally. Referral is indicated when there is lack of day centre facilities or inadequate provision for care at home.

Home Care

When attendance at a day centre is not possible it is important that some sort of service be provided both for the disabled member of the family and for those who must look after him. Sometimes the local branch of the Spastics Society* can arrange this, or the local welfare department may be involved. Other active local organisations such as the W.R.V.S.* may help. Occasional outings and holidays are often arranged. The domiciliary occupational therapist should be involved if assessment and treatment have not been adequate, but if the patient is well organised her help may not be needed. It is important not to have too many home visitors competing to give help and advice.

REFERENCES AND RECOMMENDED FURTHER READING

General

Abercrombie, M. L. J., *Perceptual and Visuo-motor Disorders in Cerebral Palsy*. Spastics Society*, London, 1964.

Ayres, J. A. (1963), The development of perceptual motor abilities. (A theoretical basis for treatment of dysfunction.) *Am. J. occup. Ther.*, 7, 6.

Ayres, J. A., *Perceptual-Motor Dysfunction in Children*. Ohio O.T. Ass., 1539 Shenandoah Avenue, Cincinatti, Ohio.

Blencoe, S. M., *Cerebral Palsy and the Young Child*, Edinburgh and London, 1969.

Bobath, B., *Abnormal Postures Reflex Activity Caused by Brain Lesion*. London, 1971.

Brereton, B. le G. & Sattler, J., *Cerebral Palsy: Basic Abilities*. Spastics' Centre, 6 Queen Street, Mosman, N.S.W., Australia, 1967.

Cotton, E., The integration of treatment and education in cerebral palsy. *Physiotherapy*, 56, 1970.

Critchley, M., *The Parietal Lobes*. London, 1953 (U.S. reprint 1969).
And see: Occupational therapy in athetoid cerebral palsy. *Occ. Ther.*, 35, no. 10, 1972.
Finnie, N., *Handling the Young Cerebral Palsied Child at Home*. London, 1968.
Frostig, M. & Jakeman, D., *Sensory Motor Development*. (Using the Frostig Programme). Special Edition, June 1968.
Frostig, M. & Home, D., *The Frostig Program for the Development of Visual Perception*. Chicago.
Gilmour, A. M. (1967), Paediatric aspects of cerebral palsy (and note Bibliography). *Scot. J. Occup. Ther.*, 70.
Gunzberg, H. G., *Primary Progress Assessment Chart of Social Development, and Progress Assessment Charts I and II*. National Ass. for Mental Health*.
Holt, K. S., *Assessment of Cerebral Palsy*. Book I. London, 1965.
Holt, K. S. & Reynell, *Assessment of Cerebral Palsy*. Book II. London, 1966.
Illingworth, R. S., *The Development of Infant and Young Children*. Edinburgh and London, 1972.
Illingworth, R. S. (Ed.), *Recent Advances in Cerebral Palsy*. Edinburgh and London, 1958.
Jenkins, R. M. D. (1967), P.O.S.M. for a 6 year old. *Am. J. occup. Ther.*
Kindermans, D. J., *The Montessori Method in Cerebral Palsy Schools*. P.O. Box No. 10173, Johannesburg, S. Africa.
Loring J. & Jorgensen., *Assessment of the Cerebral Palsied Child for Education*. Spastics Society*, London, 1968.
Smith, I. M., *Spatial Ability*. London, 1964.
Montessori, M., *The Secret of Childhood*. London (1936).
Morgentein, M. & F., *Practical Training for the Severely Handicapped Child*. Spastics Society*.
Monfraix, C. & Tandien, G. C. (1961), Disturbances of manual perception in children with cerebral palsy. *Cerebr. Palsy Bull.*
Monfraix, C. & Tandien, G. C. (1961), Development of manual perception in the child with cerebral palsy. *Cerebr. Palsy Bull.*

For Industrial Work
See reference 17, chapter 20, this book.
Seymour, W. D., *Industrial Skills*. London (1966).
Seymour, W. D., *Industrial Training for Manual Operations*. London (1954).
For Information on Residential and Work Centres apply to the Spastics Society*.
And see the Magazine of this Society, particularly copies August 1966, November 1966, February 1968, re Industrial work.
The Assessment Charts on pp. 374-376 of this chapter have been reproduced by the permission of the Centre for Spastic Children, 61 Cheyne Walk, London S.W.3.
* See *Glossary*, pp. 454-6.

An Occupational Therapist, Miss Hilary Schlesinger, has been appointed by the Spastics Society to investigate certain aspects of the employment of spastics in a work centre environment, on the following lines:

(1) To detail the spectrum of disability of handicapped persons, currently attending Work Centres, i.e. physical and mental disabilities and including other handicaps such as epileptic fits, spatial perception, co-ordination and concentration, etc.
(2) To recommend (if thought to be necessary) a standard form of assessment to be used by Work Centres, and to devise a format for comparing a handicapped person's performance with that of a non-handicapped person.
(3) To tabulate the types and variety of work provided by Work Centres and to list the advantages and disadvantages in relation to:

(a) Job satisfaction.
(b) Long-term sheltered employment.
(c) Training within the unit (and supervision).
(d) Training for those spastics thought to be suitable for outside employment.

(4) To comment on the present types of machinery, jigs, fixtures, etc. in use at Work Centres, expressing the desirability of any changes in the industrial equipment, with regard to the further involvement of the more severely handicapped spastics attending.

(5) To suggest alternative forms of day employment, i.e. non-manual work and investigate the practicability of such employment in existing work centres.

(6) To discuss practical possibilities of recreational and sports activities for the spastic employees.

Miss Schlesinger has been working in Latin America and has made a study of standardised procedures and guide lines for job and task analysis, as a basis for the evaluation of work capacity of the disabled, under the following headings:

1. Work factors
2. Format for job analysis
3. Definition of factors
4. Variables intervening in the analysis of factors
5. Criteria for grading work requirements
6. Work tests
7. Evaluation forms
8. Lists of equipment

(It is hoped that both these studies may be available to occupational therapists in the not too distant future.)

A. PHYSICAL ABILITY CHART

OCCUPATIONAL THERAPY DEPT.

NAME..

DATE OF BIRTH..

DIAGNOSIS...

....

....

....

....

· SELF HELP IN DAILY LIVING.
COMMUNICATION BY WRITING.

Handedness..

Normal •Years			YEAR							
		Preparatory	MONTH							
			DAY							
12/52	1.	Absence of grasp reflex R								
,,	2.	,, ,, ,, L								
20/52	3.	Stretch for object at arm's length R								
,,	4.	,, ,, ,, L								
	5.	Stretch for object above head R								
	6.	,, ,, ,, L								
24/52	7.	Pick up 1″ cube R								
	8.	,, ,, L								
28/52	9.	Transfer cube, R to L								
,,	10.	,, ,, L to R								
	11.	Pick up billiard ball R								
	12.	,, ,, L								
44/52	13.	Release 1″ cube R								
,,	14.	,, ,, L								
	15.	Release billiard ball R								
	16.	,, ,, L								
	17.	Place cotton reel on fixed dowel R								
	18.	,, ,, ,, ,, L								
15/12	19.	Build 2-cube tower R								
	20.	,, ,, L								
	21.	Place peg in peg board R								
	22.	,, ,, ,, L								
	23.	Pick up 6d. piece between thumb and index finger R								
	24.	,, ,, ,, ,, ,, ,, L								
21/12	25.	Build 5-cube tower R								
	26.	,, ,, L								
	27.	Supinate actively R								
	28.	,, ,, L								
	29.	Pronate actively R								
	30.	,, ,, L								
		Daily Living								
	31.	Fasten zipper on board								
1½	32.	Remove socks								
2	33.	Remove shoes when untied								
3	34.	Remove pullover								
3	35.	Remove dress								
3	36.	Remove cardigan								
3	37.	Remove trousers or pants								

*Approximate age at which normal child might be expected to
achieve ability (after Gesell).

CHART A—*continued*

Normal Years			YEAR MONTH DAY
3	38.	Put on shoes and socks	
3	39.	Put on pullover	
3	40.	Put on dress	
3	41.	Put on cardigan	
3	42.	Put on trousers or pants	
	43.	Undo large buttons on board	
	44.	Undo small buttons on board	
	45.	Do up large buttons on board	
	46.	Do up small buttons on board	
	47.	Fasten press studs on board	
	48.	Fasten hooks and eyes on board	
	49.	Fasten buckles on board	
4	50.	Lace shoes	
4	51.	Wash and dry face and hands	
	52.	Blow nose	
6	53.	Tie bows on shoes	

Toiletting

2¼	54.	Bowel control	
3	55.	Bladder control	
3	56.	Toilet self	

COMMUNICATION BY WRITING

13/12	57.	Initiate stroke with crayon	
	58.	Colour in single outline picture	
	59.	Draw line between two given points	
3	60.	Copy circle	
5	61.	Copy letters	
	62.	Communicate by writing	
	63.	Communicate by typing	

| Co-operation | |
| Tested by | |

Chart to be filled in in **RED** where ability is attempted with aid of appliance.

APPLIANCES

Date	Appliances in use	Date taken out of use

B.   PHYSICAL ABILITY CHART

NAME...
DATE OF BIRTH...............................

DIAGNOSIS...
....
....
....

KEY to CHART

Ability

☐	Not tested.
◹	None.
◩	None, but tries hard.
▧	Poor, Intermittent, or Very Slow.
◼	Moderate, or Slow.
■	Good.

(Darker Chart shows better ability throughout)
Chart filled in in **RED** where ability is attempted with aid of appliance.

PHYSICAL SUMMARY

Handedness................................

Ability to :

	YEAR
	MONTH
	DAY

1. Dress self
2. Toilet self
3. Sit on ordinary chair
4. Get around on feet
5. Get around otherwise

6. Feed self
7. Use hand for writing
8. Speak intelligibly
9. Hear

*10. See

CHAPTER 20

Occupational Therapy for Geriatric Patients

Principles involved in occupational therapy for geriatric patients, and aims of treatment, are similar to those for cases in any general hospital, but owing to the higher average age of the patients, there are certain differences. Among these are a higher rate of long-term disabling illness, a natural slowing down of mental and physical activity, poor motivation, marked feelings of uselessness and loneliness, and general frailty. In the majority of patients multiple disabilities are present, making an arbitrary division into physical and psychological conditions inapplicable. Instead, it has proved useful to employ what has been termed the Dynamic Quadruple Assessment. The four assessments involved are the primary three of psychological, physical and social, and the fourth and most important, that of residual disability after the others have received treatment. Dynamic assessment implies that the approach must be an active one, and that there is a need to reassess from time to time in the light of the patient's response to treatment and alterations in his environment. The assessment is the responsibility of the doctor, but the occupational therapist may contribute to it and must be aware of it, if she is to play her part efficiently in the treatment of the patient.

The Therapeutic Team

The geriatric team, working under the leadership of the doctor includes the clinical psychologist, nurse, physiotherapist, occupational therapist, chiropodist, speech therapist, dietitian, medical social worker, as well as surgical appliance and hearing aid specialists, and voluntary and other agents who may be called in if necessary. Cooperation is essential if the patient is not to be confused by too many interviews, and possibly conflicting treatments, or is to be prevented from playing off one department against another in an attempt to gain sympathy and special attention. Under supervision of qualified staff, unqualified staff form an essential part of the team.

Progressive Patient Care

In some geriatric hospitals, patients are grouped according to their functioning ability, with appropriate staff and equipment provided. This involves patients being moved progressively between units. On admission to hospital emphasis is on medical assessment and treatment, and nursing care. Here the patient has a passive role. The next stage provides for active participation and is started as soon as the patient is able to respond. Occupational therapy begins, and the aim is gentle encouragement and stimulation, some movement and diversion, and above all the prevention of apathy and depression. With the return of reasonable resilience, a programme of activity of daily living begins, with occupational therapy applied to any specific disability, mental or physical, on an individual and group basis. More energetic activities are used and plans for resettlement are much to the fore. For those who must be independent the next vital move for a few days or weeks is to an intensive activity of daily living unit, where domestic retraining is included. This is sometimes followed by a period of living independently, but still in hospital: hospital staff are only available if essential. This accustoms the patient to real independence. In these last stages, occupational therapy is the predominant treatment, and nursing care becomes minimal.

On return to the community, treatment may be entirely in the hands of the domiciliary team. The domiciliary occupational therapist may be involved, or responsibility may be shared by the occupational therapist at the hospital. In the latter case, the patient may attend the out-patient departments or a day hospital. With this programme only very few patients remain in long-stay wards. It is especially important that the link is made with the domiciliary workers in good time before discharge. The careful selection of furnishings and planning of buildings including all the places the patients use is of great importance. The occupational therapist has special knowledge to offer the other members of the team on these points, and should foster good relationships, so that use can be made of the knowledge when plans for new equipment and buildings are contemplated.

On the whole the occupational therapy service can be most effective when this system, based on progressive functioning ability, is used. Communication between and within the different treatment teams is essential. Plans, control and contact are usually maintained through weekly ward rounds, case conferences, clinics and by written reporting, although much informal contact takes place continually.

Approach to the Patient

In dealing with elderly patients, the most important factor is the approach to the individual. Many old people have decided opinions, while others

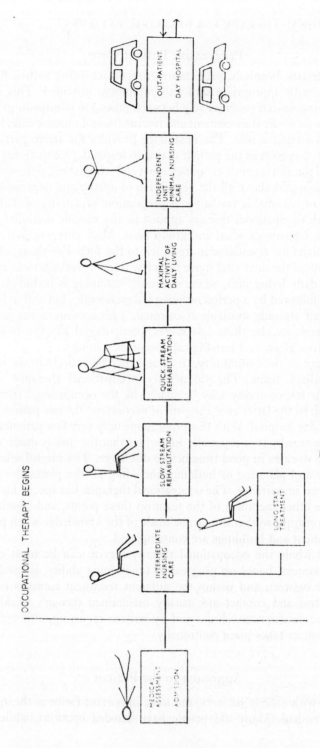

FIG. 30. Progressive patient care.

have mental changes, and some are confused. The majority need to be approached carefully if their cooperation is to be gained. There are several factors to be remembered.

Excuses

At first most patients will make excuses such as, 'It's my eyes, Miss!' or 'I've worked all my life, and I've come here for a rest'. It is essential in dealing with these, to have confidence, backed by an adequate medical prescription, and to be able to say, 'The doctor has asked me to give you this treatment, or this thing to do'. In most cases the reluctance to start springs from a fear of failure, probably well founded in past experience, and a desire not to risk further disappointment and perhaps ridicule.

These patients must be assured that the therapist is there to see them safely through any activity they undertake, and that she will not ask them to do anything too difficult. It is important that the first result should be a success, however much supervision this involves. A simple activity well done should be the aim at this stage, and more difficult tasks should be introduced only as confidence improves. It is best not to take excuses too seriously, but if they persist it may be necessary to discuss the problem with the doctor.

Decisions

Many elderly people, and especially the mildly confused, find it difficult to make decisions (except the negative one, that it is safer to do nothing). At first it is usually best for the occupational therapist to make the decisions herself, or to give a choice between two simple alternatives. Multiplicity of choice often leads to confusion, and results in complete rejection of all activity. As confidence increases more complicated choices can be offered with increasing opportunity to make decisions.

Motivation

Motivation is of great importance for geriatric patients. Many have little to look forward to after discharge, and in some cases their disability provides them with their only feeling of security. The medical social workers may be able to help by introducing alterations to their previous home environment. Patients, frightened by their inability to perform their personal chores, will regain confidence through retraining in mobility by the physiotherapists, and in carrying out activities of daily living under the occupational therapists' guidance. The will to get better can be developed through social activities, and in the mixing of in- and out-patients. Seeing others with similar disabilities managing at home with only a home-help and a weekly visit to hospital, is excellent for morale. Noting that help is given where it is needed, patients feel secure, and incentives towards recovery begin to take effect.

Motivation is also important in the sphere of creative activities. No work, however simple, should be given to a patient without a reason he can understand. 'Giving him something to do' is not enough. Patients who have no relatives for whom to work, who have little money, and whose own needs are basic, may still get great satisfaction in helping other patients, making something for the department, fulfilling an order, or working for a 'sale of work'. In predominantly physical cases the desire to get better may be motive enough, but even in these cases more interest is shown if the work is really needed by someone. Praise and appreciation are important and should not be neglected.

The 'Hostess Approach'

When patients show some degree of confusion, they may not remember the workshop from day to day and so are faced with the unknown every time they attend. This produces reluctance to enter until a feeling of familiarity has been achieved, but these patients almost invariably respond to what might be termed the 'hostess approach'. If met at the door and greeted as visitors (and if possible offered a cup of tea), they generally realise that they are expected, that the occasion is a friendly one, and that as guests they should behave well. This approach usually helps the patient who has most difficulties to settle down quickly and happily, and saves time, argument and persuasion.

Conversation

One of the greatest needs of the elderly is the opportunity to talk to a sympathetic listener. In the hospital as a whole few have the time to satisfy this need, and it could be argued that the occupational therapist is no exception, but time spent talking to these patients is rarely wasted. In conversation while working many underlying emotional and social problems are disclosed quite naturally, and can then be referred to the appropriate person for attention.

Dysphasic, deaf, aphasic, some parkinsonian and cerebral palsy patients share the experience of loneliness through lack of speech. In cooperation with the speech therapist, the occupational therapist should encourage expression through conversation while occupational therapy is in progress. Local and current events should be introduced and a conscious effort made to speak to these patients whom it is easy to neglect. Thought should be given to seating arrangements to stimulate social exchanges.

Frustration

Among the senile patients there are many who, though forgetful and slow, are still happy and well adjusted, while others, with lesser degrees of mental impairment, become difficult or aggressive, or tend to wander. Great patience is needed in handling the latter, and any sort of frustration should be avoided if the patient's cooperation is to be won. On the first visits such patients should be returned to their wards or homes as soon as they show signs of restlessness, so that they avoid any feeling of constraint. A feature of these people is a tendency to ask the same question again and again. It is pointless to say, 'I told you that before', because the patient has forgotten, and really wants to know again. The answer should be given as often as the question is asked, as only in this way can fear and lack of confidence be avoided. Similarly it is undesirable to tell these patients to sit down if they become restless. So long as they are not harming themselves or other patients it is good for them to wander around and use some of their excess energy. When they are tired they will gladly accept a chair offered as a courtesy, and with solicitude. When taking one of these patients to another room, or to the ambulance, it is very much better to offer your arm to him than to take his. The first action is associated with help, and the second with restraint. If, despite kindness, tact and guile, the patient tries to wander, no attempt should be made to turn him round and bring him back the way he came. A forwards movement around a table, or tree, or even a corridor will achieve results more quickly, and will leave the patient in a more manage-able frame of mind. If the patient can be left to wander safely alone he can then be 'met' and greeted as an old friend, and will usually return quite happily, and even with relief at seeing a friendly and vaguely familiar face. The use of a patient's name is extremely important in gaining his confidence, and so is an ability to control surprise at being called 'Mother', 'Aunty', or 'our Lil'!

Teaching Techniques

With increasing age there is usually a slowing down in the processes of understanding, reasoning, remembering and learning, and this may be combined with failing vision or hearing. Though it is not true that 'you can't teach an old dog new tricks', these difficulties make it essential for the therapist to have a sound knowledge of teaching techniques and a good deal of patience. In a few cases encouragement of greater speed may be indicated, but the best results are generally obtained when the patient is encouraged to take his time, or even to work more slowly. This applies to the patient's approach to toilet, dressing and eating, to walking and domestic activities, as well as to crafts and hobbies. To lose patience and to hurry an elderly patient is to lose his confidence and possibly his cooperation. Most of these patients are capable of high standards if tasks are carefully selected and properly supervised. Bad workmanship is usually the result of failure in one of these aspects. As a rule work for the elderly is better if linked with the patient's past activities and interests although it is important that he

14

should not be depressed by failing at something he used to do easily. For instance an old carpenter may polish a tray base successfully for another patient, but not do well trying to use his former tools; similarly, it may be wiser for a housewife to prepare a cold salad than to try to cook a hot meal.

Progression

Where progressive patient care is used, the complexity and type of activities used in occupational therapy will be governed by the condition of the patients in each unit. With a group on long term treatment there is danger of a patient getting into a rut, because he is apparently contented. Regular reviews should be carried out, as changes in occupation, although not always welcomed, may prove valuable. Not infrequently improvement occurs, and resettlement becomes a possibility.

Deterioration

However much treatment is given, it must be accepted that deterioration will take place in certain cases, either as an accompaniment to increasing age, or in the course of a progressive disease. For such people, although cure cannot be looked for, occupational therapy still has a part to play. In fact, when other treatments have been discontinued, it may increase in importance from a humanitarian viewpoint. Final deterioration can take a long time, and carefully graded occupation can shield a patient from the full realisation of his failing powers and can reassure those in close contact with him. Where there is insight it may still help the patient to adjust to the situation, and to make the most of whatever faculties are left to him.

The Physical Aspect

The aims of treatment for patients with physical disability, and the techniques available to the occupational therapist in carrying them out are the same as for younger patients so long as the patient is mentally able to accept them. These are discussed elsewhere. Frequently, however, the ideal physical treatment cannot be applied because of the patient's mental deterioration. In such cases, aids and adaptations are of little help, as they tend to be beyond his understanding, or to be mislaid. Simplification is essential. Treatment should be directed towards the maintenance of bodily function, the alleviation of symptoms arising from disabilities of old age such as rheumatoid arthritis, hemiplegia and parkinsonism, and other progressive or long-term conditions including cardiac, pulmonary, neurological and visual disabilities. Specifically, the aims should be to improve the function of muscles and joints, and the circulation to the affected parts; to develop or maintain coordination, skill and dexterity; to test or increase work tolerance and to alleviate any psychological disturbance associated with the disability. In all cases attention must be given to good posture and lighting, and particularly with cardiac and respiratory conditions care must be taken to provide interest while avoiding fatigue. The right apparatus greatly facilitates the teaching of good methods of carrying out the activities of daily living: rising from and sitting in a chair; dressing; opening doors; walking up steps etc. (see chapters 6 and 7).

In elderly patients what they can do is often more important than how they do it, so, to achieve independence, 'trick' movements may be necessary and acceptable.

Rehabilitation

Rehabilitation of the elderly usually involves a return to home but possibly not to work, although the latter is sometimes possible. Important factors are maximum physical independence, cleanliness, a reason for living, understanding relatives or friends, and a feeling of security. Occupational therapy has a part to play in all these requirements although actual resettlement is primarily the medical social worker's responsibility. Maximum physical independence involves cooperation with the physiotherapist, and possibly the dietitian. The occupational therapist's part will include activities for manual dexterity, practice in self help, and for the re-establishment of domestic competence. The provision of an interest is primarily the occupational therapist's responsibility, and if it is possible to provide an activity which can be carried on at home the chances of a successful resettlement are enhanced. In certain cases, domiciliary and hospital occupational therapists may collaborate in advising on suitable aids, and on alterations to and in the home. Out-patient treatment may be arranged. Old people's clubs are also invaluable for the right patient after discharge.

Breakdown in family relationships, rather than any noticeable change in a patient's condition, often precipitates admission to hospital. Resettlement may be hindered unless the real problem is tackled. Such relatives, if asked to attend the department, may be helped by being shown easier methods of handling the physical problems, which may ease the tense relationship. Seeing the patient less helpless than he appeared and reacting well to a social situation often brings new understanding. Tactfully given advice on handling him is usually gratefully received. One daughter wrote of the improvement in her mother's response, now she had learnt to ask, rather than tell her!

Return home may be regarded with misgiving or even become impossible unless the patient has a feeling of security. The occupational therapist can help to provide this by treatment including assessment and retraining in personal and domestic competence. This is especially important for those who live alone, and for those who must adjust to residual disability. Where

appropriate, treatment should include cooking, shopping and managing a
real bus. Follow up services may help to mitigate otherwise intolerable
loneliness.

The Day Hospital

Occupational therapy is of increasing importance as patients recover from
the acute phase of an illness and reach the period preceding discharge from
hospital. It also has significance for out-patients. It is now recognised, that,
in addition to courses of specific rehabilitation, old people frequently require
maintenance therapy—that is, regular support from the hospital team over
long periods to prevent deterioration in functioning ability. Furthermore,
the majority of older patients need a service that is organised for them in
more detail than out-patient sessions in various departments of a general
hospital. These needs led to development of geriatric day hospitals.

In this setting medical, physical, psychological or psychiatric and social
problems can be handled by a full team of staff. The patients live at home, and
travel to the hospital for the day.

Referral to the day hospital is usually made by the medical staff of the
main hospital. Reasons for referral are various: some patients may require
continued treatment following discharge from the main hospital; others
may be referred from out-patient clinics to prevent admission becoming
necessary; some, through their disturbed state may be disrupting their
home, and relatives may need relief from perpetual supervision. In all
cases the medical social worker and health visitor report on home needs.

Most patients referred are likely to need the ambulance service, although
some may be able to make their own travelling arrangements. Once in the
day hospital they are occupied with activities suited to their needs, as in any
occupational therapy department. Teas are served, and social contacts
encouraged so that the atmosphere produced is like a club. A midday meal
is provided with special diets for those who need them. Where this cannot
be arranged patients bring packed lunches, the hospital providing drinks.
The lunch hour provides practical opportunities for the encouragement of
independence and the trial of self-help aids. Baths, hairdressing and similar
personal services can also be provided in selected cases.

The mixing of in- and out-patients in the workshop and for social
activities has advantages for both. Out-patients begin to think of the others
instead of themselves, and often bring them papers, flowers or small gifts.
They also find it less frightening if their own admission becomes necessary
later because they already have personal contacts among the in-patients.
In-patients find regular contact with the outside world helpful in maintaining morale, and gain hope that they too may manage on their return home,
with day hospital support.

An important function of the day hospital occupational therapist is regular, accurate observation of the patient which can be reported to the doctor and the medical social worker. This helps them particularly when admission is being considered. A relative who is closely involved is usually less objective. Minor medical complaints can be referred directly to the nursing staff and there is the chance for all difficulties encountered to be attended to before more serious problems arise. The occupational therapist, through spending the major part of the day with the patients regularly, over fairly long periods, is in a unique position amongst the hospital staff for noting changes. She is well placed to record both reduction in performance level and medical signs, which may not have been present at an interview with the doctor but have developed with fatigue or exertion. Improvements become apparent too, and the occupational therapist is needed to advise the doctor on the patient's readiness for discharge.

Holiday admissions are linked with the day hospital scheme. Patients are admitted for a short period to allow relations, who would otherwise be completely tied, to have a holiday. Many patients look upon this as a holiday for themselves as well, and occupational therapy is generally continued during the period of admission. Patients may also be admitted as a temporary measure when relatives are ill. With the help of the day hospital and these short term admissions, permanent hospitalisation can often be deferred for a number of years.

The day hospital has value to the patient in providing treatment and new interest, to the relatives in relieving some of the burden without removing responsibility, and to the community in a considerable saving in hospital beds. It also helps the hospital in providing an opportunity for assessment of the need for admission should further deterioration take place.

Occupational therapy has a vital prophylactic contribution to make to an increasingly ageing population. Its importance is becoming more fully recognised but more workers and experiments are still needed in this field.

Disorders Most Frequently Encountered in a Geriatric Unit

It is usual for geriatric patients to have multiple pathology so the effect of each problem on the others is important.

Psychiatric Conditions

Depression, anxiety states, obsessional and hysterical states, personality changes. Schizoid, manic-depressive, psychoses. (In psycho-geriatric units.)

Senile confusional states. Varying in degree from mild forgetfulness to gross dementia, and often found in combination with anxiety states as well as most of the physical disabilities.

Special Sense Defects

Auditory, visual and speech defects, either alone, or associated with other conditions. Care should be taken to avoid social isolation, and a check made that appointments made for spectacles, hearing aids and dentures have been followed up. The occupational therapist is often the first member of the hospital team to meet a real obstacle to treatment in difficulties with the special senses.

Neuro-muscular Disorders

Parkinsonism, myopathy, disseminated sclerosis, etc.

Cardio-vascular Diseases

Such as *congestive cardiac failure* and those leading to *hemiparesis,* etc., *athero-sclerosis* and accompanying symptoms.

Respiratory Diseases

Such as *chronic bronchitis, emphysema.*

Orthopaedic Problems

Rheumatoid arthritis, osteo-arthritis, osteo-porosis, fractures, etc.

Deficiency Diseases

Malabsorption, diabetes mellitus, anaemia, etc.

New Growths

Which may be at various sites, *benign* or *malignant.*

Endocrine Disorders

Myxoedema, thyrotoxicosis, etc.

Occupations and Activities Used in Geriatric Units

Personal Activities of Daily Living

Dressing, washing, doing hair, shaving, eating, drinking, managing in the lavatory and bathroom. Washing hair, manicuring, general attention to personal appearance.

Domestic Activities

Polishing silver, cleaning shoes, doing flowers, and mending. Dusting, light sweeping and tidying. Setting tables, making and serving toast and tea, collecting cups and washing up.

More advanced work including preparation and cooking of vegetables, cooking snacks and meals etc.

Bedmaking, washing 'smalls', shopping, travelling, reading and writing and housekeeping; bookwork may be included.

Craft-work and Art

(Good design and well selected materials which are easy to handle are important for the production of satisfying, saleable goods.)

Help to others in such elementary processes as wool winding, sand-papering, stuffing cushions, polishing, making chamoix window cleaners, nylon dishwashers.

Simple community jobs, such as knitting squares for blankets, sorting beads, rugwool scraps, etc.

Combined operations, e.g. a cushion embroidered by one patient, made up by another, stuffed by a third, and sewn up by a fourth.

Simple crafts which patients have done before, including plain knitting and crochet and simple embroidery.

Coarse embroidery in rug wool on canvas, using simple stitches, e.g. running stitch or tent stitch.

Weaving on a frame. Rug wool on a cotton or macramé warp, using alternate dark and light threads, or alternate thick and thin for the totally blind. Nytrim and other edging from clothing factories can be most effective.

Making dishmop heads, cut wool toys, etc., (kept within limits of staff time for finishing). Brush making by machine where applicable.

More advanced embroidery such as cross stitch on Linden canvas.

Plain sewing, children's clothes, aprons, work bags, teacosies, and similar articles. Patchwork, soft toys.

Matchstick veneer. Teapot stands, tray bases, mats, etc.

Mosaic work for similar articles, lampstands, coffee tables, etc.

Simpler processes in major crafts such as weaving, basketry, pottery, leatherwork, bookcraft, woodwork, stoolseating, rugmaking, netting, lampshade making, etc.

Art: painting, potato cuts, posters, remaking Christmas cards, Christmas decorations.

Social Activities

Parties with games (bingo remains a firm favourite), teas and community singing.

Competitive games such as dominoes, darts and adapted ball games.

Ward diary or wall newspaper.

Outings to cinema, walks, shopping expeditions and bus rides (often with the help of voluntary workers).

Entertainments—but these must be simple and visual rather than auditory for some (e.g. slides).

Percussion band.

Quizzes, discussion groups, play and poetry reading, talks, demonstrations and musical appreciation for the more intellectual people.

The most successful social events appear to be those in which the patients take an active part.

Industrial Work (see chapter 22)

Monetary incentive can produce results in effort output. Satisfaction can be derived from quantitative achievement. Repetitive tasks can be soothing and give confidence to insecure individuals. They can also be boring and limiting, so must be wisely used.

The hospital administrator will often help in setting up industrial work under contract with outside firms, or arrange for internal work, such as packaging of dressings for use by the nursing staff.

Miscellaneous

Attendance at religious services is appreciated, especially at Easter, Harvest and Christmas.

Current events, local or world, encourage thoughts of the present instead of the past.

Music: good reception wireless or record player in moderation, with or without singing or movement to music.

Light gardening: hoeing, weeding, watering and potting. Both out- and indoor.

Help to others: this may include reading to the blind, cutting up food, fetching apparatus, etc. This cooperation seems to aid the helper as much as the person helped.

READING REFERENCES

Adams, G. F. & McIlwraith, P. L., *Geriatric Nursing*. London, 1963.
Adams, G. F., McQuitty, F. M. & Flint, M. Y., *Rehabilitation of the Elderly Invalid at Home*. London, 1967.
Lord Amulree, *Adding Life to Years*. London, 1951.
Brocklehurst, J. C., *The Geriatric Day Hospital*. King Edward's Hospital Fund for London*, 1970.
Bromley, D. B., *The Psychology of Human Ageing*. Pelican, 1966.
Davies, L., *Easy Cooking for One or Two*, Penguin, 1972.
Hawker, M., *Geriatrics for Physiotherapitss and the Allied Professions*. London, 1974.
Hollings, E. M., Nichols, P. J. R. & Wilshere, E. R., *Equipment for the Disabled*, 1973, National Fund for Research into Crippling Diseases*.
Ingleby, B. & Yorath, M., *Living with Old Age*. London, 1966.
Irvine, R. E., Bagnall, M. K. & Smith, B. J., *The Older Patient*. London, 1970.

Isaacs, B., *An Introduction to Geriatrics*, London, 1965.
Jay, P. E., Walker, E. & Ellison, E., *Help Yourselves*, London, 1972.
Post, F., *The Clinical Psychiatry of Late Life*. London/Oxford, 1965.
Rudinger, E., *Arrangements for Old Age*, Consumers' Association, London, 1974.
Townsend, P., *The Family Life of Old People*. Pelican, 1963.
Welford, A. T., *Ageing and Human Skill*. Oxford, 1958.
  And see:
Section VI. Old Age. *Proceedings of the Fourth International Congress*. W.F.O.T.* London,
    1966.
The *Ulverscroft Large Print Books*, including the *Ulverscroft Large Print Songbook*. F. A.
    Thorpe (Publishing) Ltd, Leicester. Usually obtainable from public libraries.
  And see:
Importance of art to the elderly. *Occ. Ther.*, 35, no. 4, 1972.
Simple mental tests with geriatric patients. *Occ. Ther.*, 35, no. 5, 1972.
Geriatrics, a speciality. *Occ. Ther.*, 35, no. 7, 1972.
Activities for patients over 65. *Occ. Ther.*, 36, no. 7, 1973.
Home for the Week-end—Back on Monday. Queen's Institute of District Nursing, London,
    1973.
* See *Glossary*, p. 454.

Part Six

CHAPTER 21

Occupational Therapy in the Community

Occupational Therapy in the Community

Community occupational therapy owes its development to the following pieces of legislation, the *National Health Service Act (1946)* (Section 28) [1] and the *National Assistance Act (1948)* (Section 29) [2] both incorporated in the *Social Services Act (1970)* and the *Mental Health Act (1959)* (Section 6) [3] and the *Health Services and Public Health Act (1968)* (Section 12 [4]. All are affected by the *Re-organisation of the National Health Service Act (1973)*. This service can now be provided by the District Health Authorities or by the Local Authority Social Services Department, and/or by a combination of both. No single method of provision has yet emerged.

DISTINCTION IN ROLES

When the Social Services Act was implemented in 1971 the transfer of occupational therapists employed in former health and welfare departments was left to local decision, the responsibility falling, in some instances, on health departments, and in others, on social services departments. With the new legislation the following criteria are defined for the transfer of occupational therapists:

(1) Occupational therapists should transfer if they are engaged wholly or mainly in providing occupational therapy services under medical supervision for people with a condition for which they are receiving or have received medical treatment under the National Health Service*. They should remain in the social service department of local authorities if they are engaged wholly or mainly in providing social rehabilitation for conditions not requiring active medical supervision.

(2) Occupational therapists should also transfer if they would otherwise not be working in a properly structured professional setting under a senior therapist [5].

These criteria distinguish between remedial work under medical supervision in the hospital and community in an integrated health service, and the role of the occupational therapist relating to the *Disabled Persons (Employment) Acts (1944–1958)* [6] and the *Chronically Sick and Disabled Persons Act, 1970* [7]. Effective rehabilitation cannot distinguish between bureaucratic boundaries, and administrative divisions tend to create gaps in service. 'Staff with similar professional skills should be based in the same employing authority in the interests of the professions themselves and of their patients and clients . . . The area health authorities should make available to local health authorities the advice and support of . . . health services staff. In particular they should be required . . . to make such staff available to enable local authorities to carry out their responsibilities in the field of personal social services, education and environmental health. Similarly the local authorities should be required . . . to make social work skills available to health authorities to enable them to carry'out their health care functions' [8].

Since the issue of the above statements the D.H.S.S.* has issued a circular (HSC(1S)102) (December 1974) which 'asks health and local authorities jointly to review the needs for occupational therapy in their areas and to agree a co-ordinated policy on the employment of Occupational Therapists'.

This document describes the role of occupational therapists in the Health Services and in the Social Services departments and the work undertaken by them in both spheres. Reference is also made to the need for the services of occupational therapists, and the urgency of providing more trained personnel for these fields, and recommends careful deployment of those available to meet the needs under Area Health Authorities and Local Authorities. It is suggested, too, that more use might be made of craft instructors, and of aides, who could, with some in-service training, 'work under the direction of an occupational therapist and release professional time for more highly skilled work'.

The Role of the Occupational Therapist

The work of the community occupational therapist is the same as that of any other occupational therapist, except that the contact with the patient is through his home. When a patient leaves hospital with a residual disability, such as an arthrodesed knee, a hemiplegia or with tetraplegia, it is essential that, before he is discharged, the right provisions within the community are made for him so that he can become as independent as possible in his home. Otherwise the patient faces difficulties and frustrations which highlight his disability, and make him dependent on others.

To the many patients who never go into hospital except for consultation, the community occupational therapist has much to offer. For her there is the satisfaction of following the treatment through from the onset until maximum recovery is accomplished. She has the advantage of seeing the patient in his own surroundings. At home the patient is truly 'himself', and faced with the problem of dealing with his disability. There is never the need for the community therapist to invent problem situations; she meets them daily, and her work is a challenge to her knowledge and ingenuity.

Community occupational therapists must be prepared to give service in a wide range of disabilities and age groups, including children. Ninety per cent of the nation's sick are treated by general practitioners without admission to hospital. The community occupational therapist provides a service to general practitioners as well as to hospital consultants.

It is important that the limitations of occupational therapy are clearly recognised, so that time is not wasted in attempting the impossible. Furthermore, the occupational therapist must not take upon herself the functions for which the health visitor, the medical social worker, and other members of the team have been trained and appointed.

Administration of a Community Occupational Therapy Department [9]

The head occupational therapist should have an office in the main administrative buildings of her employing authority. The machinery of local government is complex, and the therapist will find the help and advice of the senior administrative officer invaluable in many matters, such as points of law, drafting of committee reports and implementing administrative details which may be peculiar to a particular authority. Good administration is essential if a service is to run smoothly and efficiently and is to give the greatest benefit to the patient.

Finances

The senior therapist is expected to submit an estimate of income and expenditure for her department for a period of twelve months. After consideration in Committee, adjustments in the money available may be made, and she should check at the beginning of each financial year what sums have been spent from her annual allocation. She will then be expected to keep expenditure within these limits. If unexpected further expenditure becomes necessary, further authority will be needed. Planning in advance ensures that decisions are not hastily or badly made. All monies are subject to audit, and a book-keeping system agreed jointly by therapists and auditors should be followed and careful records kept. (For general accounting methods see chapter 23.)

Records

Records should be kept of all cases visited, including those where the occupational therapist has been unable to gain access. Detailed records are especially necessary when there is more than one occupational therapist on the staff, as each has her own case load, and no two are fully conversant with each others' cases. It should always be possible to obtain from the case notes a clear picture of the patient, his background and treatment. In a department of more than one therapist, a system of filing case loads separately is recommended. It excludes the possibility of 'losing' a case in the belief that someone else is dealing with it, and makes it comparatively easy for a new therapist to take over an area.

Cooperation with other Personnel

Whenever possible therapists should be in the office at a regular time each day or week, so that others know when to contact them. It is also important that they should meet and discuss case problems with other therapists and members of different community or hospital services. The community occupational therapist should make it her business to know the members of all the services of the local authority with whom she may come in contact. A personal approach may be time consuming but usually pays dividends. A knowledge of the functions of other departments is essential to avoid overlapping, and to obtain good service for the patient.

Aids, Adaptations and Equipment [10]

It is important to know which departments supply different types of equipment, e.g. the District Health Authority may provide home nursing equipment such as special beds, commodes, backrests, mobile hoists, and also walking aids, while the Social Services Department may provide more permanent hoists which have to be fastened to ceiling joists, geriatric chairs and other aids and adaptations. Materials for home alteration may be supplied through one or other local authority department, or, if related to contract work, by the local contractors. Some authorities will pay the full cost of these, while others require the patient to pay a proportion.

All aids and materials for treatment taken to the patient's home should be signed out in the occupational therapy office and the items entered on a card which the patient signs as having received. If the article is to be bought by the patient he may like to have a copy of the issue card so that he can check entries and receipts. The auditors may either arrange for the bank to supply a special paying-in book and for the therapist to be responsible for paying the money into the bank regularly, or else for the money to be paid into the accounts section of the relevant authority.

Timetabling

A therapist working in a town or city may find it convenient to start each morning in the office, writing up the previous day's case notes, preparing work for the day, contacting other departments when necessary and dealing with other items of administration.

Therapists working in a county area are usually attached to a division, or area office and visit this office at a set time each day. Those who travel long distances between home and office may find it convenient to visit patients on the way to the office, and in some instances it may be best to work from home and only visit the office once a week. In this case, it is vitally important that this visit shall be at a regular time so that patients, departmental officials and colleagues can contact her. Times should also be considered in relation to the needs of the clientele.

Referrals

Cases may be introduced to the therapist from many different sources, e.g. hospitals, general practitioners, health visitors, social workers, district nurses, home helps, friends and relatives of the patient, and even by the patient himself. It is recommended that referral cards be deposited at local hospitals and with general practitioners for easy referrals, but that cases introduced from other sources be visited initially to decide whether or not occupational therapy is needed. There is still some confusion about the functions of an occupational therapist, and it is wise to get the facts right before discussing the case with a busy doctor. It is important, however, that no examination and/or treatment be undertaken until the doctor has given his instructions and signed a referral form.

Aims of Community Occupational Therapy

A good domiciliary service should cover all types of cases and all age groups [11]. It has been said that the greater part of this work is with chronic conditions where the aim is to overcome the disability rather than lessen it and, not least, to try to deal with its psychological results. The therapist aims to help her patients to be independent in their personal lives, to work if possible, and to enjoy recreation. The methods used to carry out these aims will be developed in the following paragraphs.

Types of Cases

The four commonest problems referred to community occupational therapy centres are:

(1) Diseases and disorders of bone and organs of movement.
(2) Diseases and disorders of the nervous system.
(3) Diseases and disorders of the circulatory system.
(4) Psychiatric, psycho-neurotic and personality disorders [12].

And the four commonest referred for active rehabilitation are fractures, strokes, osteo-arthrosis, and backache (with or without sciatica) [13].

Adults. Many people referred to the therapist are permanently handi-capped, although physically fit, i.e. those with congenital deformities or traumatic paraplegia. Once these people have been provided with aids and adaptations, they are able to live relatively normal lives, going to work, and participating in sport and social activities quite independently. Only when asked for help should the occupational therapist visit again.

Many of the diseases listed above are degenerative. The patient should be kept active and useful for as long as possible, and different aids and adapta-tions, and new activities, will be needed as the disease progresses. Gradually the emphasis will move from helping the patient, to helping the relatives to be able to nurse the patient. Advice about suitable aids and techniques, in cooperation with the district nurse, should enable the patient to be looked after at home for the maximum time.

Much can be done to help arthritic and hemiplegic patients to be independent despite their disabilities. The provision of aids alone is not enough; careful training is needed in their use, and any which are not used should be withdrawn. Kitchen training is of special importance to the hemiplegic housewife, and, while it may be convenient to assess and train the patient in a rehabilitation unit, it is in her own home that she has to put her training to use. It may be necessary to spend a whole day working with such a patient. This is time well spent, if it convinces both the patient and her family that independence can be achieved.

Liaison with the rehabilitation team at the hospital or special unit will help the community therapist to prepare for the severely disabled patient such as the paraplegic or tetraplegic, before he is discharged. It is valuable for her to see the patient's home to assess the need for adaptations or rehousing, and to visit the patient in hospital. She can discuss problems with the hospital team and have an opportunity of assessing the attitude of the patient's family towards him and his disability. She can reassure the relatives and indicate to them how they will be able to look after the patient when he is discharged from hospital. This is often a source of great anxiety to them and they may need instruction and support before, as well as after, the patient returns home.

The psychological aspects of treatment of the physically disabled should always be considered, as some community occupational therapy services include the mentally as well as the physically ill. Since the Chronically Sick and Disabled Act [14] also covers the mentally ill, authorities are increasingly aware of the need to provide for them. Occupational therapists have still to formulate their role and clarify their objectives of treatment in this area [15].

Children. Handicapped children should be helped to be independent and as they grow up to try to solve their own problems. Children should be helped to be mobile in the home with walking aids, or wheel-chairs, so low that they can reach objects on the floor, the normal play-level of a child. This also enables them to explore and investigate, essential factors in mental and physical development. Paraplegic children will need to develop arm and chest muscles in order to lift themselves about, and they should be taught to use a hoist.

Occupational therapists should be ready to give their help and encouragement to other organisations for the handicapped; there may be a large number within their working area. One session spent with, for example, a toy library, can save some individual visiting, and help both parents and children in the development of normal relationships.

Cooperation with the school medical officer, the health visitor, the district nurse and social workers is essential. Regular meetings should be held to plan for the child's treatment and care. Mothers can become confused by conflicting advice from too many people. It has been found useful to hold clinics where pre-school aged children and their mothers meet together with the community team. There is opportunity of giving the children exercise through play, and of assessing their mental and physical progress, while the district nurse and the health visitor can weigh and measure the children and discuss problems with the mothers. These children benefit greatly from mixing with other children, and mothers become less apprehensive about letting their children move about. A variety of walking aids and runabout trollies should be available to encourage mobility, as should a selection of sense training toys for mental development and hand–eye coordination [16].

Types of Occupation

Patients in their homes, needing to be as independent as possible, will first concentrate on activities of daily living [17], including those household activities which they can achieve. If wholly occupied by these, their main need will be for social contact and recreation.

To maintain activity and interest, and, where possible, earning capacity for those unable to do much in the home, hobbies, crafts, small contract assembly work or study courses may be indicated. Small day groups may be organised on an informal basis for either work or social activities, for which patients may be brought from home by Local Authority or voluntary transport. After careful assessment and with continued occasional direction and advice, the help of aides, and craft or other instructors may be sought. If items are made for sale they should be of a high standard. Some authorities have their own shop for disposal of work done by the disabled and blind. The help of the Handcrafts Advisory Association* or the Preparatory Training Bureau* may be called for here (see chapter 4). Working alone is uncongenial for many, and new occupation, good colours, new designs and fresh incentives help to stimulate interest, and samples, books and photographs are particularly useful. Competitions, to which as many patients as possible are transported, are helpful, if held fairly frequently, and accompanied by an exhibition and prize-giving ceremony with good publicity. Regular visiting breaks up definite periods into units during which a specified amount of work may be expected of the patient, the achievement of which provides a measure of his success.

Home Visiting

The initial visit to the patient's home is important in establishing the right relationship with him and his family. The therapist should introduce herself, explain why she has come, and who has asked her to visit. The patient is encouraged to talk about himself and his difficulties, giving the therapist a chance to sum up his attitude to his disability and also that of his family. She observes the type of home, and notes any obvious barriers to independence such as steps, outside lavatory, unsuitable chairs, steep stairs, etc. She should first help with whatever the patient and his family consider to be their greatest difficulties and tackle other problems later.

The therapist must have the correct mixture of friendliness and professionalism. The situation is the reversal of that in a hospital where the patient is the visitor. The community therapist can only suggest and advise, and if necessary try to persuade the patient to accept treatment. Even so she must always be in control of the situation, for instance she must never allow herself to be persuaded to provide equipment which she feels is unnecessary.

There is a need to be careful in conversation with patients, relatives and neighbours, as words may well be remembered and repeated, and may take on a meaning which was never intended. This is especially true in the case of lonely people with too much time to think. It is unwise to make promises unless it is certain that they can be fulfilled. Neighbourly interest and support should be encouraged but care must be taken never to divulge private or unnecessary information.

Any visitor from the local authority is expected, by the patient, to know all the regulations and facilities supplied, not only by the local authority, but also by the hospital and social security services, as well as by the voluntary organisations. The community therapist should know how to advise the patient to get in touch with the right department.

Some patients and their relatives insist that they 'know their rights', especially in such matters as the provision of equipment, adaptations, and housing. When making recommendations in respect of these, therapists should be sure of their facts and the rightness of their decisions. It is always wise to discuss controversial points with a senior officer of the employing authority.

Although the aim is to deal with essential matters first, i.e. rising from bed and chair, managing toilet, feeding and dressing, these cannot all be taught in one visit. The provision of a simple aid such as a 'pick-up' stick may help to increase the patient's feeling of independence and optimism immediately. It is wise to help with one thing at a time and let him master one particular movement before going on to another. Patients and families can become confused by having to remember too many instructions. Some patients are reluctant to admit that they cannot do certain things, such as managing the toilet unaided, and it may be some time before it is possible to discuss such matters freely.

The duration of visits cannot be standardised. Some take only a few minutes, others may require an hour or more and it is not possible to finish work at a set time each day. It is unwise to promise to be at a house by a certain time unless absolutely necessary, as both patients and relatives may be either disappointed or annoyed if the arrangement has to be changed. On the other hand, in country districts, with long distances to travel, it is best to be sure that the patient is at home before calling. If a therapist cannot gain admission to a home, she should leave an official visiting card, and record the call in the case notes.

The community occupational therapist will have to call on patients in many different types of accommodation. She will have to find addresses across fields or by riding in a lift to the top floors of multi-storey flats or by climbing stairs where there are no lifts. Some homes may be dirty, and the therapist will find it useful to keep washing materials in her car for personal use after visiting. Clothing should be simple and practical and easily washed or cleaned. Although there are no regulations about it, some community therapists find uniform useful, while others prefer the more casual approach of everyday clothes.

Assessment [18]

The task of helping a patient to be independent in his home starts first with assessment of his physical and mental capabilities, helping him to exploit his full potential. The therapist must be competent in assessing the following:

(1) The mental capacity of the patient, and his attitude towards his disability.
(2) The patient's physical ability and disability.
(3) The psychological aspects of the illness, if any.
(4) The attitude of the family to the patient and his disability.
(5) The suitability of the accommodation and furniture in relation to the disability.

Certain items can be assessed informally in discussion. After consideration of all these factors, the therapist should be in a position to decide if and how she can help the patient. More detailed forms of assessment may be needed later, e.g. for dexterity, for kitchen and work assessment, etc.

Rehabilitation

Exercise and occupation may form a necessary part of the mental and physical stimulus needed to start the patient on the road to rehabilitation. This is especially true of patients who have become inactive through being left to sit at home for months and who feel that life no longer holds any meaning for them.

Not only the needs of her patient, but also the limitations in the home conditions, and the attitude of the family must be considered. Where the patient is loved and respected, inconveniences will be accepted, such as making room for a typewriter, sacks of leather, bath seat, and walking aids, etc. Where the patient is barely tolerated every possible objection will be raised to the introduction of apparatus and materials and nothing will be done to protect it from damage. It will be a difficult decision whether or not to issue equipment to such a home. Where provision is essential for the good of the patient, it should be given but a close watch kept on it.

Activities of Daily Living [19]

The range of aids now available is extensive, and care should be taken to ensure that new ones appearing on the market are tested carefully before being issued.

Some patients are referred for treatment while they are still in bed, the primary aim being to encourage mobility. For this the therapist must have a knowledge of kinetics, and should know the various types of special beds which are available for the patient who is unable to help himself. He can still be given a modicum of independence if he can bring himself into a sitting position by pressing a button, moving a lever or pulling on a rope. A board placed under a sagging mattress may make the difference between a patient lying helpless in a hollow and being able to turn on one side and get out of bed. Once on his feet he may be relatively mobile.

Many patients are immobile, however, simply because they cannot get up and down from sitting. The simple device of extending the legs of a chair or putting it on a platform may help. Those with painful joints may find a spring-assisted seat helpful [20]. An audio bell will save the frustration of struggling to the door. Bells which flash a light instead of ringing are helpful to deaf patients [21].

It is better to adapt furniture already in the home than to supply extra equipment for what are often already overcrowded rooms, for example extending the legs of the patient's own bed and chairs may save the use of hospital beds and special chairs. Trollies made to the correct height, and square rather than oblong make useful carrying and walking aids (see plates 16, 21 and 22). Many handicapped people eat their meals standing at the draining board simply because they cannot carry dishes into the living room.

Bath aids are important, but before deciding that a patient needs these, make sure that he has a bath in his house. Each bath should be measured carefully for seats, boards and rails, and each item supplied must be checked to ensure that it is secure before the patient is taught to use it. Patients must be warned to run the water, turn the taps off and test the temperature before getting in. A non-slip mat gives greater security inside the bath, and a small damp towel over the edge prevents the hand from slipping. Provision of a mobile or ceiling hoist may make the difference between a patient being nursed at home or being admitted to hospital. In the future an increasing number of patients will be nursed at home, and some form of hoist will be essential.

In small rooms where narrow passages preclude the use of a standard self-propelling wheel-chair, a *model 9 transit chair* may be useful. The patient can pull himself about by holding on to furniture or can get useful non-weight-bearing exercise by 'walking' or pushing with his feet. This chair has brakes, it folds for transit purposes and having swivel castors in the front, it is easy to manoeuvre. A strong metal framed chair with castors can serve for indoor use. If the right height, and fitted with a lavatory seat, the chair can be propelled directly over the lavatory thus avoiding the need to transfer.

When the patient must be carried up and down stairs, an ambulance chair is the easiest to use although two people must carry it. Most patients prefer being carried by chair rather than being lifted bodily.

Production, Study and Hobby Activities

A patient who is as mobile as possible but still radically homebound will need some occupation within his abilities. The provision of these has been discussed on p. 417 of this chapter. Occupational therapists should keep up to date with schemes organised through the Department of Employment, which is now providing more services for home workers.

Day Centres

Whenever possible, occupational therapy services should include day units staffed by occupational therapists and a technician, and visited regularly by a medical consultant. After assessment at home and consultation with his doctor, written permission for a patient's attendance is obtained. A form giving a clear picture of the patient, his family and his accommodation and also the aims of referral is made out for use by the day centre staff.

Attendance may be recommended for any of the following reasons:

(1) Provision of activities impossible within the limited confines of the home.
(2) Assessment for use of equipment before its supply or installation in the home.
(3) Assessment for work or retraining [22].
(4) Resocialisation.
(5) Relief for the family.

A multi-purpose centre offers the best facilities for the patients and should include workrooms, assessment room, including equipment likely to be used by patients at home, a rehabilitation kitchen, bath and hairdressing rooms, and facilities for chiropody, a library, a room for social activities, and facilities for sports and gardening. Some take contract work from local firms and are able to make small payments to those who do it. This type of centre may include offices for social workers and other allied professional staff so that a patient can participate in a wide variety of activities and also meet and discuss with the people most able to help him.

Housing [23]

In addition to understanding the physical problems of the severely handicapped in their homes, especially those confined to wheel-chairs, it is important to understand the problem from the local authority angle. Patients who feel that their housing is not satisfactory, can ask their doctor for a medical form of recommendation to go through the Housing Committee to the Area Health Authority for housing consideration. The domiciliary community therapist may be asked to report on the patient's ability, as well as his disability, and his present accommodation. A clear picture should be given of the patient's limitations, age and sex of other members of the household, type of present accommodation, and any further relevant information, as well as some recommendation on the type of accommodation which would be suitable, and also, if adaptations are likely to be necessary.

The use of a form giving information briefly and to the point is recommended. The therapist may be asked to view any proposed accommodation and advise on its suitability for the patient, or if adaptations are needed. Alteration to the present home may be preferable to rehousing if this would mean separation from relations and friends whose proximity may be of great importance to the whole family, both as a means of support and assurance that help is available if needed, and to ensure continuing social contacts.

If no suitable accommodation is available, the therapist may be asked to consult the architect's department about accommodation which can be adapted while still at the drawing-board stage, especially before bathroom and kitchen fixtures are installed. Plans for heating, positioning of light and power switches and of meters are also important as is the hanging of doors which can affect access to rooms, and approach paths, thresholds, etc. This allows for greater flexibility and usually such adaptations cost less than to existing buildings, but it may mean a far greater delay. Committee permission will be needed for payment of the cost of the alterations. Some authorities have been able to build purpose designed bungalows, which are obviously the answer to most of the housing problems of the disabled.

In many areas, local authorities may have a system of 'housing points'. Points are given for size of family, degree of overcrowding, and for medical reasons, and only families with a certain number of points will be eligible for corporation housing. Should the medical officer feel that a particular case requires urgent housing, he can recommend that special priority be granted on medical grounds. In this case, a family may be given suitable housing immediately, and jump the queues of people who have often waited years for corporation housing. Therapists should therefore be very sure of the facts before requesting 'special priority' for a patient. A great deal of experience of home visiting is necessary before it is possible to obtain a true standard of conditions in an area. Housing which is considered very bad in one town may be considered reasonable in another, because the latter has a much larger housing problem.

Recreation

Achievement of as normal and full a life as possible includes the encouragement of social activities, shopping, church attendance and holidays and sports. Patients who have been confined to house or hospital for long periods are often frightened or shy of joining in activities with the general public. They may be persuaded to join a club, or go shopping or on holiday, if they know that someone will be there who understands their problems. For this reason, domiciliary occupational therapists may find it useful to organise these activities with the object of giving the patient confidence in the first place, and then encouraging him to join ordinary clubs, etc., later.

There are a number of basic points which should be observed when taking out parties of handicapped people.

(1) Visit the premises personally, meet the management and discuss the proposed visit.
(2) If there are steps, ask if ramps are available.
(3) Insist on seeing every part of the premises which will be used by the handicapped people; those not used to dealing with the disabled have little idea of their limitations.
(4) Measure the width of all doorways through which wheel-chairs will have to pass, and width of the passages that lead to them.
(5) Assess suitability of both male and female toilets. This may be the

deciding factor as to the suitability of the place. If the entrance to the toilets is suitable, but the cubicles too narrow for a wheel chair to enter, an ambulance chair is useful, the patient transferring on to it before entering the cubicle. It is always advisable to take a bedpan and a bottle on any excursion with handicapped people.

Clubs

These, run by occupational therapists, should provide mental and physical stimuli and the accent should be on patient participation. If purpose designed accommodation is not available, it is important to choose a building with easy access for wheel-chairs, where there is parking space for invalid cars, and where patients can enter and leave transport safely. Toilets should be accessible to all patients, and, if the cubicles are too small for a wheel-chair to enter, a sani-chair which can be run over the toilet should be provided.

Holidays

Many domiciliary occupational therapists arrange holidays for patients in their care. If taken without their relatives, it not only gives them a holiday, but gives the relatives a much needed rest as well. If help is limited, then the number of severely disabled people taken must also be limited, the numbers being made up of those who require only a little help with dressing, toilet and feeding. It is unfair to take the disabled away from their homes into unfamiliar surroundings unless skilled helpers are available (this is not the time for willing but inexperienced people to learn how to help them). Some holiday camps and seaside hotels and boarding houses arrange special holidays at non-season dates and rates, and these are much appreciated. It is important for the therapist to learn about the whole area in which she functions. Patients can then be told how and where to obtain information for themselves.

It is generally advisable for an occupational therapist to have experience in a hospital department before going into community work. This is because a community therapist works single handed when on the job, although she may have the help and support of a large department and of a number of colleagues. Above all the community therapist should be a mature person capable of dealing with the varied situations which will confront her. The work appeals to people with a spirit of adventure and to whom the problems of the disabled are a challenge which must be met.

REFERENCES AND RECOMMENDED FURTHER READING

1. This gave permissive powers to local authorities to make arrangements for the prevention of illness, the care and after-care of those with disease or disability, mental illness or defect.

2. A local authority was hereby authorised to promote the welfare of the blind, deaf or dumb, and others substantially and permanently handicapped by illness, injury, congenital deformity, or other disabilities. #
3. This act extends # above.
4. This act gives more direction than permissive powers re the above #.
5. See Ref. 8 below—and Occupational therapy in the community. *Occ. Ther.*, 36, no. 1, 1973 and N.H.S. reorganisation transfer of staff. *Occ. Ther.*, 36, no. 11, 1973.
6. See Chapter 1 and *The Employment Service, plans and programmes.* Manpower Services Commission, H.M.S.O.* 1974. p. 17.
7. See *Help for Handicapped People*, D.H.S.S.*, H.B.1. 1972.
8. See *A Report from the Working Party on Collaboration between the N.H.S. and Local Government*, 2.24. pp. 13.14. H.M.S.O.*, 1973.
9. See chapter 23, this book.
10. See chapter 7, this book.
11. See chapters 17, 18, 20, this book.
12. See chapters 12, 13, 14, 15, this book.
13. See chapters 5 to 11 inclusive this book.
14. See ref. 6 above.
15. See ref. 11 above.
16. See chapters 17–18 this book.
17. See chapter 7 this book.
18. See chapter 7 this book.
19. As 16, 17 above.
20. See Plates 1 and 2, this book.
21. See chapters 6–13. 20.
22. See chapter 7, this book.
23. Goldsmith, S., *Designing for the Disabled*, R.I.B.A.*
    Walton, F., *An Introduction to Domestic Design for the Disabled*, Disabled Living Foundation*.
    Help for the Handicapped, D.H.S.S.*, H.B.1, 1972.
    Coping with Disablement, Consumers' Association, 1974.
* See *Glossary*, p. 454-6.

CHAPTER 22

Industrial Work in Rehabilitation

The use of activity in rehabilitation has, in the last decades, extended into the field of industrial work [1], and the concept of the rehabilitative value of work has also found wide acceptance in the hospitals, local authority and special centres [2]. These all cater for sheltered work or for retraining or rehabilitating for fitness for outside employment. Industrial work must never, however, be used to the exclusion of other, and in some cases more necessary, methods of treatment. Its purpose in rehabilitation is for the benefit of the worker, and not for extending production.

The Purposes of Industrial Work in Rehabilitation [3]

These fall under the following headings:

(1) *Rehabilitation of the medium and long term patients*

(Short term patients seldom need this, except for assessment.)

(*a*) To encourage development of work habits.

(*b*) To help retention or increase of speed and capacity for work.

(*c*) To introduce new skills to those who cannot return to former work.

(2) *Maintenance of work habits in long term patients*

(*a*) To encourage a normal 'daily life' pattern for the patient.

(*b*) To encourage a degree of communication and reciprocity and the formation of relationships.

(*c*) To offer an opportunity of gaining an appropriate reward/payment and consequent satisfaction.

(3) *Sheltered work for the mentally or physically handicapped*

(*a*) To enable those who have the ability to work, but who need special care, to feel a part of a working community.

(*b*) To offer relief to families who need to work and live their own lives, by providing care for their disabled relatives in constructive conditions.

Types of Cases for whom Industrial Work is Suitable [4]

Both physical and psychiatric patients can benefit from industrial work as a therapeutic measure, provided it is used with discretion. Although there can be no set rule for prescribing industrial work, it is not generally considered suitable for psychiatric admission patients.

Certain local authorities have experimented with centres for both physically and psychiatrically handicapped. In some the two groups are kept separate, dining at different times and having their own staff. In other centres patients work and dine together, sharing recreational facilities and staff. This latter seems a more satisfactory method, as all staff then know the working of the whole unit. When different disabilities are mixed it also serves to help the patients to accept each other's handicaps, and to appreciate the problems of their fellows. Constant review of the group as a whole is important, as disproportionate numbers of psychiatrically ill patients can affect the atmosphere and perhaps the falling off in attendance of other workers. One important aspect of industrial work is that it provides a natural situation in which the staff can work *with* the patients rather than in an entirely supervisory capacity.

Industrial Work for Psychiatric Patients

Chronic schizophrenics are perhaps the ones who will derive most benefit from industrial work, whether they belong to the long-stay category or that of the 'chronic readmission' [5]. Wing [6] and Wadsworth [7] have shown that chronic schizophrenics are capable of productive work and sustained effort, and many are sufficiently emotionally stable to return to useful jobs which will satisfy their need for recognition. The work itself, and contact with the firms' representatives when they call, all contribute to this. In a work situation, institutional symptoms from long hospitalisation are often easier to overcome than psychotic ones [8], although paranoid schizophrenics often do well in jobs in open industry [9]. Leucotomised patients do not usually make such good progress [10]. Similarly, industrial work is widely used and valuable in the treatment of *subnormal patients* [11], and if well chosen, patients can achieve a high standard and prove reliable and faithful workers.

Alcoholics make good workers, and when sufficiently well stabilised, can help the less well preserved of their fellows. *Psychopaths* may have a disruptive influence on a unit. They rarely, if ever, benefit from the satisfaction of industrial work, and although they may need the discipline of a well organised workshop at some stage in their treatment, it may, perhaps, be too sheltered to offer the best setting for the final stages of their rehabilitation. If *epileptics* are given suitable jobs and observed carefully but unobtrusively, they can provide a nucleus of able workers who are regular attenders and capable of performing the more complicated operations that will ensure a steady flow of work for the less able patients.

Industrial work can also be useful when a patient is said to have problems with his work-mates. The staff can see him in a setting akin to that in which he worked before, or which may have precipitated his illness, and his real ability to work consistently and with others can be tested in the work unit setting.

Industrial Work for Physical Patients [12]

Hand injuries benefit from repetitive industrial work such as assembling and packing. This must provide sufficient variety to necessitate an increase of range of movement and muscle strength as the hand improves. Work can be positioned in elevation for oedematous hands. *Shoulder and elbow* work can be given with power drills and hand planes. Assembly work can be so positioned as to exercise in the required range. *Lower limb* work, particularly for static quadriceps and the ankle, can be provided on adapted power drills and hand planes. Prolonged standing practice prior to return to work can be graded with increasing periods of industrial work. *Back injuries* can be given work at differing heights for increased flexion or extension. Lifting practice can also be incorporated. *Head injuries* can be assessed for concentration and level of ability.

Long-term patients can benefit from realistic work. They frequently require retraining in work habit and are stimulated by the interaction of the group. When assessing such patients, some will get bored with repetitive work, others will be too slow for outside employment, but both the patient and the occupational therapist will get a clearer picture of the former's ability in relation to normal work.

In a physical hospital there may not be sufficient patients attending the department to justify taking on work from industry, but simple jobs such as making plaster rockers for the orthopaedic clinic, articulated crocodiles cut out of scrap wood on the fretsaw, painted and assembled by hand, rubber stamping, folding and putting 'follow-up' reports into envelopes, or preparing new patients' folders can all be usefully adapted to a production line.

Patients in physical hospitals are seldom paid for their industrial work as this would create too many problems. Such money is usually put into some form of benevolent fund so that all the patients may benefit from it.

Industrial Work for the Cerebral Palsied

Because of the specialised nature of this work, it is described in the chapter relating to these conditions (see chapter 19).

Staffing an Industrial Rehabilitation Unit [13], and Necessary Outside Contacts

Treatment and Work Specialists

There are many different types of industrial units and as many different ways of staffing them. It is an accepted fact that a doctor shall be the *medical director* of the unit. Ideally an occupational therapist, with the appropriate additional training and experience should, under the doctor, be the *occupational consultant* for treatment and rehabilitative aspects of the work. That she should be the manager of it from the industrial and productive point of view is debatable.

It is essential that the staff should work as a team, particularly as they have responsibilities in fields as widely differing as industrial practice and occupational therapy.

The occupational therapist in charge of, or consultant to, an industrial unit should have a practical understanding of *work study*, have worked in a factory, and have studied important current literature on the subjects of *kinetics, ergonomics, industrial training*, etc. She should also study the facilities and possibilities in the area in which she works.

It may be best to have an *industrial manager* in charge of production, who can seek contracts, and, in consultation with the occupational therapist, arrange layout and equipment, instruct the workers and supervise the work. He should be responsible for maintenance of standards and arrange for collection and return of work, if sub-contracted. In a unit of any size he should have an assistant who can share these responsibilities with him. Both should be conversant with the relevant factory acts, local trade union attitude, fire regulations, safety precautions, and know what to do in the case of an accident.

The social problems of the workers may be dealt with by a specially employed *social worker*, or by some agency or worker linked with the hospital or local authority centre. In large units there may be facilities for regular *medical clinics* with visiting *doctors* and/or *nurses*. In hospital units this attention would be given by the hospital itself.

In industrial units *aides*, recruited locally and trained on the job can take responsibility under the manager or occupational therapist consultant, for such things as mistakes in the work, which the patients can be helped to rectify, and the maintenance of standards. It is part of the job of the aides to teach patients to count, stack and pass on the correct work to the next worker or supervisor.

Clerical help is needed. Accounting should preferably be centralised and an office assigned to the personnel dealing with it. Clerical helpers should be able to act as the secretariat of the unit, relieving the industrial manager of routine jobs. Selected clerical work can sometimes be done by patients, under supervision, and office accommodation adapted suitably to patient/ staff needs. A *storekeeper* may also be needed in a large unit.

Outside Contacts

Contacts with the disablement resettlement officer will be important for any unit through which vocational assessment, training and 'toughening up', are given, leading to resettlement of the worker. Links with local branches of the Chamber of Commerce, Trade and Rural Industries, and with managers of local firms can be most valuable; it is important, in the interests of the workers, to encourage community support.

The workers' relatives have an important part to play in successful industrial rehabilitation. The worker may live at home and conditions there may need investigation and/or adaptation. The relatives' interest in, and appreciation of, the workers' efforts to earn, and encouragement of regular attendance, can be vital factors in the success of the resettlement.

If the patient still lives in a hospital or in a hostel or residential work unit, appreciation, cooperation and understanding of *wardens, nursing supervisors* and other 'home makers', can, similarly, be of great importance.

Setting up Industrial Units

Careful thought needs to be given to the setting up of industrial work units for the disabled, in whatever setting they are to be placed. The following are important considerations:

(1) Are there enough people needing this form of sheltered work to justify setting up the workshops?
(2) Will the workshops fill a need which cannot be satisfied in any other way?
(3) Can they be equipped and managed on a proper business basis?
(4) Is transport sufficiently near—public or special?
(5) What outwork is obtainable in the area, or should the unit have a production line of its own?

In the setting up of industrial work within a hospital, usually a psychiatric hospital, or institute for the mentally subnormal, there may be more certainty of success than in centres outside, because the development can be slower, and suitable modifications and adaptations made as plans progress. Certain industrial processes, such as small assembly work, or the making of simple items (e.g. cardboard windmills on sticks) can be introduced into non-specialised occupation centres. Contract assembly work might have to be completed in a limited time; the latter could be organised to suit the workers' own rate.

If there are several units within a small area, competition for work may be keen and the unit will have to maintain high standards to keep in business. This will apply particularly in an area where types of industry are not ideal for sub-contracting or the factories are few in number.

In some areas, the industrial units have formed associations or independent companies to facilitate cooperation and avoid price cutting. The hospital authorities concerned have recognised these even if not directly connected with their boards. These companies or associations are properly constituted with rules and membership fees; and meet at regular intervals. This liaison is useful in that any unit which cannot accept jobs either because they are unsuitable or because it is too fully committed, can pass them to another.

Obtaining Work [14]

If the unit employs patients with varying physical and psychiatric disabilities, light assembly work, trimming of plastic goods, and packing is usually the most adaptable type of work for the greatest range of patients.

The industrial manager should be familiar with the firms in the area who can supply suitable work. Reference to a classified directory or advertisements in the local paper may help. A high standard of work produced by the unit is its best recommendation. Clean, colourful and attractive products are more stimulating than dull and dirty ones, particularly with the long term disabled. In rural areas, where the patients are mostly from agricultural communities the type of work available will be different from that found in or near towns. Open air activities can include car washing, clearing football grounds of rubbish after the weekly games, fruit picking groups and railway van loading and unloading. Breeze block making, day-old chick and seed box assembly, fruit and vegetable packing and grading are further examples of the type of work to be found in rural areas.

Costing and Payment [15]

Careful accounting, including costing, is essential if patients are to have a fair reward for the work. Whatever the product, the basic principles of production management, work layout (i.e. organisation and methods), costing and quality control, are similar. It is therefore necessary to break down the job into its component operations, and cost it for a trial run before finally accepting it.

The therapist and/or manager will know what the labour force is capable of doing, so that jobs which cannot be finished on time are not accepted. It is unlikely that the labour force available at any one time will be the total number on the register. It is not realistic to expect the contractor to be interested in helping the patients. He may well be, but primarily he wants to know that the work will be returned on the specified delivery date, finished to the required standard.

Costing

When the offer of a job has been obtained it is necessary to cost it before finally accepting the contract. There are usually three ways in which a price is determined:

(1) By the firm asking for a price.
(2) By the firm offering a price.
(3) By negotiation with the factory manager on comparative rates within the factory.

Inexperienced managers may be too willing to accept work, no matter how little is offered for the effort, under the impression that any work is better than none. This is unwise. Most units base prices on a 50–70p. per norm hour minimum.

(1) *To give the firm a price* it is necessary to obtain several samples of the product and its components to be assembled, trimmed or packed, and with the assistance of a stopwatch, ascertain the time needed for completion of the task. To arrive at a reasonable quotation it is useful to have two or three staff members or patients doing a trial run. Assuming that a unit is working to 50p. per hour, if it has taken three minutes to produce one item it will take approximately one hour to produce 20. The cost of the job therefore, will be 50p. for 20, or, to make it into workable amounts for invoicing, £2.50 per 100.

All movement must be taken into account, such as unloading, undoing parcels, tying up and loading.

(2) *When the firm offers a price*, this will be based on the costing out at the economical price that it can afford to pay. The foregoing test should also be applied in the unit. If the price is too low the manager should try to negotiate a more economic one. When a price is arrived at to which the unit can work economically, this should be adhered to. Furthermore, this should be a workable price agreed to if necessary by other units in the area.

(3) *Prices based on comparative rates in the factory.* When dealing with a firm where there is a trade union, the union may wish to be consulted in price discussion. If the payment rate is 50p. an hour, and the production is 100 ergs per hour, the basic figure is 50p. per 100, but in doing this work, the unit is saving the factory such overheads as space, clerical work, insurance, lighting, heating, etc., so in consideration of this advantage normally costed at 100 per cent and offsetting transport cost, the onus of which is generally on the factory, 33 per cent is added, making a total of 67p. per 100. This usually works out satisfactorily for both sides and is in most cases the highest rate of pay earned in industrial units.

Payment to Workers [16]

A patient working in hospital is limited in the amount he can earn per week without complications connected with National Insurance arising. The Department of Health now authorises payments up to £4.50 in certain circumstances.

Payment may be on a *piece rate*, with a separate, higher rate for those who check and pack. It is advisable to show a percentage of the unit's earnings for those who check and pack, even if it has sometimes to be done by the staff. (This will provide a reserve fund for the lean times which occur in any unit.) Payment may also be made on a *time rate* to which can be added allowances for regular attendance, punctuality, etc.

Another payment method is on an *effort rating system*. Patients are graded, normally on a 5-point scale, according to the effort they have put into the job, irrespective of output. Each grade carries a particular sessional rate and the actual week's payment is worked out by multiplying the price for the grade by the number of sessions for the pay week. This latter scheme is the more generally favoured but unless the unit is a large one, it is easy to overestimate the income from the work done, so there should be regular balancing of the accounts. It is important to use a clocking-in system and wherever suitable to make the patients keep a record of their production on a work card. This is handed to the supervisor at the end of each pay week. It is good practice even if the effort rating system of payment is in use in the unit.

Planning and Organising an Industrial Unit [17]

Accessibility and amenity planning for the workers must be a first consideration. This should follow recommendations made for the planning of living and working conditions for the disabled. Maximum use of available space is important.

It is advisable to employ the techniques of O & M* for the layout of the buildings as well as for jobs. This may initially necessitate flow charts, so that the floor space of the whole unit is utilised to its maximum, and unnecessary walking is eliminated.

Storage

Space required for storage of components and finished articles may take up a third of the floor area available. It should be separate from the working area, but adjacent to it, with easy access on the same level. If a proprietary brand of angled aluminium is used, the storage space can be adapted for the different jobs that may be available: the depth and size of shelves can be changed. When seasonal work is undertaken, it can then be stored easily, at the appropriate time. The storekeeper will have jurisdiction over this area and

15

will receive, sign for and check the components on delivery. He will despatch outgoing work, obtaining the carrier's signature for the amount loaded. Insurance has lately been discussed between representatives of sub-contracting firms and the National Health Service*. Those in charge of industrial units should check current regulations.

Accessibility

Doors should be a standard size that can swing, or have stops to lock them in the open position. Trolleys must go through the doors easily.

Loading and Lifting

The loading bay should be sited so that:

(1) It is accessible from both ingoing and outgoing parts of the store.
(2) It has sufficient run-in to take a van or articulated lorry without obstructing the roadway.
(3) The road to it is wide and straight enough to manoeuvre at least a three ton van, preferably an articulated lorry, and will take the heaviest vehicle likely to use it.

The loading bay must be a suitable height to allow a trolley to be run into standard bodied vans when the tail gate is down. A block and tackle is also useful as it makes the loading and unloading of heavy packages and equipment feasible with the minimum of manpower. It is inadvisable to have this on runners as it can be a source of accidents if left imperfectly secured or, being outside the building, if tampered with when the unit is unattended. Also it should be remembered that many firms supply goods on pallets. These are stacked on the lorry at the factory by means of a fork lift truck. If it is at all possible, therefore, this item should be included in the equipment of the unit. If such a truck is not available, the goods loaded on pallets will have to be manhandled and this will involve a considerable waste of manpower and time for which payment is not usually forthcoming. For preference, all access points should have roofing so that neither patients nor goods suffer from rain.

Transport

Some units prefer to run their own transport so that they are independent of manufacturers. Others prefer to rely on the suppliers of work so they do not have to arrange for servicing vehicles, replacements and employing a driver.

Job Layout

The layout of a job is most important. Without correct sequence the whole operation can become arduous, uninteresting, slow and incorrectly finished. Managers must be capable of designing, and in some cases, making, simple jigs, to assist in the assembly of components, so that the work can be done more easily and quickly.

In a factory, the least number of movements are employed in assembly, but in an industrial unit it is often necessary to break down a task to a greater number of movements, so as to simplify each. If there is a holdup on the line, the way to increase output may be to divert more help to an over-burdened section. Each particular job may require special modifications in layout.

Quantity and Quality Control

Having accepted work from a factory the industrial manager has assumed a dual responsibility, to the factory and to the patients in his care. He is responsible, too, for the security of the materials. The factory must be made aware that no government department (i.e. in a hospital) carries insurance. The factory may wish to undertake this itself. With psychiatric patients, it is often noticed that the higher the standard set, the higher the quality of the goods will be, but much will depend on the relationships between staff and patients, and undue stress in any form must be avoided. Working patients need to learn to meet some stress, however, and the industrial unit can provide for this in a controlled situation. Here they can be conditioned to some pressures, and assessed for the degree of strain they can tolerate.

Industrial work in rehabilitation, if properly used, can provide a series of situations similar to, but never the same as, those found in normal working conditions. Patients must be given encouragement and oppor-tunity to take as much responsibility for the efficient running of the unit as is possible. Like all occupational therapy, industrial work is only a medium for helping the patient to become as competent as possible. It can provide a bridge for return to outside life for many long-term patients, and helps to maintain normal contacts for those on medium or short-stay treatment.

Although considered valuable as a rehabilitative agent, considerable study and assessment of its results are needed before it can be said that industrial work pays dividends in treatment successes. Preferences of the patients for whom it is prescribed may have to be considered. In an experiment and survey made of payment to patients for this type of work and, to a control group who did craft-work, the latter were the more appreciative. This sug-gests that the incentive of earning may have more influence in some of these industrial situations than the work itself. There is for some a normalising discipline, however, in doing productive work, or for others, a satisfactory routine which in its repetitiveness, gives opportunity for indulgence in their own thoughts.

REFERENCES AND RECOMMENDED FURTHER READING

1. See Willmott, P., *Social Services*. Pelican, 1967, and chapter on *Resettlement*, p. 40 this book.
2. Willmott, P., *op. cit.*, p. 188.
3. See King's Fund* Report, *Industrial Therapy in Psychiatric Hospitals*, p. 6. London, 1968.
   Lemmings, P. E. (1965), Industrial techniques in occupational therapy. *Occ. Ther.*
4. *Op. cit.* (3 above), pp. 26-27
5. Douglas, A. D. M., Conway, S. & Beeby, G. J. (1966), A personal survey of industrial therapy in the psychiatric hospitals of the Sheffield region. *Brit. J. Psych.*, 112, 1013–1017.
6. Wing, J. K. & Giddens, R. G. J. (1959), Industrial rehabilitation of male chronic schizophrenic patients. *Lancet*, ii, 505–507.
7. Wadsworth, W. V., Wells, B. W. P. & Scott, R. F., *The State of Industrial Therapy in the Mental Hospitals of England and Wales*. (Private circulation to Mental Hospitals.) 1963.
   (1962), The employment of chronic schizophrenics. *J. Ment. Sci.*, 108, 300–305.
   (1962), The organisation of a sheltered workshop. *J. Ment. Sci.*, 108, 780–785.
8. Gittleson, N. L. (1966), The schizophrenic rehabilitee. *Brit. J. Psych.*, 112, 201–202.
9. Early, D. F. & Magnus, R. V. (1968), Industrial therapy organisation (Bristol, 1960–65). *Brit. J. Psych.*, 114, 335–336.
10. Nicholas, M. (1967), The rehabilitation of long-stay schizophrenic patients. *Brit. J. Psych.*, 119, 155–158.
11. See Gibson, J. & French, T., *Nursing the Mentally Retarded*, pp. 120–121. London, 1974.
    Hallas, C., *The Care and Training of the Mentally Subnormal*, pp. 112–113, 116, 150. Bristol, 1974.
12. See chapters 5 to 11 inclusive on Physical Conditions.
13. *Op. cit.* (3 above), pp. 42 to 51, and 64–68.
14. *Ibid.*, pp. 56-61.
15. *Ibid.*, pp. 28–34.
    And see:
    The Netherne industrial pay scheme. *Occ. Ther.*, 35, no. 4, 1972.
    Occupational and industrial scheme in N. Ireland. *Occ. Ther.*, 36, no. 2, 1973.
    Survey of rating scales in psychiatric hospitals. *Occ. Ther.*, 36, no. 5, 1973.
16. *Op. cit.* (3 above), pp. 56–63.
17. The occupational therapist involved in industrial work should see:
    Bass, B. M. & Vaughan, J. A., *Training in Industry*. London, 1967.
    Currie, R. M., *Work Study*. London, 1972.
    Edholm, O. G., *The Biology of Work*. London, 1967.
    Hill, M. (1967), The development of industrial therapy in Britain. *Am. J. Occ. Ther.*, 21, 3.
    Maier, N. R. F., *Psychology in Industry*. London, 1965.
    Tredgold, R. F., *Human Relations in Modern Industry*. London, 1963.
    Pamphlets *Ergonomics for Industry*. Information Division, Dept. of Science and Industrial Research, London.
    Introduction to Work Study. I.L.O.* Geneva, 1965.
    She should also note that a *National Ass. of Industrial Therapy* has been in existence since 1971.

* See *Glossary*, p. 454.

CHAPTER 23

Communication and Management relating to an Occupational Therapy Department

Good management is essential in occupational therapy, because of the contribution it makes to the successful treatment of the patient, and because it ensures that the treatment service takes its place smoothly among other services. It is also important because the service is so diffuse and has so many facets, that it, more than many, could easily become unorganised and disorientated. Management is a means to an end and not an end in itself. It involves foresight, the ability to plan and organise, the ability for sympathetic understanding and leadership, and a knowledge of facts and objectives. Without the ability to form satisfactory relationships and to cooperate with all other departments the full value of the occupational therapy service cannot be developed. Although details of planning and methods of achieving objectives vary between the different specialised fields, there are certain basic principles which underlie organisation in any field[1]. The art of good management lies in discovering the best method of applying these principles to suit the particular circumstances [2].

The aspects to be considered in this chapter are:

(1) Planning of treatment.
(2) Departmental planning and organisation.
(3) Control of equipment and stock.

Planning of Treatment

All patients should be accepted on medical referral of some kind. This is a part of the professional undertaking of the occupational therapist, and although this may be difficult to achieve, referral or prescriptive instructions should be obtained before treatment is started, even if they are brief and given in the least time-consuming form.

Provision of Facilities for Treatment [3]

The form in which referral is received by the occupational therapist varies between hospitals, centres or organisations. The essential information to be included has already been discussed [4].

An important factor in treatment planning is that the occupational therapist should anticipate and arrange for provision of facilities for the activities and techniques likely to be required, taking into consideration the district in which the department is situated, and the types of disabilities for which it caters. The centre may be in an industrial area catering for a number of accident and injury cases; heavy workshop facilities are, then, essential, as well as lighter treatment activities. If the majority of cases are housewives, office and clerical workers, shop-keepers or cleaners, suffering from neurological, arthritic or cardiac conditions, other facilities may be needed, including kitchen and domestic units, and lighter practical activities, such as dressmaking, typing and shorthand. To ensure that progress is maintained, the necessary follow-on equipment is essential.

Coordination and Communication with Other Departments

Other professional members of the team vary according to the type of hospital or treatment centre [5]. Although an occupational therapist works directly under medical supervision, she may be answerable administratively to some other form of administration.

Hospital Management Committees, as such, have ceased to exist, under the reorganisation of the National Health Service*, but, in many hospitals management teams have been set up to deal with internal policy making, including treatment management, departmental organisation, and priorities. These committees vary from hospital to hospital as they are not a part of the prescribed new structure of the National Health Service* [6]. The increase in multi-disciplinary management in hospitals means that a head occupational therapist must be prepared to attend such meetings and to put forward her department's needs and policy in succint terms. These needs must be seen in relation to those of the whole hospital, and co-operation should be shown over priorities [7]. Occupational therapists may also be called upon to give evidence to the Health Care Planning Teams [8], established within Districts.

Many occupational therapists have been able to attend 'Middle Management Courses' run locally by the National Health Service*, and these have been most valuable in encouraging co-operation with allied workers and in increasing understanding and recognition of the work and problems of different groups [9].

The occupational therapy staff should be large enough to give *adequate* treatment to all patients referred to them. It is right that nurses, specialist instructors, and trade department supervisors should share in the application of the treatment, but it is only in the centre where, under able medical direction, all team members are welded in the service of the patient, and where all work placement is a matter of inter-consultation and has a therapeutic aim, that it can be said that the purpose for which the treatment centre exists, is being fulfilled.

No occupational therapist, in any centre, should be content to limit her work only to the actual treatment of the patient. She must also take time to develop the coordination, personal and administrative, which will prevent overlapping, promote cooperation, and ensure that her contribution is an integrated part of the whole treatment scheme for each patient [10].

Communication is the key to understanding, and it should be clear, concise, and, where possible, incapable of misinterpretation, in spoken and written reports, letters and directives. Different opinions and some compromise must be accepted. The occupational therapist should also be aware of non-verbal communication, and its importance in group and individual treatment situations. This also occurs between staff and sometimes gives a useful indication of problems which may be beneath the surface.

Preparation of Work and Adjustment of Apparatus and Equipment

The occupational therapist must work in an organised way, planning carefully and allocating time economically. She must discriminate between urgent jobs and those which can wait; those which can be done by an individual patient or by a group of patients, with benefit to them, and those which she must do herself. All work should be adequately prepared for or by the patients: apparatus and equipment should be kept in working order, and required materials should be available. Time may be needed for adjustment of apparatus.

Most commercially produced equipment designed for treatment is adjustable and can, therefore, be used in quick succession by patients with varying treatment needs. The occupational therapist must understand its scope and learn how to adjust it. Accurate adjustment ensures the following:

(1) A correct starting position, e.g. one which re-educates balance by progressive reduction of support; or one which, by providing maximum support, conserves energy for the work itself.

(2) Activity appropriate to the aims of treatment and to its duration, e.g. increase of muscle power, mobility or dexterity in a half-hour's daily treatment; or good production without fatigue in a two hour work period, e.g. a housewife using an adjustable stool, a specially designed adjustable trolley [11] and kitchen utensils individually selected or adapted.

If tables, work tops, chairs, stools and beds, etc., are adjustable, much time is saved and improvisation is less often necessary. In some departments there is a need for a section of strong overhead mesh, minimum width 4 foot, and optimum height, 8 foot. This provides secure and adjustable positioning for sling suspension equipment and other treatment adjuncts. A strong stable stool 2 foot high on which to stand is an essential item of equipment.

Patients' Work and Progress Reports [12]

The first essentials regarding reports are that the forms should be agreed with the doctor and other members of the team, to whom the report should be of use, and that they should be presented in medical terms, relating only to matters of importance regarding the patients' progress. If an activity is referred to, it should be referred to only as indicative of its intrinsic value as treatment or for assessment or resettlement purposes. Reports should be brief and clearly written, but should contain sufficient detail to be understood by another member of the staff treating the patient, whether immediately afterwards or at a much later date, e.g. on readmission of the patient.

The frequency of reports depends on the rate of recovery or change in the condition of the patient. The average interval is once a week, but in some cases daily reports are required, in others, i.e. long-term mental conditions, monthly reports are sufficient. Care should be taken not to repeat previous information.

A definite time should be set aside for writing reports. This should be as soon as possible after treatment, in the case of frequent reports, or small details with a definite bearing on the case may be forgotten. In the case of monthly reports brief reminders in the form of daily notes including any incidents of importance should be kept to facilitate the writing of adequate reports. Such 'log books' will show who comprises the working group, how they react to fellows and staff, and, will, perhaps, furnish reasons for deviations in behaviour. Adequate reports will also be of value in research projects.

Departmental Planning and Organisation

Space, Necessary Services and Amenities

Obtaining adequate space for an occupational therapy department often presents a problem, particularly in hospitals where accommodation is insufficient to allow for the inclusion and development of the many medical services. Before assessing the space required for work in a particular centre, the occupational therapist should consider:

(1) The types of disability for which the patients in that centre will require treatment, and whether this will be given mainly in the

hospital wards or treatment rooms, or as out-patient treatment in an occupational therapy department.

(2) The approximate numbers of in-patients and out-patients who will be requiring treatment, whether mainly in groups or individually.

(3) The type and size of equipment to be used.

(4) Adequate space for assessment of and training in A.D.L.* [13].

It is essential to point out quite clearly that certain needs cannot be fulfilled without adequate space, and that it is of no use to embark on an ambitious programme of treatment without the minimum number of square feet in which to carry it out. At other times, good work can and should be done from a limited base. If the occupational therapist is willing to show reasonable cooperation at first, she may be offered more facilities as her work extends, but she should indicate clearly the minimum necessary, and the further extensions which may soon become essential.

If building or planning is contemplated, the occupational therapist should be viewed as a specialist in her field, and be consulted in the matter. The interested authorities, including the occupational therapist, should visit similar centres with recently built departments and draw up schemes incorporating the most appropriate sections of each. Where practicable, movable partitions and sound proofing can increase adaptability of space. The former, made up of storage units, and built on a modular system are excellent as they can then fulfil two functions. Kitchens, bathrooms and heavy workshop areas with special fixed apparatus and flooring problems will require most careful consideration.

It is beyond the scope of this book to give detailed plans of departmental buildings [14]. These may be converted, or purpose built, and should comprise:

(1) Treatment rooms, with patients' waiting area and cloakroom facilities.

(2) Administrative areas, with offices, store and cloak rooms, and rest and locker space for staff, and students, if there are any of the latter.

The occupational therapists' office should be situated where she can see her patients but not necessarily be seen by them, as it is often not in the patients' best interests to have too much attention or supervision. Treatment rooms would in most cases include heavy (more noisy) and light (quieter) workshops. In physical centres a quiet room and rooms for assessment and training for the activities of daily living would be necessary. In both physical and psychiatric centres a domestic unit is important. In a psychiatric hospital, which is usually large and with long distances between different sections, several centres may be needed.

16

Architectural points to remember:

(1) Accessibility: (*a*) single storey or split level;
              (*b*) ramps, stairs, lifts;
              (*c*) covered entrance for patients coming by ambulance or car;
              (*d*) relation to other departments, especially if building is separate from main structure.
(2) Type of flooring in general and fixed areas.
(3) Coving of skirting and ceiling (for ease of cleaning).
(4) Sliding, 'push-bar' or swinging doors both for entrance and storage.
(5) Movable and stackable furniture, including storage units.
(6) Depth of shelving.
(7) Height of seating and tables (high and low).
(8) Type of lighting, fixed and supplementary.
(9) Heating (should be able to regulate from within the department).
(10) Ventilation (cross draughts, fan lights, venetian blinds if large areas of glass are employed).
(11) Power supply: 13-amp ring main for general purposes. Triple phase 440 volts A.C. for heavy machinery and industrial units.
(12) Non-inflammable building materials—particularly for roofing.
     The Ministry of Health building notes do not specify this but it is extremely dangerous when disabled people are being treated with a staff/patient ratio that is adequate for treatment but not for speedy evacuation of a building in case of fire.

No occupational therapy department should be started without the necessary services of water, light, heat, drainage, etc. Plumbing is expensive and therefore careful planning is needed to ensure installation at minimum cost at all points required throughout. It can be installed with built-in, blanked-off outlets with suitable flooring so that, as requirements increase, these additional outlets can be opened up.

An electric power supply is important [15]. This is now available in a console unit which can be mounted centrally in the department and can carry links for a variety of plugs and connections. The height of these connections should relate to the position of the work and patient. Good working light is also essential.

Central heating provides a good basic working temperature controlled within the department with additional heaters where needed; electricity or gas are preferable to solid fuel, remembering the necessary safety precautions. The department should be kept at an even temperature and aired well at frequent intervals. Venetian blinds are essential where there are large areas of glass, unless anti-glare or anti-heat glass is used [16].

Accessibility of the wards, workshops, etc., is important, and should be considered in the light of the work to be undertaken and of the type of patient to attend the department. This should not be too far from the rest of the buildings or it tends to become isolated and may be difficult for some patients to reach or out of touch with the medical and other staff. If noisy activities are to be included, it is advisable that these should not be too close to wards or departments which would be disturbed.

Important structural details include adequate windows to allow ventilation and daylight, accessibility, with doors that are wide enough to admit wheel-chairs or beds if necessary and, in such cases, of a type which can be opened by the patients attending, e.g. swing doors. If large equipment is to be used, it must be possible to get this into the department. Care should be taken that all fittings and fixtures are placed at suitable heights, and if hoists are used these should be well secured to avoid accidents.

The furniture and furnishings required will depend on the type of disability. Varying types and height of chairs and tables may be necessary and, in some circumstances, these may be most useful if of a kind which can be moved easily and stacked. The room has sometimes to be used for a dual purpose, but this is not ideal. Reasonable comfort and attractiveness should be the aim, but it should be remembered that in some cases it is important to maintain a 'working atmosphere', and so, where there is space to do so, it is often best to have a more 'social' treatment room as well.

Choice [17] and Deployment of Staff and Staff Welfare

This is an individual matter for individual hospitals or centres, and will depend on the layout of each, the type of patient and the amount of ward or department work. These factors will influence the head occupational therapist's decisions when interviewing staff [18] and when discussing their suitability with administrators and consultants. The special interests and qualifications of such staff will affect the planning and overall timetabling of departmental responsibilities, covering staff duties such as ward rounds, attendance at clinics, work in the department, and home visits, where necessary. Consideration should also be given to the most suitable times for patients to attend for treatment. The convenience of specialists and of other treatment sessions should also be considered. Administrative work should not interfere with patients' treatment, but is an important factor to be catered for by the head occupational therapist and her staff.

Many departments include activity specialists and technical instructors on their staffs, and these should be included in the regular staff meetings to co-ordinate treatment and organisation. A department may also be responsible for providing clinical experience to occupational therapy students. It is wise to appoint an occupational therapist on the staff to plan and supervise their programmes: it is also important to advise the qualified staff how to train and use them effectively.

Staff welfare is the responsibility of the head occupational therapist. She will, by her attitude to patients, colleagues, and departmental responsibilities, set the tone of the department, and help to develop an atmosphere

conducive to successful treatment. She should be given the support and
loyalty of her staff.

Office Administration [19]

A comprehensive filing system is essential. The criterion of a good system
is that it should be simple, convenient, and easily understood by all members
of staff. The information likely to be kept in an occupational therapy
department includes matter concerning patients, their disabilities and their
treatment; matter concerning activities used in treatment, names and
addresses of institutions and people who can supply information on specialised subjects, pamphlets on social services, and timetables of transport
arrangements, etc.; names and addresses of those supplying self aids
materials and equipment, etc., with catalogues and price lists. It will also
include any special subjects which form a section on their own, for example
the plans and details of a new department, stocktaking, or industrial projects

Each section of a filing system may have to be subdivided and cross
referenced, and the equipment and space required depend upon the amount
of information to be kept. It is useful to have a particular colour for occupational therapy referral and reports, so that records are distinctive among those
of other treatments. All methods need careful planning and indexing [20].

The simplest equipment is a metal filing cabinet, with suspension files, or
a lateral filing system [21]. Information concerning the patients and their
treatment may be divided according to the type of form or report; for
example, all referral cards may be kept in one division and all progress
reports in another, or it may be more convenient to keep all the information
concerning an individual patient on one card or in one file. Each form or
each file should be kept in alphabetical order in its particular section. Box
files may be more useful than manilla covers for storing instruction leaflets,
or patterns. These should be kept in the place where they are most frequently used. Care must be taken that confidential information is kept in a
safe place, preferably locked. Correspondence, whether internal or in
connection with individuals or firms outside the centre, should be filed in
date order. Official correspondence should be typed or written with a carbon
copy which can be retained in the appropriate file. Replies should be stapled
or pinned to the letter concerned.

Care of Accommodation and Equipment

It is normal to have some domestic help in an occupational therapy department, and this should be deployed carefully. The cleanliness of the rooms,
careful storage of stocks, and care of tools and equipment are essential. First
aid equipment should be available. Tools should be kept in shallow, locked
cupboards, preferably with shadow boards for easy checking after each

session. Patients should be taught to use the tools correctly and to put them away safely. In certain centres they should only be issued to responsible patients. An occupational therapy department should comply with the safety regulations which operate in factories and should be equipped for fulfilment of the centre's fire precautions. Fire precautions should be adequate, fire drill regular, and the use of appliances clearly understood. Where gas-fired appliances are used there should be provision for unimpeded air flow as a precaution against misadventure or suicide [22].

A series of master switches on the console unit mentioned above, in the office and in the entrance to the department, ensures complete control for emergencies, as does a similar series of gas tap controls. Power driven equipment and moving belts should be guarded, and it may be necessary for patients to wear some items of protective clothing. Water should not be used near electric switches. Defects, such as intractable locks, loose nosings on stairs or trapdoors, faulty electric switches or frayed cables, etc., should be reported immediately, to avoid serious accidents. Faulty equipment should be covered or removed until it can be repaired. For such items as electric potters' wheels, washing machines, printing presses, etc., contract servicing may well be arranged.

The working space needed for a patient may be greater than for the able bodied, and furniture and equipment should be placed with care. Sticks or crutches lying on the floor are dangerous, and difficult for their owners to retrieve. The provision of hooks and terry clips will help to stabilise work, and hold sticks, etc.

Care of accommodation and equipment should include the regular checking of the inventory of furniture, apparatus, tools and domestic items. It is advisable to mark equipment so that it can be found easily and re-claimed if mislaid. Additional equipment received should be added to the inventory and an entry made of losses, condemned or replaced articles.

Control of Equipment and Stock

It is the responsibility of the occupational therapist to arrange for the provision of equipment and materials to be used in treatment. It is also her responsibility to make sure that they are properly looked after and used in the most economical way. Accurate records of all financial transactions should be kept and it is strongly advised that stock of both equipment and materials be checked at least once a year, whether this is asked for by the authorities or not. Interim checks are also advised.

Selection

The careful selection of equipment and materials is essential to ensure satis-factory treatment and avoid wastage. It is advisable to consult catalogues and obtain samples where possible before a choice is made, and in the case of tools or machinery an inspection should be made before purchase. If the occupational therapist is not familiar with certain types of equipment she should consult a colleague, a technician, or obtain advice from the maintenance officer or a suitably qualified member of staff. It may be necessary to convince the hospital authorities that the cheapest article in a particular range is not necessarily an economical purchase. Equipment must be well made and strong enough to stand up to constant use and must be safe. Materials must be of a suitable quality to produce a satisfactory result and to ensure that there is little waste due to flaws.

Budgeting and Purchasing

Agreement to the purchase of materials and equipment usually has to be obtained from the supplies officer, or through the administrative authorities. This may be done in the form of an agreed sum to be spent during the financial year, which involves the submission of an estimate of requirements, or a list of requirements may have to be submitted for authorisation as equipment is needed. Many departments are now required to submit major future requirements, in order of priority, to the Administrator, usually about 6 months before the end of the financial year, so that all Annual Estimates can be considered and a hospital budget drawn up. It is important to retain some freedom of choice within the terms of the budget. Authorisation for normal replacements in usually given against presentation of the condemned item.

Methods of ordering by the occupational therapy department vary between individual centres. It is usual to send a requisition to the supplies department which may be in the hosptial or at District or Local Authority headquarters. If this method does not prove satisfactory the occupational therapist should ask to draft the order herself. Her request is more likely to be granted if she can show that she does not order indiscriminately and that she keeps accurate and careful records of use.

Goods received in the department should be checked against the order and the delivery-note or invoice, and the information then entered in a loose leaf ledger from one of the approved suppliers of stock control systems. If everything is in order, buying routine will probably require that the invoice shall be certified as correct by the head occupational therapist and returned to the finance office for payment; if there are omissions or discrepancies or damage, the main stores will have to be informed. These procedures may vary in detail from one centre to another.

Quantities

When ordering equipment to start a new department, or a new activity, it is necessary to consider the number of patients likely to be using each item, taking into consideration such factors as continual or only occasional use.

Under present conditions it may be wise to order as large a quantity as can be stored reasonably. This avoids constant price increases and cuts delivery charges which are also subject to V.A.T.* It is a mistake, however, to overstock in any particular item as, if the total value of stock in hand is high, authority may not then be given to order other items which are required. Also, some materials deteriorate when stored too long, and sufficient quantities to last only a given time, should be bought. Quantities again depend on the number of patients likely to be using the particular materials, and their estimated speed of working.

Storage Methods and Care of Materials

A well run department gives time for good treatment. It is sometimes argued that valuable time is taken in dealing with administrative work, but if the habit of orderly work is developed, it soon becomes satisfactorily automatic, and if a good system of storage and filing is followed, considerable time is saved in finding material or information when required. It is advisable to have a good store room. The size will naturally depend upon the amount of material which is carried and, however small it may be, it must be well ventilated and dry, but not too hot. The occupational therapist should be aware of the best methods of storing different materials. Some materials are subject to special regulations when in store or in use. Fire Safety Officers should be able to advise on appropriate precautions [23]. Air should be allowed to circulate round lengths of timber, by using bricks or similar blocks as supports between horizontally placed planks: wool should be stored away from strong sunlight and kept free of moth.

If the store room is in a position where the materials will not be exposed to dirt, open shelving is adequate. Otherwise, cupboards with closing (sliding) doors, or covering curtains may be necessary. Shelves should be of varying widths and depths and movable partitions are helpful. The store room should be kept strictly for raw materials and finished work, a running stock being kept in the treatment rooms themselves.

For some materials, bins or strong boxes may be more suitable and, if chests of drawers are used, shallow drawers are usually more useful than deep ones. All bins, cupboards, shelves and drawers should be kept tidy.

Waste of material can be prevented by using that which is most suitable for a particular article, by care in cutting out, as of leather, or calculating requirements, such as in the length of a warp, and by adequate storage facilities for scraps, ends, or remnants. Ingenuity in the saving and use of scraps is also most important.

Selling

Except in special circumstances, it should be the aim of the occupational therapist to cover the cost of materials by the sale of articles. Exceptions to the recovery of cost include arrangements which may be made with the doctor and administrator, for example in centres where a group of patients are working on a project such as puppetry, or making and repairing articles for the centre's use, or, in some psychiatric or children's hospitals or others, where the making of *saleable* articles is not part of the treatment. There are also times when it may be important to treatment that the patient can buy the finished article at a price within his means.

If articles are to be sold, the following points should be borne in mind:

(1) If sold to the maker, the charge is made at (material) cost price. (The price is based on materials used with a percentage added for wastage.) Carriage and postage should be included in the charge to the patient.

(2) If sold to a person other than the maker, or disposed of at a sale of work, a higher price should be asked. Care should be taken that the cost is not above the normal market price of the articles, taking into consideration the standard of work. The profit on articles thus sold may be given to the maker, to a special patients' fund, or be paid into the department's funds to offset the cost of materials used in other ways.

If the majority of articles are not bought by the patients who make them, or are not '*converted*' in the terms described below, it may be necessary to arrange periodic sales of work, to obtain orders, or to find markets for particular types of work. In all circumstances, the therapeutic aspect must be accepted as more important than the business aspect, and in some cases the value of materials or articles may have to be written off. The terms conversion or transfer are used to describe material converted into therapeutic uses but not necessarily saleable, i.e. into items of A.D.L.* equipment for permanent loan, such as a plate buffer lent to a patient for use in the ward or at home. Conversion also covers supplying and/or making articles for use in hospitals or institutions for which no charge is made.

Book-keeping

It has already been stated that purchases should be entered in a *stores ledger* or *purchases book*, and a record kept of all materials used. These two sets of records, together with records of income from sales, form the basis of book-keeping required in an occupational therapy department.

Details of book-keeping vary between the different hospitals or health authorities, but the basic principles underlying any method are the same. Broadly speaking, the value of stock at the beginning of a given period, plus the purchases made during the period, should balance with the stock in hand at the end of the period, plus the value of materials shown as used in treatment, but not sold, and the amount of cash received for sale of articles. This may however, be affected by the wastage allowance or other similar adjustments, and old stock may have to be revalued at a lower rate because of depreciation.

In a large department with its own store room for bulk stock it may be necessary to keep a *stores ledger*. This may be in the form of a page for each type of material, or several types may be included on one page with a double column for each. Purchases are entered on the left or debit side of the page, or the left hand column, and issues are entered on the right, or credit side. *Stock cards*, which are kept in a special box or filing drawer, may be used in the same way.

Some firms allow *discounts*, for prompt payment, or if goods are bought in quantity, or because the purchaser is a hospital. These price reductions may be handed to the patients in the form of a reduced price for materials purchased from the department, or, as is frequently the case, the normal price can be charged, and the discount retained by the department as a cover against losses or wastage. In the former case, the *nett* value of the goods (i.e. the value after deduction of the discount) would probably be entered in the books, while the *gross* amount would be shown if the discount is not to be passed on to the patients.

Patients' accounts may be kept in the form of *invoices* or *work record cards*. Again, methods vary. In some departments sufficient material to make an article is issued to a patient and entered on the invoice; on completion, any material over is weighed or measured and credited on the invoice; the amount used is the cost of the article. In other departments an article, including the materials to be used, is entered on the work record card, and on completion the amount of material used is weighed or measured, and priced. If the latter method is used a percentage should be added to the cost of the article to cover wastage and sundries.

When a patient pays for an article he has made, he should be given a *receipt*, and the receipt number should be entered on his invoice or work record card. (To avoid difficulties it is wise to retain money in the hand until the receipt and change are given.) If an article is not bought by the maker, its disposal should be recorded on the invoice or card, i.e. 'stock' or 'shop'. It is advisable to allot a serial number to articles which are to be offered for sale and enter them in a finished stock book, so that their final disposal can be traced, if required, by the auditors.

An *official receipt book* should also be kept in the occupational therapy department, and a receipt given to anyone paying money for articles or materials used.

At the end of a given period, usually every day, the value of all receipts which have been issued should be entered in a *cash book* unless the receipt book is designed to cover both. This should be totalled at convenient intervals, weekly if possible depending on the amount received, and paid into the finance office. The signature of the clerk receiving the money should be obtained against the total in the cash book. A good cash box is essential in a department.

Records concerning the use of materials which have so far been discussed, deal with saleable articles only. A separate book should be kept to record materials used in repairing or making articles for the hospital. Articles, such as adaptations, which are made for the occupational therapy department, should be entered in the inventory. Those made for other departments should be signed for when delivered.

Where out-work or industrial projects are used in treatment it is vital that a system should be worked out to record the obtaining of 'orders' and conditions relating to these, the work done by each patient and the amount and method of payment for the work. The success of industrial projects also depends on careful organising and recording of transport and control of materials or parts for assembly, and of completed work.

In some centres, material used in recreational activities may be accounted for in a similar way. In others, requirements for these activities have to be supplied out of social club or committee funds, which have been collected through fund raising activities or by subscriptions.

Petty cash or some form of provision for incidental purchases is important for an occupational therapy department, and accounts must be kept, the amount which may be spent being limited by the allowance made in a particular centre. These accounts are usually for the purpose of cash purchases of small expendable items. One procedure is to obtain the given sum, e.g. £5, at the beginning of the month, and record this amount on the debit page of the *petty cash book*. Purchases are entered on the credit side, and the receipts kept until the end of the month. When the book is balanced the receipts should be handed into the finance office, together with the money over, to bring the amount in hand up to the original sum, and a new issue be requested. Similar accounts can be kept for special expense allowances. It is also possible at times to obtain an 'open requisition order' for a specific quantity at a shop where the centre has an account, for such items as dress fabrics, giving the patients wide choice of single lengths. With new computing methods incidental items can now be paid for and a receipt obtained. This is then signed by the Supplies Officer and the computer code added. The receipt is then presented to the Cashier who will repay the money.

It has been contended that valuable time is taken up in the keeping of financial records, which could be used to better advantage in treating patients. The advantages of giving time to develop a simple and effective system of book-keeping cannot be too strongly stressed. Once a practical system is developed, the time consumed is relatively little, provided entries are kept up to date, and the ensuing efficiency of the department is well worth the time spent. Ideally, a clerk/book-keeper should be employed in a busy department, thus saving the time of the occupational therapist for the work for which she has been specially trained.

Stocktaking

Stock should be taken annually of all materials in the department. Expendable items do not need to be accounted for as they are written off automatically by being classed as such, although a charge is made for them in the price of any article made. Findings should be checked against the recorded stock in hand, and the stocktaking sheets forwarded to the administrative office. In some centres, it is the practice to have a member of staff from the administrative office present as an independent checker. It is advisable to close the department during stocktaking to enable this to be done with greater accuracy and speed.

Authority for increased facilities and development of the department involving additional expense is more likely to be given if it can be shown that existing facilities are being used to full advantage, and no unnecessary expense is incurred. Occupational therapy can be an expensive form of treatment if not adequately controlled, and businesslike administration in all facets of the work is of direct benefit in the treatment of patients.

In this chapter the basic principles underlying the management of an occupational therapy department in hospitals or similar units where in-patients or out-patients are treated have been discussed. Those relating to industrial and community occupational therapy are included in the chapters on these aspects.

REFERENCES AND RECOMMENDED FURTHER READING

1. Breck, *Principles and Practice of Management.*
   See Warham, J., *An Introduction to Administration for Social Workers.* London, 1967.
2. See this book, chapters 4 to 11 inclusive, for setting and requirements for *Physical Treatment*; chapters 12 to 17 inclusive, for *Psychiatric Treatment*; chapters 17 to 19 inclusive, for *Treatment of Children;* chapters 19 to 20 inclusive, for *Treatment of Patients with Special Problems;* chapters 21 to 23; for *requirements in special settings.*
3. For samples of *Referral Forms* indicating treatment required, see chapter 2.
4. See chapter 6, *Assessment and Reporting,* and in all chapters, *Aims of Treatment.*
5. Note *variations* in those listed in the *Treatment Teams for Physical and Psychiatric Patients of all types and age groups.*
6. See chapter 1.

7. See chapter 2.
8. See chapter 1.
9. Occupational therapy students are now receiving instruction in theories of management.
10. This is particularly emphasised in *Group Treatment* in psychiatric work.
11. See Plates 1, 2, 16, 21, 22.
12. See chapter 6, *Assessment and Reports* and chapter 12, *Check List*, regarding employment of psychiatric patients.
13. See chapter 7.
14. See *The Council for Codes of Practice: British Standard Institution*, CP 96; Part I, 1967. *Access for the Disabled to Buildings*, Part I, General Recommendations. Goldsmith, S., *Designing for the Disabled*. London, 1967.
    Health Service Design Note 3. A Guide to User Activity Measurement in Health Buildings. H.M.S.O.*, 1969.
    Appropriate Pamphlets: *Information Service for the Disabled*. Disabled Living Foundation*.
15. For further information on electrical installations and precautions see:
    Macfarlane, J. E., *Electricity in the House*. London, 1965.
    Wilman, C. W., *Electricity*. London, 1964.
    Chapman, J. M., *Basic Electricity*, 5 vols. London, 1960.
    Warring, R. H., *Beginner's Guide to Electronics*. London, 1966.
16. Information on sandwich glass—(the vacuum between two sheets acting as insulator without excluding light), can be obtained from J. Clark and Eaton Ltd., Scoresby House, Glasshill Street, London S.E.1. and Pilkington Brothers, St. Helen's, Lancs. 'Antisun' glass with a greenish tinge is also available, for places where good light without glare is needed.
17. See chapters 1, 2, and advice in specialist chapters for qualities needed in the occupational therapist herself, and for the use of specialist and 'aide' help in the treatment teams.
18. In some hospitals Personnel Officers have been appointed and, although they may advise the head occupational therapist, it is not satisfactory for them to take the final responsibility for staff selection and welfare.
19. Firms which supply a full range of office equipment from whose catalogues useful ideas can be obtained:
    Roneo Ltd., Alexandra House, Kingsway, London W.C.2.
    Sanky Sheldon Ltd., 20 Kingsway, London W.C.2.
    Shannon Ltd., Imperial House, Kingsway, London W.C.2.
20. The Middlewood Hospital, Sheffield, has developed an interesting method of planning indexing and cross references of reports.
21. See ref. 19 above.
22. See Ministry of Labour and Central Office of Information, Pamphlet no. 35: Basic Rules for Safety and Health at Work. H.M.S.O.*, 1967.
23. Copies of regulations are available from H.M.S.O.*, London.
* See *Glossary*, pp. 454-6.

General Bibliography

Anatomy and Physiology

Abrahams, A., *The Human Machine*. Pelican, 1956.
Glaser, E. M., *The Physiological Basis of Habituation*. Oxford, 1966.
Kapandji, I. A., *The Physiology of Joints*. Edinburgh and London, 1970.
McNaught, A. B., *Companion to Illustrated Physiology*. Edinburgh, 1970.
McNaught, A. B. & Callender, R., *Illustrated Physiology*. Edinburgh, Rev. 1970.
Nathan, P., *The Nervous System*. Pelican, 1969.
Perrott, J. W., *Anatomy for Students and Teachers of Physical Education*. London, 1970.
Ross, J. S. & Wilson, R., *Foundations of Anatomy and Physiology*. Edinburgh, 1974.
Rowe, J. W. and Wheble, V. H., *Anatomy and Physiology Applied for Orthopaedic Nurses*. Edinburgh and London, 1973.
Rowett, H. G. Q., *Basic Anatomy and Physiology*. London, 1966.
Sinclair, D., *An Introduction to Functional Anatomy*. Oxford, 1970.
Smout, C. & McDowell, R., *Anatomy, Physiology, Pathology and Bacteriology*. London, 1968.
Taverner, D., *Physiology for Nurses*. Edinburgh, 1972.

Psychology and Sociology

Anastasi, A., *Psychological Testing*. New York, 1961.
Aranguren, J. L., *Human Communication*. London, 1967.
Bass, M. B. & Vaughan, J. A., *Training in Industry*. U.S.A., 1966.
Beard, R. M., *An Outline of Piaget's Developmental Psychology*. London, 1969.
Brown, R., *Social Psychology*. U.S.A., 1966.
Drever, J., *A Dictionary of Psychology*. Penguin, 1952.
Gillis, L., *Human Behaviour in Illness*. London, 1972.
Hall, C. S. & Lindzey, G., *Theories of Personality*. New York, 1970.
Kahn, J. H., *Human Growth and Development of Personality*. Oxford, 1971.
Kretch, D. & Crutchfield, R. S., *Theory and Problems of Social Psychology*.
Leonard, P., *Sociology in Social Work*. London, 1966.
Myrdal, A. & Klein, V., *Woman's two Roles, Home and Work*. London, 1968.
Sherif, M. & C. W., *Social Psychology*. New York, 1969.
Sjodahe, L., *Elementary Industrial Psychology*. London, 1966.
Smythies, J. R., *Brain Mechanisms and Behaviour*. Oxford and London, 1970.
Storr, A., *Human Aggression*. London, 1968.
Timms, H., *A Sociological Approach to Social Problems*. London, 1967.
Welford, A. T., *Fundamentals of Skill*. London, 1968.
Brown, J. A. C., *The Social Psychology of Industry*. Pelican, 1954.
Cathercole, C. E., *Assessment in Clinical Psychology*. Penguin Science, 1968.
Eysenck, H. J., *Check your own I.Q.* Pelican, 1966.
Eysenck, H. J., *Know your own I.Q.* Pelican.
Lorenz, K., *On Aggression*. London, 1966.

General

Bingham, W. Van. D., *Aptitudes and Aptitude Testing*. New York, 1936.
Carter, M., *Into Work*. Pelican, 1966.
Davis, J. E., *Principles and Practice of Rehabilitation*. 1944.
Farrer Brown, L. & Warren, M. D., *Public Health and Social Services*. London, 1965.
Fraser, R. Ed., *Work 1. Twenty Personal Accounts*. Pelican, 1968.
Fraser, R. Ed., *Work 2. Twenty Personal Accounts*. Pelican, 1969.
Perry, E. L., *Ward Administration and Teaching*. London, 1968. (Good references to the treatment team.)
  Some Aspects of Rehabilitation. National Fund for Research into Crippling Diseases. 1968.
  Social Services in Britain. H.M.S.O., London, 1967.
  Rehabilitation and Care of the Disabled in Britain. H.M.S.O., 1965.

* Glossary, Some Useful Information and Addresses

A.D.L.	Activities of daily living
B.A.O.T.	British Association of Occupational Therapists
B.M.A.	British Medical Association
C.P.	Cerebral palsy
C.S.P.	Chartered Society of Physiotherapists
D.L.F.	Disabled Living Foundation
E.C.T.	Electro-convulsive therapy
E.S.R.	Erythrocyte sedimentation rate
H.A.A.	Handicrafts Advisory Association
H.M.S.O.	Her Majesty's Stationery Office
I.L.O.	International Labour Organisation
I.Q.	Intelligence quotient
N.A.M.H.	National Association for Mental Health
N.H.S.	National Health Service
O. & M.	Organisation and methods—a work study term
O.T.	Occupational therapy, or occupational therapist
P.I.L.O.T.	Patient Initiated Light Operated Tele Control. A system in which a light beam activates photo-electric cells. (See *Rehabilitation*, British Council for the Rehabilitation of the Disabled, 63, Oct./Dec. 1967)
P.N.F.	Proprioceptive neuromuscular facilitation
POSSUM or P.O.S.M.	Patient Operated Selector Mechanisms. The equipment is produced by the Research Unit, under R. G. Maling. The term is derived from the Latin *possum*, which means 'I can' or 'I am able'. It can also be referred to as P.O.S.M. (See *Rehabilitation*, British Council for the Rehabilitation of the Disabled, 63. March/June 1968) *Possum unit P.S.U. 1*, available on the N.H.S. *Possum unit P.S.U. 2*, not available on the N.H.S.
R.I.B.A.	Royal Institute of British Architects
R.N.I.B.	Royal National Institute for the Blind
R.N.I.D.	Royal National Institute for the Deaf
V.A.T.	Value added tax
W.C.	Water closet (toilet)
W.F.O.T.	World Federation of Occupational Therapists
W.R.V.S.	Women's Royal Voluntary Service
Zambette	Zambette System 7 (not available on the N.H.S.). includes: patient operated light-weight chair, radio and TV controls, telephone connection, fan heater, intercom systems

D.H.S.S.	Department of Health and Social Security
R.H.A.	Regional Health Authority
R.A. or R.A.O.	Regional Administrator or Regional Administrative Officer
R.M.O.	Regional Medical Officer
R.N.O.	Regional Nursing Officer
R.T.	Regional Treasurer
R.W.O.	Regional Works Officer
A.H.A.	Area Health Authority
A.H.A.(T.)	Area Health Authority with a teaching hospital in the area
A.A.	Area Administrator
A.M.O.	Area Medical Officer

A.N.O. Area Nursing Officer
A.P.O. Area Pharmaceutical Officer
A.T. Area Treasurer

D. District
D.C. District Council
D.M.C. District Medical Committee
D.M.T. District Management Team
D.A. District Administrator
D.C.P. District Community Physician
D.F.O. District Finance Officer
D.N.O. District Nursing Officer

C.H.C. Community Health Council
F.P.C. Family Practitioner Committee
F.P.S. Family Practitioner Services
J.C.C. Joint Consultative Committee
P.A.C. Professional Advisory Committee
H.C.P.T. Health Care Planning Teams. These consist of general practitioners consultants, paramedical staff and representatives of Local Authority social and other services departments

In Scotland
S.H.H.D. Scottish Home and Health Department
A.H.B. Area Health Board
D.E.C. District Executive Committee

THE EMPLOYMENT SERVICE
(as reorganized 1974)

C.O.D.O.T. Classification of Occupations and Directory of Occupational Titles
C.Y.E.E. Central Youth Employment Executive
D.R.O. Disablement Resettlement Officer
E.S.A. Employment Service Agency
I.R.U. Industrial Rehabilitation Unit
J.I.M. Job Information Manual
L.E.A. Local Education Authority
M.S.C. Manpower Services Commission
O.G.U. Occupational Guidance Units
P.E.R. Professional and Executive Recruitment
R.D.P. Register of Disabled Persons or Registered Disabled Person
T.O.P.S. Training Opportunities Scheme
T.S.A. Training Services Agency

Forms issued by the employment service
D.P.1 A confidential medical report, giving recommendations for industrial rehabilitation
D.P.17 Application for entry of name in the R.D.P.
D.P.32 Confidential medical report to support an application to register or to renew a registration with the R.D.P.
D.S.2 Claim for an attendance allowance, issued by the D.H.H.S.
Part III Provision of accommodation for the elderly and disabled
For further information, see:
 Attendance Allowance for Adults and Children. Leaflet NI 205. H.M.S.O.
 Department of Health and Social Security Index of Leaflets. Leaflet NI 146. H.M.S.O.
 Employment and Training Government Proposals. H.M.S.O.

Help for Handicapped People. HB1. D.H.S.S. *Industrial Injuries—Disablement Benefit.* Leaflet NI 6. H.M.S.O.
The Employment Service—Plans and Programmes, ELP 14. H.M.S.O.
The National Health Service Reorganisation Act 1974.
The Reorganisation of the National Health Service 1974, Regional Health Authority, Oaklea, 47 Whitehall Lane, Buckhurst Hill, Essex.

SOME USEFUL ADDRESSES

Bell and Howell Language Master, Rank Audio-Visual Ltd, P.O. Box 70, Great West Road, Brentford, Middlesex.
British Association of Occupational Therapists, 20 Rede Place, London W2 4TU.
British Council for the Rehabilitation of the Disabled, Tavistock House, Tavistock Square, London, WC1H 9LB.
British Epilepsy Association, 3–6 Alfred Place, London WC1E 7ED.
British Medical Association, BMA House, Tavistock Square, London WC1H 9LB.
Central Council for the Disabled, 34 Eccleston Square, London SW1V 1PE.
Chartered Society of Physiotherapists, 14 Bedford Row, London WC1R 4ED.
Consumer's Association, 14 Buckingham Street, London WC2N 6DS.
    For publications: Caxton Hill, Hertford, Herts.
Disabled Living Foundation, 346 Kensington High Street, London W14 8NS.
Handicrafts Advisory Association, c/o The Greater London Association for the Disabled, 183 Queensway, London W2 5HL.
King Edwards' Hospital Fund for London, 14 Palace Court, London W2 4HT.
King's Fund Centre, 24 Nutford Place, London W1H 6AN.
National Association for Mental Health, Harmont House, 22 Harley Street, London W1N 2ED.
National Book League, 7 Albermarle Street, London W1X 4BB.
National Foundation for Educational Research Publishing Company, 2 Jennings Buildings Windsor, Berks.
National Fund for Research into Crippling Diseases, 1 Springfield Road, Horsham, Sussex RH12 2BR.
National Society for Mentally Handicapped Children, Pembridge Hall, 17 Pembridge Square, London W2 4EH.
Possum Controls Ltd., 63 Mandeville Road, Aylesbury, Bucks. HP21 8AE.
Preparatory Training Bureau, c/o British Council for the Rehabilitation of the Disabled, Tavistock House, Tavistock Square, London WC1H 9LB.
Royal Institute of British Architects, 66 Portland Place, London, W1N 4AD.
Royal National Institute for the Blind, 224/6/8 Great Portland Street, London W1N 6AA.
Royal National Institute for the Deaf, 105 Gower Street, London WC1E 6AH.
Spastics Society, 12 Park Crescent, London, W1N 4EQ.
Zambette Electronics Ltd, 3 Avon Way, Shoeburyness, Essex.
For details of other societies, etc., see *A Handbook of Organisations Relating to the Health and Social Services.* Health and Social Services, 1973. Available from the King's Fund Centre.

Guide to Activities Used in Treatment

(but not curative in themselves)

Note:

The activities which are concerned with:

    (1) Assessment for A.D.L.
    (2) Assessment for return to work
    (3) Speech therapy reading and writing practice

are not listed separately because they are so often used and occur too frequently in the text to make indexing useful.

Activities used in:

    (1) The treatment of children are listed on pp. 347, 367, 373–4
    (2) The treatment of geriatrics are listed on pp. 406–8

and see throughout for recommended activities under special conditions.

Index